# WHEN LIFE IS IN JEOPARDY FROM

# COMPLICATIONS OF CANCER

**A book written for everyone, providing detailed questions and answers about serious complications of common cancers**

**Stephen Garrett Marcus, M.D.**

ISBN: 1-4664-8285-0
ISBN-13: 978-1-4664-8285-2
LCCN: 2011919790
CreateSpace, North Charleston, SC

*To my family*
*and in loving memory of my parents*

# TABLE OF CONTENTS

# INTRODUCTION

Complications of cancer are common, and become more frequent and severe if cancer progresses or spreads. Early identification and prompt treatment of these complications unquestionably prevents much suffering and saves lives. Several years ago, it became apparent to the author that no book or central source of information was available that thoroughly discussed these critical complications, some of which affect virtually every person who develops a life-threatening cancer. *Complications of Cancer* provides easy to understand, comprehensive and candid information about these life-threatening conditions.

The book has three sections: "Life-Threatening Cancers", "Complications of Cancer," and "Clinical Trials."

The first section, "Life-Threatening Cancers" provides a detailed overview of the 15 most common life-threatening cancers, including information about symptoms, making the diagnosis, determining the extent, if any, to which the cancer has spread, initial surgical and medical treatments, prevention and treatment of progression or recurrence, and treatment available to reduce discomfort if the cancer is not adequately controlled. This overview provides a framework for understanding the complications that can develop.

The second section, "Complications of Cancer," discusses 50 serious complications or complicating illnesses that can occur as a direct result of cancer, another underlying illness, or as a side effect of medical or surgical treatments. These complications are the direct cause of the great majority of events that endanger the life and health of people with cancer.

The effectiveness of current treatments of many types of cancer is inadequate. Facing this, people often seek experimental treatment that could provide a chance for survival and recovery. The third book section, "Clinical Trials", gives information about how new treatments are tested by responsible medical researchers and how to enroll in a clinical trial of an experimental or innovative treatment.

The focus of this book is on medical and surgical treatments of cancer and on complications of cancer that can develop. Although it would be preferable to prevent cancer rather than treat it, preventive measures are usually beside the point once cancer has struck. Prevention discussed in this book emphasizes prevention of disease recurrence or progression, and prevention of complications of cancer or its treatment.

The treatment of cancer and its complications is steadily improving. No medical book can be written which will be entirely current by the time it is available on the internet, reaches the shelves of a bookstore, or when it is transmitted to a handheld reading device. Differences of opinion exist between competent physicians. The reader must be aware that information in this book is not a replacement for the decisions about medical care made by medical professionals responsible for a person's treatment.

The most common questions a person will have when facing a cancer are "how can I fight this disease", and "what can I expect to happen". *Complications of Cancer* discusses the essential medical tools used to fight cancer, and stresses that prompt recognition and treatment of complications is one of the most critical aspects of fighting cancer, and plays a central role in determining outcome. By thoroughly reviewing the most common cancers and their critical complications, this book seeks to provide the reader with a vital weapon in the fight for life and good health: information.

# IMPORTANT NOTICE TO THE READER

The information contained in this book is informational assistance only. The information is not medical advice for individual conditions or treatment and is not a substitute for a medical examination or for the medical advice and care rendered by a personal physician.

The author of this book makes no guarantee regarding the completeness, accuracy, or reliability of the information in this book. The author and the publisher do not assume any responsibility or liability for damages, direct or indirect, or for any damages, however caused, that result from the use of any information contained in this book. Internet links to websites suggested in this book are independent of the author of this book and the author does not warrant the thoroughness, accuracy or objectivity of the information provided by these websites.

Seek the advice of medical professionals to evaluate the accuracy, comprehensiveness, and utility of any information, opinion, advice, or other content available in this book. The information in this book does not replace the need for a person's physician who must make an evaluation of a person's medical condition and prescribe a safe and effective treatment for each individual person.

# THE MOST COMMON LIFE-THREATENING CANCERS

# BLADDER CANCER

## DEFINITION

### What is bladder cancer?

Bladder cancer is a cancer that begins in the cells that line the inside of the bladder. Unless the cancer remains confined to the bladder, there is a high risk of spread of the cancer throughout the body.

## SYMPTOMS

### What are the symptoms of bladder cancer?

The most common symptom of bladder cancer is blood in the urine. The urine may appear quite bloody, then clear up after a few days, then appear quite bloody again. Pain with urination, as well as increased frequency of urination, are occasional early symptoms of bladder cancer.

## MAKING THE DIAGNOSIS

### How is the diagnosis of bladder cancer made?

A "cystoscopy" makes the diagnosis of bladder cancer.

A cystoscopy is a procedure in which a physician puts an instrument with a light on its end called a "cystoscope" up the urethra and into the bladder. With the cystoscope, the physician can examine the entire inside wall of the bladder and take biopsies from any area that appears suspicious for cancer. The biopsies will establish or rule out the presence of cancer.

Examination of the urine under the microscope can sometimes identify cancer cells, especially those arising from the form of bladder cancer, discussed below, called "carcinoma in situ". This test, known as "urine cytology", in conjunction with cystoscopy, provides critical information when there is a suspicion of bladder cancer.

## What information will the biopsy give about the bladder cancer?

The appearance of the cancer cells under the microscope, the size of the visible cancer seen by the physician, and the depth to which the cancer has invaded into the wall of the bladder can give a good indication of the level of danger posed by the cancer. Cancers that are "low grade" have a lower tendency to spread deeply into the wall of the bladder and to other areas of the body. Cancers that appear to be "high grade" have a much higher tendency to spread deeply into the bladder or to other areas of the body.

There is a particular type of bladder cancer called "carcinoma in situ" in which a thin layer of highly malignant bladder cancer cells covers a rather large area of the inside surface of the bladder. Carcinoma in situ of the bladder is a dangerous form of bladder cancer that requires intensive treatment.

# DETERMINING WHETHER
# THE CANCER HAS SPREAD

*How is the extent, if any, to which bladder cancer has spread, determined?*

A first important step in planning treatment is to determine whether the bladder cancer has spread into the wall of the bladder or beyond the bladder.

Biopsies of one or more areas of the bladder, done during the cystoscopy, can determine whether the bladder cancer has invaded beneath the superficial cell layer and into the muscular wall of the bladder. An intravenous pyelogram, in which the kidneys excrete a radiologist's dye, can determine whether the cancer is blocking the normal flow of urine from kidney to ureter to bladder to urethra.

Bladder cancer that invades into the muscle of the bladder wall has a high tendency to spread elsewhere in the body. Blood tests, a chest x-ray, and a CT or MRI scan of the abdomen and pelvis will look for evidence of spread of the cancer beyond the bladder. If the person has recently noticed pain in any bones, a bone scan will look for evidence of spread of the bladder cancer to the bone.

## SUPERFICIAL BLADDER CANCER

*What is superficial bladder cancer?*

When physicians refer to superficial bladder cancer, they mean a bladder cancer confined to the cells lining the inside surface of the bladder and that has not invaded deeper into the bladder muscle or spread to any other part of the body.

## TREATMENT OF SUPERFICIAL BLADDER CANCER

### *What is the treatment of superficial bladder cancer?*

Superficial bladder cancer is treated by snipping the bladder cancer off the inside wall of the bladder through a cystoscope (this procedure is called "endoscopic resection"). To do this, the physician will, with anesthesia, put the scope up through the urethra into the bladder, and then carefully examine the entire visible inside of the bladder. Abnormal areas will be biopsied to determine whether they are cancers, and, if they are cancers, how large they are, and how deeply they extend into the wall of the bladder. To the extent possible, the physician will attempt to remove all visible cancer at the time of the endoscopic resection.

### *How successful is endoscopic resection in treating bladder cancer?*

The success of endoscopic resection will vary, depending on whether the tumor was high grade or low grade. High-grade tumors are far more likely to recur after endoscopic resection than low-grade tumors and, if a high-grade tumor is present, physicians are likely to recommend some additional treatment after the endoscopic resection to help prevent recurrence.

When the bladder cancer recurs after endoscopic resection, the recurrence will usually show up within 12 months. Once there has been one recurrence after endoscopic resection, it is far more likely that there will be another recurrence after another endoscopic resection.

### What treatment can reduce the risk of recurrence of low-grade bladder cancer after endoscopic resection?

A single dose of chemotherapy given directly into the bladder ("intravesical chemotherapy") can reduce the risk of recurrence of the bladder cancer. If the bladder cancer does recur, endoscopic resection can be repeated, followed by approximately six weekly doses of "intravesical chemotherapy" or by "intravesical BCG" as described below.

### What treatment can reduce the risk of recurrence of high-grade bladder cancer after endoscopic resection?

BCG is a strain of bacteria that causes an intense bladder inflammation when put directly into the bladder. This inflammation is associated with shrinkage or disappearance of superficial bladder cancer and with a reduction of risk of bladder cancer recurrence after endoscopic resection. "Intravesical BCG" is treatment of bladder cancer by putting BCG directly into the bladder. Side effects of intravesical BCG include burning with urination and a feeling of having to urinate frequently.

Several chemotherapy medications, such as Mitomycin C, when put into the bladder after endoscopic resection, will reduce the risk of recurrence. These chemotherapy medications may be somewhat less effective than BCG in controlling high-risk bladder cancer.

## *How do physicians put BCG into the bladder?*

Physicians put BCG into the bladder through a tube (a "catheter") inserted through the urethra and into the bladder. A commonly used treatment regimen is to administer BCG into the bladder every week for 6 weeks. For those people with superficial bladder cancer which is "high risk", physicians commonly recommend "maintenance therapy" in which three once-a week doses are given at 3 and 6 month intervals after the first course of treatment, then every six months thereafter until three years have elapsed from the first treatment.

## *How does the physician check to see if the cancer has recurred?*

At three to six month intervals, the physician can examine the inside of the bladder with the cystoscope to see if there is evidence that the cancer has recurred. When there are suspicious areas, the physician may scrape off some of the superficial cells or take biopsies so that the presence or absence of cancer cells can be determined under the microscope.

## *What happens when the superficial bladder cancer keeps recurring or persists despite endoscopic resection and BCG?*

Failure to control superficial bladder cancer with endoscopic resection and BCG puts a person at risk of developing a dangerous invasion of the bladder cancer into the muscular wall of the bladder. If there is failure to control superficial bladder cancer or if invasion into the muscular wall of the bladder occurs, surgical removal of the part of the bladder containing the cancer or of the entire bladder is a common recommendation.

### What is the treatment of carcinoma in situ?

Carcinoma in situ tends to involve a large area of the inside lining of the bladder. For this reason, endoscopic resection is very difficult.

Administration of BCG directly into the bladder can cause the carcinoma in situ to disappear about 70% of the time. Those people who have complete disappearance of the carcinoma in situ have about a 50-50 chance of having their carcinoma in situ remain in complete remission four years or more after treatment.

If carcinoma in situ recurs after endoscopic resection and BCG, it places the person at considerable risk of developing bladder muscle invasion. If carcinoma in situ recurs, another try at BCG, or an attempt at the use of an experimental medication are considerations. Many physicians will feel, however, that the risk for developing spread of the bladder cancer beyond the bladder is so high that the most appropriate treatment for the person with recurrent carcinoma in situ is surgical removal of the bladder.

### Is surgery to remove the bladder required if the cancer has invaded the muscle in the bladder wall?

Surgical removal of the bladder is a very effective method of reducing the risk of bladder cancer spreading to other areas of the body. The surgery is, however, a life-changing event after which normal urination is not possible.

Depending on the size and location of the bladder cancer and the extent to which "endoscopic resection" through the cystoscope was possible, non-surgical treatment with radiation and chemotherapy may control muscle-invasive bladder cancer. If this non-surgical treatment is chosen, careful follow-up by the urologist and other medical professionals will be required, with cystoscopy and biopsies of the bladder at regular intervals, to be sure that cancer in the bladder has not recurred. Most, people receiving this treatment are able to maintain their intact bladder without having progression of their cancer 2 years or more after treatment. The long-term effectiveness of this combination of radiation and chemotherapy is still under evaluation.

## SURGICAL TREATMENT OF BLADDER CANCER

*Is it necessary to remove the entire bladder when a person has a superficial bladder cancer that is resistant to endoscopic resection and BCG?*

There is an operation called a "partial cystectomy" which will remove only a part of the bladder. This operation is for those people whose bladder cancer is relatively small and for those circumstances when the urologist feels there is a good possibility of removing the entire cancer from the bladder.

There is some controversy about whether or when it is a good idea to attempt to cure a person's bladder cancer with a partial cystectomy. Many urologists feel that a partial cystectomy exposes the person to the risk of incomplete removal of the bladder cancer, along with a higher risk that the cancer will recur in a way that will not be curable by surgery.

## What is a total cystectomy?

A total cystectomy removes the entire bladder and, in addition, may remove lymph nodes on both sides of the bladder.

Normally, the ureters, which carry urine from the kidneys, drain their urine into the bladder. When we urinate, the bladder drains urine into the urethra and the urethra drains urine from the body. With removal of the bladder, the ureters will need attachment elsewhere so that they can drain urine from the kidneys. The most common way of doing this is to attach the ureters to a segment of small intestine. Drainage of urine is through the segment of small intestine sewn to the skin on a person's side. The urine collects into a bag and discarded several times a day.

A number of newer procedures divert urine in a way that an external collection bag is not necessary. For example, an artificial bladder created from a piece of small intestine and attached to the urethra allows a person to urinate more normally. Much of the surgical expertise into these new procedures for cystectomy is in the top medical centers.

## Can a man remain potent after a cystectomy?

Cystectomy can damage the nerves that control a man's ability to get an erection and can cause impotence. There have been some recent improvements in the technique of cystectomy such that nerves are not as damaged and potency might be preserved. Although there may be a temporary loss of potency after the cystectomy, about half of men will regain potency after the cystectomy. Medications such as Viagra can help sexual potency after a cystectomy.

### How effective is cystectomy at curing the bladder cancer?

The effectiveness of the cystectomy will depend upon how deeply the bladder cancer invaded the wall of the bladder at the time of the operation.

Most people with superficial bladder cancer have a cure of their bladder cancer after cystectomy.

When the bladder cancer has penetrated into the muscle of the bladder, the chance of cure after cystectomy will depend upon how deeply the cancer has penetrated into the muscle, and whether the cancer has spread into the local lymph nodes. Because of the risk that the cancer will return when it has extended into the muscle of the bladder, physicians often recommend chemotherapy prior to surgery in an attempt to prevent recurrence after the surgery. This type of chemotherapy is "neoadjuvant chemotherapy".

### What type of neoadjuvant treatment is given?

The most commonly used chemotherapy regimen consists of a combination of four drugs—Methotrexate, Vinblastine, Adriamycin and Cisplatin. These four drugs given together have the nickname "the MVAC regimen".

### What are the side effects of the MVAC regimen?

The most serious side effect is suppression of production of white blood cells by the bone marrow (see chapter "Bone Marrow Suppression"). Because the white blood cells are essential for fighting infection, this can make a person very susceptible to serious, and life-threatening infections. Other important side effects of MVAC include sores in the mouth (see chapter "Severe Oral Mucositis"), and nausea and vomiting (see chapter "Nausea and Vomiting"). Most of the time, the side effects, though very distressing, can be managed with anti-nausea medicines, extra fluid by mouth or by vein, and, when necessary, by reduction of doses of the drugs in the MVAC regimen.

### What is adjuvant chemotherapy?

In contrast to the neoadjuvant therapy given before surgery, adjuvant therapy is chemotherapy given after surgery to reduce the risk of return of the cancer.

### Is adjuvant chemotherapy useful after a cystectomy?

When cystectomy removes a bladder with cancer that has spread to the tissues surrounding the bladder or to lymph nodes beyond the bladder, adjuvant chemotherapy may slightly reduce the risk of recurrence of the bladder cancer. There is, however, a lack of definitive proof of this benefit of adjuvant chemotherapy confirmed by large randomized trials comparing adjuvant treatment to no adjuvant treatment. This has led to some disagreement among experts as to the value of adjuvant chemotherapy after cystectomy.

## TREATMENT OF METASTATIC BLADDER CANCER

### What happens if bladder cancer recurs after cystectomy?

Bladder cancer that recurs after cystectomy usually recurs in distant body organs. Recurrence of bladder cancer in distant body organs is "metastatic bladder cancer".

## *What is the treatment of metastatic bladder cancer?*

The treatment of metastatic bladder cancer that has some proven ability to shrink the cancer or delay its growth, and extend survival, is with chemotherapy.

A commonly used chemotherapy regimen consists of the same "MVAC" combination of four drugs used for the neo-adjuvant treatment described earlier. With this combination, approximately half of people will get a temporary shrinkage of their cancer, which generally lasts for under a year.

A newer combination of medicines consists of "Gemcitabine" (brand name is "Gemzar, manufacturer's product website is www. gemzar.com) and "Cisplatin". With this combination, the response rate and the durability of the response is about the same as with "MVAC", although with less side effects. In particular, the combination of Gemcitabine and Cisplatin appears to cause fewer problems with suppression of white blood cells necessary to fight bacterial infection.

## *What chemotherapy is useful if the person recurs after MVAC or Gemcitabine + Cisplatin?*

There is no standard, proven effective treatment if the initial chemotherapy treatment for metastatic bladder cancer is no longer effective. Additional chemotherapy drugs may produce a temporary response in less than one-fourth of people, although it is not clear that this treatment increases the odds of surviving longer.

## *What is the outlook for a person with metastatic bladder cancer?*

Metastatic bladder cancer is rarely curable. Regression or disappearance of cancer after chemotherapy is most commonly temporary. Those people who have complete or partial disappearance of their metastatic bladder cancer survive longer than those people who do not have shrinkage of their cancer with chemotherapy. On average, and taking into consideration that some people may live much longer than average and some much shorter than average, and that some people are healthier at the time they begin chemotherapy than others, the average survival time from the time a person with metastatic bladder cancer begins chemotherapy is a bit over a year.

An important option for a person with metastatic bladder cancer is to seek a clinical trial testing a new form of treatment.

# BRAIN CANCER: GLIOBLASTOMA

## DEFINITIONS

### What is brain cancer?

Brain cancer is a rapidly growing, extremely dangerous malignant brain tumor. If the growth of this tumor is not under control, it can spread to vital areas of the brain and cause damage to an extent that is incompatible with life.

Although "brain cancer" is the more common name for the disease in the media, the name more commonly used by physicians is "malignant brain tumor".

### Are there different types of malignant brain tumor?

Malignant brain tumors fall into two major categories: "primary malignant brain tumors" which begin in the brain and "metastatic brain tumors" which begin elsewhere in the body and spread to the brain.

Most primary malignant brain tumors in adults are a highly malignant type of tumor called a "glioblastoma" (sometimes referred to by its full name "glioblastoma multiforme" or by its initials "GBM"). Its close relative, the "anaplastic astrocytoma", is less common and less fast growing. Physicians often combine glioblastoma multiforme and anaplastic astrocytoma together in one category and call them "malignant gliomas".

This chapter will discuss glioblastoma. Discussion of "metastatic brain tumors" is in the complications section of this book in the chapter entitled "Brain Metastasis".

## SYMPTOMS

### What are the symptoms of a glioblastoma?

The first symptoms a person has as a result of a glioblastoma will vary depending on where in the brain the tumor is located and how fast the tumor is growing.

Headache is a common early symptom. The pain may awaken the person in the middle of the night and become quite severe by the morning.

Neurologic function, which reflects the area of the brain where the tumor is located, may be affected. For example, if the tumor involves an area of the brain that controls movement of one side of the body, there may be weakness of that side of the body. If the tumor involves the area of the brain that controls vision, there may be visual disturbances.

Personality changes may occur which are at first quite subtle. Friends, family and co-workers may notice strange or out-of-character, or even embarrassing behavior. The person may become irritable and easy to anger, or quite the opposite, lethargic and apathetic.

Seizures occur in approximately one-third of people with a glioblastoma (please see chapter entitled "Seizures"). The ability to move, to sense, to think, to speak, or any of the countless functions performed continually by the normal brain can be severely affected.

## MAKING THE DIAGNOSIS

*How is the diagnosis of a glioblastoma made?*

When a person has symptoms that are suggestive of a glioblastoma, a CT scan or a MRI scan of the brain will generally be the key test that a physician will recommend. These scans will show a tumor, or in medical language, a "mass lesion" wherever it is located in the brain. The scans cannot define the precise nature of the "mass lesion", although the appearance of the mass lesion can raise a high suspicion of the presence of the highly malignant "glioblastoma", or in contrast, a benign and curable tumor such as a "meningioma".

If a CT or MRI scan indicates the likely presence of a malignant brain tumor, it is important to try to determine whether the tumor started in the brain (as a "primary brain tumor") or spread to the brain from a cancer elsewhere in the body (and is a "brain metastasis", also called a "metastatic brain tumor").

A medical history, a physical examination, routine blood chemistry panels, and a chest x-ray, can sometimes identify the presence of cancer outside of the brain. If this brief evaluation fails to identify a cancer outside of the brain, consideration will be given to having a surgeon remove a piece of the brain tumor for examination under the microscope, that is, of obtaining a "brain biopsy".

There are important differences in the way the different types of primary malignant brain tumors are treated. A biopsy of the brain lesion makes the precise diagnosis.

*Is a brain biopsy always necessary when the CT or MRI scan suggests the presence of a malignant brain tumor?*

People with cancer of the lung, breast or other organs who have already had a confirmed spread of their cancer and who develop a malignant brain tumor usually have a metastatic brain tumor. In these circumstances, a biopsy may not be necessary to make a reasonably definitive diagnosis.

There are times, especially in children, when the malignant brain tumor is located in an area of the brain that is extremely difficult and risky to biopsy. In these circumstances, the appearance of the tumor on CT or magnetic resonance scan may be adequate to make the diagnosis and guide therapy.

Largely, unless the malignant brain tumor is almost certainly metastatic or unless surgical removal of a piece of the tumor is too risky, the biopsy is an essential tool to the planning of appropriate therapy.

*How does a neurosurgeon obtain a brain biopsy?*

A neurosurgeon performs this procedure. Depending on the location and size of the tumor, as well as the probability, based upon the MRI scan, that the tumor is the highly malignant "glioblastoma", the goal of the neurosurgeon may not only be to perform the biopsy, but to remove as much of the tumor as possible. In order to perform this procedure, a "craniotomy" (in which the neurosurgeon makes a hole in the skull and operates on the brain) may be performed with the goal of making the diagnosis and removing as much of the tumor as possible in the same operation.

There are circumstances where the neurosurgeon believes that removal of the tumor is too dangerous or where it is not clear that removal of the tumor is necessary or possible. A procedure called a "stereotactic biopsy" may be done in which a very tiny hole is made in the skull and a fine needle is passed deep into the brain with the guidance of a CT or MRI scan. Using this technique, the neurosurgeon is usually able to remove enough tumor tissue to allow a pathologist to examine the tissue under a microscope and make a precise diagnosis.

## MEDICINES TO CONTROL SYMPTOMS

### What medicines control the symptoms of glioblastoma?

A steroid medicine called "dexamethasone" is particularly effective in shrinking some of the swelling that usually exists around the glioblastoma. This reduction in swelling will reduce the size of the mass lesion in the brain and, therefore, reduce some of the symptoms. Because dexamethasone, when given for many months, may lead to loss of calcium from bones and "osteoporosis", dietary supplementation with calcium and Vitamin $D_3$ may be helpful.

If seizures have occurred, anti-seizure medicines (called "antiepileptic medications") will be useful. An antiepileptic called "levetiracetam", (brand name is "Keppra XR", and manufacturer's product website is www.keppraxr.com) is a common choice for a person with a glioblastoma who requires antiepileptic medication.

## SURGICAL TREATMENT OF GLIOBLASTOMA

### Can surgery cure a glioblastoma?

Glioblastoma is incurable by surgery. Even after removing the entire visible tumor and a large area of normal appearing brain around the tumor, glioblastoma cells remain in the brain. The neurosurgeon can, however, cut out a good portion of the tumor, and, by doing so, considerably relieve or prevent symptoms, and delay or prevent early, life threatening expansion of the tumor into critical zones of the brain.

### How critical and difficult is it for the neurosurgeon to remove as much of the glioblastoma as possible?

Although glioblastoma is not curable by surgery, the extent to which the surgeon removes the glioblastoma can have an impact upon relieving existing symptoms, delaying development of disabling neurologic symptoms, and can improve the odds of a longer survival by reducing the amount of tumor ("debulking" the tumor) such that radiation or chemotherapy can be more effective. The goal of the neurosurgeon will be to remove as much of the glioblastoma as possible without damaging areas of the brain that govern essential neurologic functions.

Maximal removal of tumor without harming normal brain function is complicated surgery and requires great skill and experience on the part of the neurosurgeon and the team of physicians and medical staff who will care for the person after the operation. For this reason, it is good to have this "debulking surgery" done in a highly specialized hospital with extensive experience in performing this complex surgery.

## ADJUVANT THERAPY OF GLIOBLASTOMA

### *What is adjuvant therapy of glioblastoma?*

Adjuvant therapy of glioblastoma is treatment administered after surgery has removed as much of the tumor as was surgically possible. Adjuvant therapy treatments available with proven effectiveness are radiation and chemotherapy.

## ADJUVANT RADIATION THERAPY OF GLIOBLASTOMA

### *What is the adjuvant radiation therapy of glioblastoma?*

Because glioblastoma begins to grow back immediately after surgery, additional treatment is necessary. Roughly 90% of the time, when glioblastoma recurs, the recurrence is within two or three centimeters of the "margin of resection", meaning the edges of the area from which the surgeon removed all or part of the tumor. For this reason, radiation therapy administered focuses on this area after surgery

Radiation therapy to the site of the tumor slows its growth and extends survival time. New radiation therapy techniques that concentrate the dose of radiation delivered to the tumor, called "involved field radiation therapy", focuses the radiation on the tumor and the two or three centimeter margin of the brain immediately surrounding the tumor that is likely to contain glioblastoma cells. This maximizes the effect of the radiation on the glioblastoma, while minimizing radiation exposure of normal areas of the brain. The radiation daily, five days per week, for a period of six weeks.

### How important is it to begin radiation therapy immediately after surgery?

People with glioblastoma, who have a short delay between surgery and radiation, may have an improved chance of longer survival as compared to people who begin their radiation within two weeks of the surgery. Therefore, some delay may be good and it may be unimportant and unhelpful to have the radiation therapy begin within two weeks of the surgery. A common recommendation is for initiation of radiation within four to six weeks of surgery.

## ADJUVANT CHEMOTHERAPY OF GLIOBLASTOMA

### What is adjuvant chemotherapy of glioblastoma?

Adjuvant chemotherapy of glioblastoma is with a medication called "temozolomide" (brand name is "Temodar", manufacturer's product website is www.temodar.com) and is given daily along with the radiation therapy, and then five days per month for roughly six months after radiation is completed. Temodar adds, on average, several months of survival, increasing average survival time from approximately 12 months to approximately 16-20 months with a better than two-fold improvement of the odds of survival two years after diagnosis.

## GAMMA KNIFE: STEREOTACTIC RADIOSURGERY

### *What is the gamma knife and is it effective?*

The gamma knife, also known as "stereotactic radiosurgery", is a method of delivering a highly focused beam of radiation to the tumor in one or a very few treatments. The benefit derived from gamma knife as opposed to more conventional surgery and radiation is highly controversial when considering possible side effects and lack of clear evidence of benefit, with regard to either tumor control or survival. The gamma knife can have severe damaging effects on normal brain by causing swelling of the radiated area that, in turn, causes injury to the surrounding brain.

## RECURRENT GLIOBLASTOMA

### *What is recurrent glioblastoma?*

Despite the best available treatment, glioblastoma usually recurs, with the recurrence becoming evident, on average, 7 months or so after completion of radiation. Most of the time, this recurrence is within two or three centimeters of the area from which the original tumor was surgically removed and irradiated. The technical definition for recurrence or progression is an increase in tumor size by 25%, based upon MRI scans, or the appearance of a new area of the brain that is involved with tumor.

### *What is pseudoprogression?*

The MRI scan that evaluates glioblastoma includes the injection of a radiologist's dye called "gadolinium". Because blood vessels inside a brain tumor are leaky, this gadolinium leaks from the blood vessels into brain tissue and is visible with the MRI scan as a whitish area called a "gadolinium-enhancing lesion". Measurements of the changes in the size of the gadolinium-enhancing lesion help physicians evaluate the response of the glioblastoma to treatment.

After radiation to the brain tumor and surrounding brain, the destruction of brain tumor cells can induce a condition called "radiation necrosis", in which the dead tumor cells cause some inflammation of surrounding brain, and some additional leakiness of local blood vessels. This can produce a "gadolinium-enhancing lesion" that is indistinguishable from tumor progression. As a result, physicians call this "pseudoprogression".

Although pseudoprogression may be associated with brain swelling and new neurologic symptoms, it often is completely without symptoms and harmless.

## How can physicians tell the difference between progression and pseudoprogression?

No simple test can tell the difference. If new symptoms do not appear, and especially if the questionable progression occurs shortly after completing radiation treatment, physicians continue treatment with Temodar, repeating the MRI scan every month or two, to see whether the MRI changes stabilize or improve, or whether the changes evolve in a way that make the diagnosis of progression or pseudoprogression obvious.

# TREATMENT OF RECURRENT GLIOBLASTOMA

## *What is the treatment of recurrent glioblastoma?*

Depending on the size and location of the recurrence, and associated new symptoms that have developed, an operation to remove as much tumor as possible may transiently regain control of the tumor and relieve symptoms. Examination of the tissue removed during the operation can also confirm whether there has been tumor progression or radiation necrosis with pseudoprogression.

A very novel therapy, the "Novo-TTF device" has recently become available for people with recurrent glioblastoma. This device, through electrodes on the scalp, creates a low-intensity electric field that disrupts the machinery inside the glioblastoma cells that drives them to multiply. The FDA has approved the Novo-TTF device for use in recurrent glioblastoma, based upon the finding that survival for people using the Novo-TTF device is roughly equal, at six months, to that of people receiving chemotherapy. The big and impressive difference, however, in reported clinical trials between the Novo-TTF device and chemotherapy is that the Novo-TTF device is not associated with significant side effects, and that roughly 8% of people with recurrent glioblastoma treated with the Novo-TTF device survive four years or longer with treatment, as compared to no patients treated with chemotherapy. Preliminary results also suggest a slightly better survival for people treated with the Novo-TTF device compared to treatment with bevacizumab, as described below.

The biotechnology medication "bevacizumab" (brand name is "Avastin", manufacturer's product website is www.avastin.com)

inhibits the growth of blood vessels that a malignant brain tumor needs to feed its growth. Avastin improves the odds of survival for a few months longer if glioblastoma has progressed after chemotherapy. There are however, serious potential side effects of Avastin, including perforation of the stomach or intestines and internal bleeding. In addition, there is a recent report that some people with glioblastoma treated with bevacizumab may be predisposed to developing damage to the nerve in the back of the eye that transmits information from the eye to the brain. The association of this condition, called "optic neuropathy", with bevacizumab and glioblastoma is still under evaluation and uncertain, but appears to affect approximately one person in forty with glioblastoma getting this medication and can result in serious loss of vision in one or both eyes.

The unfavorable long-term outlook for people with glioblastoma encourages many people and their families to seek new or innovative treatments of glioblastoma immediately after making the diagnosis.

## EXPERIMENTAL TREATMENT OF GLIOBLASTOMA

### Who is doing the research on glioblastoma?

The most innovative glioblastoma treatment and research programs are at large medical centers or in hospitals specializing in cancer care or the treatment of neurological diseases. Physicians who specialize in the treatment of malignant brain tumors are "neuro-oncologists", and, along with neurosurgeons with a special interest and expertise in treating malignant brain tumors, coordinate much of this research.

# BREAST CANCER

## DEFINITION

### What is breast cancer?

Breast cancer is a cancer that begins in the breast. Unless eradicated in its earliest stages when confined to the breast, breast cancer can spread to other major organs in the body.

## SYMPTOMS

### What are the symptoms of breast cancer?

The most common first symptom of breast cancer is a new hard lump (referred to by physicians as a "mass") in the breast. Cancer in the breast can tug on tissue inside the breast, and can cause breast skin to dimple and the nipple to flatten or invert or deviate to one side or the other. A bloody discharge from the nipple always raises the suspicion of breast cancer and requires evaluation.

With the current mammography and other screening tools available to identify breast cancer in its earliest stages, it is common, at the time of diagnosis, for a woman to be without symptoms suggestive of breast cancer.

## <u>MAKING THE DIAGNOSIS</u>

### *How is the diagnosis of breast cancer made?*

A first step taken in evaluating a suspicious new mass in a breast may be to perform a mammogram. This test can give important, though not conclusive information about the size and location of the mass, and give clues, which are only clues, as to whether the mass is benign or malignant.

An ultrasound examination of the breast, performed by a physician (usually a radiologist) with special training in evaluation of breast masses, uses harmless sound waves bounced off the breast. Signals produced by these sound waves, sent to a computer, generate images that permit physicians to evaluate the size, shape, and consistency of masses that are present in the breast.

It is very important to understand, however, that a negative mammogram or an uncertain finding with the ultrasound test does not eliminate the possibility that a woman has breast cancer. If there is a suspicion that a mass is a cancer, it should be biopsied.

A diagnosis of breast cancer can usually be made by "needle aspiration" in which, based upon the mass that can clearly be felt, or using ultrasound images for guidance, a needle is passed into the breast mass, a small piece of tissue is sucked out ("aspirated") and sent to a pathologist for examination under the microscope. An "excisional biopsy", in which a piece of the mass is cut out with a scalpel and looked at under the microscope, is an alternative way to make a diagnosis. Because, compared to an excisional biopsy, the needle biopsy is equally accurate, much easier to perform, less painful, less expensive, leaves almost no scar, and is associated with a much faster recovery time, it is, in the great majority of circumstances, the preferred and most appropriate test to determine whether a new mass in the breast is a breast cancer.

## What information can the laboratory obtain from the biopsy?

By looking at the cells under the microscope, the laboratory can determine whether cancer is present, and if it is, draw conclusions about how likely it is that the cancer will rapidly grow, invade local tissues, and perhaps spread elsewhere.

An additional critical test is to look at "predictive" aspects of the cancer, that is, at aspects of the cancer that can predict a response to some specific treatments. The three most important "predictive" tests will look for the presence or absence of "estrogen receptors", "progesterone receptors" and "HER-2 overexpression" in the breast cancer cells. "HER-2 expression" indicates whether the cancer has too many copies of a gene called "HER-2". This gene is responsible for production of a protein that stimulates growth and spread of breast cancer cells. The presence or absence of "estrogen receptors", "progesterone receptors", and "HER-2 overexpression" provides extremely critical information about the likelihood that a woman will respond to important medications.

# DETERMINING WHETHER THE CANCER HAS SPREAD

*What tests, after making the diagnosis of breast cancer, determine whether the cancer has spread beyond the breast?*

Once the diagnosis of breast cancer is established, the immediate priority is to determine whether the cancer has spread beyond the breast. This "staging" of the breast cancer is essential in determining the next steps in therapy.

A careful evaluation of bodily symptoms and a thorough physical examination can identify evidence of spread of the cancer beyond the breast. Blood tests may show evidence of spread of the cancer to bone or liver. A chest x-ray may suggest that the cancer has spread to the lung or to other places inside the chest. If, based upon these tests or a person's symptoms and physical examination there is a suspicion of spread of the cancer beyond the breast, further evaluation could include CT or MRI scans or a bone scan.

*How commonly has breast cancer already spread beyond the breast into the bones or internal organs at the time of first diagnosis?*

Breast cancer that has spread beyond the breast into the bones or internal organs is "metastatic disease" or "metastatic breast cancer". Approximately 5% of women with breast cancer have metastatic disease at the time of first diagnosis.

## DUCTAL CARCINOMA IN SITU ("DCIS")

### What is ductal carcinoma in situ (DCIS)?

Breast milk, produced in the breast in "lobules", travels to the nipple through "ducts". Ductal carcinoma in situ, commonly abbreviated as "DCIS", is a cancer that involves the lining of the ducts that carry milk to the nipple. Although this cancer is localized and generally curable at the time of diagnosis, it can grow and invade adjacent breast tissue and become dangerous, if not properly treated.

### What tests confirm the presence of DCIS?

DCIS usually produces no symptoms. Routine mammography can raise the suspicion of DCIS based upon the identification of small deposits of calcium called "microcalcifications". If mammography raises a concern about the possible presence of DCIS, physicians will commonly perform a "percutaneous core biopsy" in which a needle, placed through the skin and into the breast, removes a small cylinder-shaped piece of tissue. A percutaneous core biopsy removes a somewhat larger piece of tissue than can be removed by a needle aspiration biopsy, and allows the pathologist examining the biopsy to confirm a diagnosis of DCIS, as opposed to the more aggressive "invasive cancer" described below.

## INVASIVE BREAST CANCER

### What is invasive breast cancer?

In contrast to DCIS in which the cancer only involves the cells lining the ducts, invasive breast cancer, which usually started in the ducts or lobules, has spread, or in medical terms, "infiltrated", into the tissues of the breast that surround the ducts or lobules. The most common invasive breast cancers have the names "infiltrating ductal carcinoma" and "infiltrating lobular carcinoma".

## TREATMENT OF BREAST CANCER THAT APPEARS TO INVOLVE ONLY THE BREAST

### *What is the treatment for breast cancer that appears to involve only the breast?*

The paramount objective of early breast cancer treatment is to eliminate the cancer from the body and to cure the disease.

There are two major approaches to achieving a cure of early breast cancer. The conservative approach will remove only the area of the breast containing the cancer and leave the remainder of the breast intact. Total breast removal ("mastectomy") is a more intensive choice used in selected circumstances.

### *How is the choice of treatment made?*

Years ago, surgeons almost universally believed that the treatment of choice was a radical mastectomy that removed the entire breast, chest muscle beneath the breast, and local lymph nodes. This procedure, called the "radical mastectomy" is no longer the standard of care of women with early breast cancer. It is now clear, that the proper initial treatment of breast cancer depends upon the size and location of the cancer within the breast and upon the appearance of the cancer under the microscope.

# SURGERY THAT DOES NOT REMOVE
# THE ENTIRE BREAST

## What is the surgical treatment of very small breast cancers?

Women with very small breast cancers can often have their cancer treated in a way that will largely preserve the breast. The breast-conserving procedure commonly used is a "lumpectomy", that is, surgical removal of the "lump" in the breast and a bit of surrounding tissue. A pathologist examines the lump and surrounding tissue under the microscope, and determines whether the "margins", that is, the interface between where the cancer was located in the breast and the immediately surrounding and outer edges of the surgically removed tissue, are clear of cancer. If these "margins" contain cancer cells, a physician may attempt to eliminate remaining cancer cells by surgically removing a bit more tissue from the area surrounding the location of the previously removed breast lump. This often results in a "clean margin", not containing cancer cells. If the margin, however, continues to have cancer cells, mastectomy may be required to give the best odds of curing the cancer.

Although breast-conserving surgery has the major advantage of an improved cosmetic appearance of the chest after the treatment, some women prefer to have their breast cancer treated with a mastectomy. For these women, the surgery performed will be a "modified radical mastectomy" in which the entire breast and some lymph nodes in the armpit are surgically removed.

# MASTECTOMY: SURGERY THAT REMOVES THE ENTIRE BREAST

*Are there times when a mastectomy is
more effective than a breast-conserving procedure?*

Women who have cancer involving several different areas (a "multicentric" tumor) have a better chance of having all the cancer removed by a mastectomy than by a breast-conserving procedure. Similarly, if the mammography shows small areas of calcium deposits (called "microcalcifications") that have the appearance of cancer throughout the breast, mastectomy is more likely to cure the cancer than breast conserving surgery.

Because radiation is essential after a lumpectomy, mastectomy is an appropriate treatment for women with a localized breast cancer who are in their early stages of pregnancy. The only safe alternative to the fetus when a woman chooses to have a lumpectomy will be to delay radiation therapy until shortly after delivery.

*What does the surgeon remove with the mastectomy?*

The mastectomy procedure will remove the entire breast, some tissue around the muscles in the chest, and lymph nodes in the armpit (the "axilla"). A "skin-sparing mastectomy", in which breast tissue beneath the skin is removed while sparing the skin itself and sometimes the nipple, can make reconstructive surgery easier to do if the woman chooses to have this done.

## THE AXILLA AND AXILLARY LYMPH NODES

*What is the axilla, what are axillary lymph nodes?*

The armpit in medical terms is the "axilla". The lymph nodes in the armpit are "axillary lymph nodes". Surgical removal of these lymph nodes is an "axillary lymph node dissection".

## EVALUATING AXILLARY LYMPH NODES

*Why is it important to determine whether cancer cells are present in axillary lymph nodes?*

The presence or absence of breast cancer cells in the axillary lymph nodes provides vital information with regard to a woman's probability of remaining free of recurrence of the cancer and is a key factor in making the decision about whether further treatment, such as chemotherapy, is needed.

*With invasive breast cancer, how commonly is cancer present in the axillary lymph nodes at the time of initial diagnosis?*

Overall, approximately one-third of women with apparently localized invasive breast cancer have cancer in one or more axillary lymph nodes at the time of first diagnosis.

*How much higher is the risk of breast cancer recurrence if the axillary lymph nodes contain cancer cells?*

The presence of cancer cells in the axillary lymph nodes roughly doubles the risk of recurrence of the breast cancer.

## What is a sentinel node biopsy and how do physicians perform it?

There is a relatively new technique available, called a "sentinel node biopsy" which has largely replaced the "axillary lymph node dissection" as a way of determining whether axillary lymph nodes contain cancer. The sentinel node biopsy greatly reduces the number of lymph nodes removed and, by doing so, significantly reduces the risk of side effects from lymph node removal.

To do a sentinel node biopsy, the physician will put a special blue dye into the tissue around the tumor in the breast, from which the dye will travel through channels called "lymphatics", to the axillary lymph nodes. The physician can then easily identify the lymph nodes that contain the dye. These are the lymph nodes where the cancer, if it has travelled, is most likely to be.

If these lymph nodes are removed, examined under the microscope, and do not contain cancer, it is very unlikely that cancer will be found in other lymph nodes.

In the past, if the sentinel nodes did contain cancer cells, physicians would commonly recommend a full axillary lymph node dissection. Based upon a recent study, it appears that full axillary node dissection does not reduce the risk of recurrence or extend survival for women who have had breast-conserving surgery and have cancer-containing lymph nodes ("positive lymph nodes") found with sentinel node biopsy. Radiation given after breast conserving surgery, and chemotherapy given when sentinel nodes are positive, (these treatments are described below), appear to be sufficient to eliminate the small amount of remaining cancer in the lymph nodes, making axillary lymph node dissection unnecessary.

## *What are the side effects of an axillary lymph node dissection?*

After an axillary lymph node dissection, a woman can develop painful swelling of the arm (this arm swelling is called "lymphedema") which can become a chronic problem. There is also a possibility of damage to the nerves in the axilla that provide sensation to the arm.

## *Is it always necessary to evaluate the axillary lymph nodes in women with small breast cancers?*

Evaluation of the axillary lymph nodes is a critical component of the care of women with localized invasive breast cancer.

If a woman has ductal carcinoma in situ (DCIS), as described above, and receives treatment with a lumpectomy and radiation, evaluation of the axillary lymph nodes often is not recommended, since they are uncommonly involved with DCIS. In the unlikely event of later identification of invasive breast cancer, sentinel node biopsy remains possible.

Women who have DCIS involving several different areas "multicentric DCIS" of the breast, or DCIS of a size or location more treatable by mastectomy, are more likely to have undiscovered areas of invasive cancer, and are at a somewhat higher risk of having spread of the cancer to their axillary lymph nodes. If the planned treatment of the DCIS is a mastectomy, physicians commonly recommend, prior to surgery, lymph node evaluation with a sentinel node biopsy since, after a mastectomy, sentinel node biopsy is not possible.

# RADIATION THERAPY AFTER SURGERY THAT DOES NOT REMOVE THE ENTIRE BREAST

## *Is radiation therapy always necessary after a breast-conserving procedure?*

The woman who does not have radiation therapy after a breast-conserving procedure appears to have a roughly two-fold higher risk for developing local recurrence of her breast cancer, and a roughly 15% higher risk of dying from breast cancer, as compared to a woman who has received radiation therapy. Most experts believe very strongly that a woman who has had a breast-conserving procedure should have radiation therapy as part of her treatment.

## *How is radiation given?*

There are some differences in the exact regimen of radiation administered in different centers. A recent very large study compared the effectiveness of a three-week course of somewhat higher doses of radiation with a five-week course of somewhat lower doses of radiation. All women enrolled in the study had breast cancer removed with breast-conserving surgery and had no lymph nodes from the axilla that contained cancer. There was no apparent difference in the risk of local recurrence of the cancer, survival, side effects, or in the cosmetic appearance of the chest after radiation, whether given at higher doses over three weeks or lower doses over five weeks.

If lymph nodes in the axilla contain cancer, there is evidence that radiation to the area of the lymph nodes in the axilla along with radiation of the breast can further reduce the risk of local recurrence of the cancer and of spread of the cancer to distant areas of the body. The major side effect of the radiation of the lymph nodes in the axilla is the risk of developing a chronic and uncomfortable swelling of the arm called "lymphedema".

## RADIATION THERAPY AFTER MASTECTOMY

*Is radiation therapy useful after a modified radical mastectomy?*

Radiation given after a modified radical mastectomy can reduce the risk that the cancer will appear again on the chest in the area of the surgery, and can reduce the risk of developing a distant recurrence, that is, a "metastasis" of the cancer.

When considering the recommendation for radiation after a modified radical mastectomy physicians will take into account the number of lymph nodes containing cancer as determined by the axillary node dissection or sentinel node biopsy, and the size of the tumor before the surgery. In general, radiation usually is recommended after a modified radical mastectomy for women with four or more involved lymph nodes and is sometimes recommended in women with fewer involved lymph nodes. Some experts will also recommend radiation when the original tumor was large, for example, if the tumor was over 5 centimeters at its largest diameter.

## NEOADJUVANT CHEMOTHERAPY

*What is neoadjuvant chemotherapy?*

Breast cancer, at the time of initial diagnosis, may be of a size or in a location, which makes surgical removal, by either a lumpectomy or a mastectomy, difficult. Chemotherapy can sometimes shrink the cancer to the point where surgery can remove all or most of the cancer. This type of treatment is "neoadjuvant chemotherapy".

## When is neoadjuvant chemotherapy most commonly used?

There are two major reasons for giving neoadjuvant therapy.

When a woman has a relatively large breast cancer that appears to require a mastectomy for its successful and complete removal, neoadjuvant therapy may shrink the cancer to a sufficient extent to allow breast-conserving surgery.

Breast cancer can sometimes grow very rapidly and, at the time of diagnosis, may be too large for surgery alone to have the potential to remove all of the cancer in the breast and surrounding tissues. These cancers, which are considered to be "locally advanced", can sometimes be reduced in size by neoadjuvant chemotherapy, such that surgical removal and local control of the cancer becomes possible.

## What does neoadjuvant chemotherapy consist of?

Neoadjuvant chemotherapy generally consists of two or more intravenous medications that are given, in various regimens, over a period of three to four months.

## What treatment is available if the breast cancer does not respond or progresses despite the neoadjuvant chemotherapy?

Most of the time, neoadjuvant chemotherapy successfully reduces the size of the breast cancer. If, however, the cancer is unaffected by the neoadjuvant chemotherapy, radiation treatment to the breast cancer, or hormonal treatment as described below, may reduce the size of the breast cancer sufficiently to permit an attempt at surgical removal.

## LOCAL RECURRENCE AFTER BREAST-CONSERVING THERAPY OR MASTECTOMY

### What is local recurrence?

Local recurrence, in the context of breast cancer, means either recurrence in the breast after breast-conserving surgery or, after mastectomy, recurrence in the area of the chest wall from which the cancer was removed. Approximately one in ten women develops a local recurrence after breast conserving surgery or mastectomy.

### When does this recurrence usually occur?

Local recurrence of the breast cancer most commonly occurs two years or more after the initial surgery.

### Why is it important for a woman who has had breast conserving surgery or mastectomy to have regular check-ups?

After a breast-conserving procedure or a mastectomy, regular check-ups are critical to the identification of early evidence of cancer recurrence. This check-up generally includes an examination of the skin on the chest wall, and of the breasts including mammograms. Recurrence in the breast (or a new cancer in the same or opposite breast), or recurrence on the chest wall, when found at its earliest stages, is more likely to be curable with treatment.

*What tests will physicians often perform when a woman develops evidence of a local recurrence of her breast cancer?*

Physicians will often perform a needle biopsy, as described earlier in this chapter, to confirm that a new mass felt with the examining fingers or identified with the mammogram is, in fact, cancer. If the mass is a cancer, the laboratory can determine whether the cancer cells are positive for estrogen and progesterone receptors, and for HER-2 overexpression. These laboratory results are important in guiding the next steps in therapy.

Because this recurrence can be associated with spread of the cancer elsewhere in the body, a full evaluation could include blood tests, CT scan of the chest, abdomen and pelvis, a bone scan, as well as other tests. If tests identify an area suspected of containing cancer, a biopsy can confirm the presence of cancer cells and the diagnosis of locally recurrent breast cancer.

*What is the treatment if the breast cancer recurs in the breast after a breast-conserving procedure or mastectomy?*

If the local breast cancer recurrence is not associated with spread beyond the breast, a total mastectomy will often cure the breast cancer and is the treatment commonly recommended.

*What is the most common appearance of local recurrence after a mastectomy?*

Local recurrence of breast cancer after a mastectomy most commonly appears as one or more round hard masses called "nodules" in the general area from which the cancer was removed (this general area is referred to as the "chest wall" and recurrence in this area is referred to as "chest wall recurrence"). Recurrence of the cancer also can occur in the lymph nodes in the armpit (this type of recurrence is "axillary node recurrence") or in the lymph nodes just above the collarbone (the medical word for the collarbone is the "clavicle" and lymph nodes above the clavicle are "supraclavicular lymph nodes"). Recurrence of the cancer in local lymph nodes can make these lymph nodes feel like small, hard, somewhat oval-shaped masses.

## How is local recurrence after a mastectomy treated?

The most effective treatment of local recurrence after a mastectomy is to have a surgeon remove, if possible, all identifiable nodules or masses that contain cancer. This surgical removal has the potential to cure the cancer or significantly delay it from returning.

If the woman has not yet had radiation to the chest wall, radiation therapy directed at the chest wall and the "axillary" and "supraclavicular" lymph nodes (as described above) could eliminate or suppress the growth of any cancer cells present in those areas. The radiation is administered over a period of five to six weeks, with five days radiation treatment during each of those weeks (usually Monday through Friday).

If the cancer is very large and difficult to remove surgically, chemotherapy can often shrink the cancer to the point where surgical removal of the local recurrence is possible.

After treatment of the local recurrence with surgery and radiation, the woman is at a significant risk for development of distant spread of her cancer. For this reason, additional therapy such as chemotherapy or hormonal therapy may be given after completion of surgery and radiation, in an attempt to prevent the cancer from returning.

## PREDICTING WHETHER THE CANCER WILL SPREAD BEYOND THE BREAST

*What best predicts whether the cancer will spread beyond the breast?*

An important factor that predicts the likelihood of whether a breast cancer will spread beyond the breast is whether lymph nodes in the axilla contain breast cancer cells. A pathologist, who will examine (under a microscope), the axillary lymph nodes removed during the sentinel node biopsy or the axillary node dissection, will perform this evaluation.

Other important factors determining the likelihood of recurrence are the size of the original cancer as well as the appearance of the cancer under the microscope. Cancers that are determined by the laboratory to be negative for HER-2 and for estrogen or progesterone receptors ("triple negative breast cancer") are somewhat more likely to spread unless further treatment is given.

## PREVENTION OF SPREAD OF THE CANCER BEYOND THE BREAST

*What are the limitations of lumpectomy with radiation or of modified radical mastectomy?*

Cancer cells which have spread to areas of the body beyond the breast at the time of the initial surgery, will be unaffected by surgery that controls the cancer in the breast and by radiation given to the breast, axilla, or chest. These cells will continue to grow unless stopped by some additional therapy. It is the distant spread of the breast cancer, the "metastatic disease", which is responsible for the life-threatening complications of breast cancer.

## What treatment can prevent the spread of cancer beyond the breast?

Treatment given to prevent the recurrence or spread of breast cancer after potentially curative local therapy is "adjuvant therapy".

Two principal forms of adjuvant therapy can reduce the risk of cancer recurrence: chemotherapy and hormonal therapy.

## Is adjuvant therapy always necessary?

Women with breast cancer that has spread to lymph nodes in the axilla are at a higher risk of recurrence. Based upon an enormous amount of information, experts believe that when cancer has spread to lymph nodes, some form of adjuvant therapy with proven effectiveness is necessary.

For women with breast cancer that has not spread to lymph nodes in the axilla ("node-negative breast cancer"), physicians will consider the size of the original cancer. If the original cancer was over 0.5 to 1 centimeter in diameter, many experts will believe that adjuvant therapy is appropriate. In addition, other risk factors which will be considered are the appearance of the cancer under the microscope, the presence or absence of estrogen, progesterone and HER-2 receptors on the surface of the cancer cells, and perhaps some of the newer tests under development that predict the likelihood that the cancer will or will not spread. This information enables evaluation of the probability of recurrence. With this information, as well as information about the reduction of risk associated with the different types of adjuvant treatment, a woman with breast cancer can make the most informed decision regarding how to proceed.

## CHEMOTHERAPY TO PREVENT SPREAD OF THE BREAST CANCER: "ADJUVANT CHEMOTHERAPY"

*If adjuvant chemotherapy is considered necessary, when does treatment usually begin?*

Adjuvant chemotherapy usually begins within 6 weeks after the surgery that removed the cancer from the breast.

*How is adjuvant chemotherapy treatment given?*

Cyclophosphamide (brand name is "Cytoxan"), doxorubicin (brand name is "Adriamycin"), paclitaxel (brand name is "Taxol") and docetaxel (brand name is "Taxotere", manufacturer's product website is www.taxotere.com) are among the medications most often used.

A common treatment regimen, especially in women who have lymph nodes that were found to be positive for breast cancer, will include Cytoxan and Adriamycin intravenously on the same day approximately once every three weeks until four "cycles" of this treatment have been given. After that, the woman receives four cycles of Taxotere, with the Taxotere administered once every three weeks, on the first day of each of four cycles.

Women who do not have lymph nodes positive for cancer, but, because of the size of their cancer or its appearance under the microscope, are at risk of recurrence, can have the risk of recurrence reduced by a combination of chemotherapy medications. Some physicians consider the combination of the medicines "Taxotere", "Adriamycin" and "Cytoxan" (the "TAC" regimen), administered once every three weeks for six treatments, as an appropriate regimen for women with "node negative" breast cancer who are at a high risk for recurrence of cancer. With this regimen, over 85% of women will be free of evidence of breast cancer six years or longer after treatment is completed.

Please see the discussion below regarding the adjuvant chemotherapy administered if a woman's breast cancer cells test positive for "HER-2 overexpression".

### What are the side effects of the chemotherapy?

The main side effects are nausea, vomiting, sores in the mouth, and hair loss. Suppression of the production of white blood cells and platelets by the bone marrow is common. Although the bone marrow usually recovers quickly after chemotherapy, the low number of white blood cells and platelets in the bloodstream will cause the woman to have a transiently higher risk for acquiring serious infections (see chapter entitled "Bone Marrow Suppression)". Adriamycin has the potential to cause significant damage to heart muscle, although the four cycles given as adjuvant treatment are generally not sufficient to cause this side effect.

Women who have not yet reached menopause may lose the hormonal functioning of their ovaries because of adjuvant chemotherapy. Since these hormones help to maintain the amount of minerals in the bone, pre-menopausal women who lose ovarian hormonal function are at an increased risk of developing osteoporosis.

## What is the commonly recommended treatment if the woman's breast cancer cells tested positive for HER-2 overexpression?

HER-2 overexpression, as discussed earlier in this chapter, is present in approximately one in four women with breast cancer. HER-2 overexpression has profound importance, since it provides a target for a critical medication.

HER-2 overexpression causes the appearance of a "receptor" on the surface of the breast cancer cells, which signals the cancer cells to grow and spread. A "monoclonal antibody" was designed that could, with great specificity, bind to this receptor, interrupting its signaling capability, and by doing so, restrain the growth and spread of the cancer. This medication has the generic name "trastuzumab" and the brand name "Herceptin" (manufacturer's product website is www.herceptin.com). Women whose breast cancer cells tested positive for HER-2 overexpression may reduce the risk of having their cancer recur by approximately 50% when Herceptin is included in their adjuvant treatment regimen.

When Herceptin is included in adjuvant treatment, a new regimen combines the chemotherapy medications "Taxotere" and "Carboplatin" with Herceptin. This regimen, known as the "TCH regimen", has an advantage over older regimens that included the medication "Adriamycin" which, when given together with Herceptin, can have damaging effects on the heart.

## How is the TCH regimen given?

The two chemotherapy medications, Taxotere and Carboplatin, are administered intravenously every three weeks. Each three-week period is a "cycle" and women receive six cycles of chemotherapy. Every week during chemotherapy, a woman will receive an intravenous injection of Herceptin. Following completion of the chemotherapy, a woman will receive Herceptin every three weeks, until she has received Herceptin injections for a total of one year.

## How serious is the heart risk in women who are receiving Herceptin?

It appears that about one woman in thirty who receives adjuvant therapy containing chemotherapy and Herceptin develops some heart failure or other heart problems and that this side effect is usually transient and not associated with major long-term problems. A cardiac evaluation before Herceptin treatment begins, along with monitoring of cardiac function during the months of Herceptin treatment, reduces the already small risks associated with the Herceptin treatment.

## How do specialists currently balance the benefits and risks of Herceptin in women with HER-2 positive breast cancer?

Women with cancer that has spread to lymph nodes or women with a large cancer in their breast at the time of diagnosis are at a higher risk of developing recurrence of breast cancer after initial surgical treatment. Herceptin clearly reduces this risk in women with overexpression of HER-2. For women who are likely to benefit from Herceptin, the risk to health associated with recurrence of the cancer is far greater than the small risk of developing heart problems from Herceptin.

## *How effective is adjuvant chemotherapy at reducing the mortality of breast cancer?*

Based upon a recent analysis of over 100,000 women with breast cancer treated with chemotherapy over the past 40 years, it appears that chemotherapy reduces the risk of death from breast cancer by roughly one-third. It is possible that the more modern adjuvant chemotherapy regimens used today reduce the risk of death from breast cancer still further.

## HORMONAL THERAPY TO PREVENT SPREAD OF THE BREAST CANCER

### *Who can benefit from adjuvant hormonal therapy?*

To benefit from adjuvant hormonal therapy, estrogen receptors must be present on the surface of the cancer cells. If these cells are "estrogen receptor negative", benefit from hormonal therapy is unlikely.

### *When is the adjuvant hormonal therapy given?*

If adjuvant chemotherapy is a required treatment to reduce the risk of recurrence of the breast cancer, hormonal therapy begins shortly after the chemotherapy is completed. If adjuvant chemotherapy is not considered to be necessary, adjuvant hormonal therapy, when required, begins shortly after surgery and local radiation treatments (if radiation is required), have been completed.

### What is the adjuvant hormonal therapy when a woman has not yet reached menopause?

The adjuvant hormonal therapy generally recommended for women who have not yet reached menopause is the medicine "tamoxifen" which blocks the ability of a women's own estrogen to bind to the estrogen receptors on cancer cells. Blocking this interaction between estrogen and estrogen receptors inhibits the growth of the cancer. Tamoxifen is a pill that a woman takes every day. Treatment with tamoxifen should continue without interruption for five years.

In some circumstances, and especially in women under 40 years of age with higher natural production of estrogen, physicians recommend "ovarian ablation" meaning surgical removal of the ovaries or irradiation of the ovaries, or "ovarian suppression", meaning suppression of production of hormones from the ovary. The medicine called "goserelin" (brand name is "Zoladex", manufacturer's product website is www.zoladex.com) blocks the ability of the ovaries to make estrogen and is a frequently used medicine for ovarian suppression.

Removal of the ovaries may be particularly appropriate in women who have the "breast cancer susceptibility gene mutation", abbreviated "BCRA". BCRA indicates susceptibility to both breast and ovarian cancer, so that removal of the ovaries can prevent later development of ovarian cancer.

Blocking estrogen production, combined with blocking estrogen binding to estrogen receptor-bearing cancer cells, may further reduce the risk of breast cancer recurrence. Clinical trials are evaluating this combined adjuvant hormonal treatment, as well as its benefit when given after adjuvant chemotherapy.

## When a woman is no longer menstruating and post-menopausal, what is the adjuvant hormonal therapy?

For post-menopausal women, a class of anti-estrogen pills called "aromatase inhibitors" is available which may be slightly more effective than tamoxifen and which has different side effects. The aromatase inhibitors that are available are "anastrozole" (brand name is Arimidex, manufacturer's product website is www.arimidex.com), "exemestase" (brand name is "Aromasin", manufacturer's product website is www.aromasin.com), and "letrozole" (brand name is "Femara", manufacturer's product website is www.femara.com). The aromatase inhibitors are more likely than tamoxifen to cause osteoporosis and associated bone fractures, and are more likely to raise blood pressure and blood cholesterol levels. Tamoxifen is more likely than aromatase inhibitors to cause hot flashes, blood clots in the legs, and may increase the risk of developing uterine cancer or other problems with the uterus. The current recommendations for women who are post-menopausal and for whom hormonal adjuvant treatment is appropriate is to either treat with five years of an aromatase inhibitor or to treat with two or three years of an aromatase inhibitor followed by two or three years of tamoxifen, for a total of five years of adjuvant hormonal treatment. Discussion of the risks and benefits of aromatase inhibitors and tamoxifen may influence a woman to choose one treatment or the other based upon an understanding of side effects expected with treatment.

The aromatase inhibitors are not considered to be appropriate for women who are still menstruating because they can stimulate a menstruating woman's functioning ovaries and somewhat counteract the effect of estrogen receptor blockade.

## Is one aromatase inhibitor more effective than the others are?

The aromatase inhibitors appear to be equally effective and to be equally likely to cause side effects. Because the aromatase inhibitor "anastrozole" has just become generic, it is less expensive, and physicians may prefer to prescribe it instead of the others.

## What effect does hormonal therapy with aromatase inhibitors have on bones?

Hormonal therapy with aromatase inhibitors can decrease the amount of minerals in the bone and weaken them. Tamoxifen has the opposite effect, slightly increasing the amount of minerals in the bone.

Loss of bone minerals and resulting loss of the structural strength of bone is "osteoporosis". Osteoporosis associated with hormonal therapy of breast cancer increases the risk of developing bone fractures after only minor trauma. Because of this, many physicians will recommend a simple and painless "bone mineral density test" at the beginning of therapy and at regular intervals so that the effect of the treatment on the strength of the bones can be followed closely.

## Are there ways to prevent osteoporosis during aromatase inhibitor therapy?

Dietary supplementation with calcium and Vitamin $D_3$, to some extent, can be helpful. Exercise, and especially resistance exercise, can be helpful. The medications called "bisphosphonates", which are discussed in the chapter entitled "Bone Metastasis", may also inhibit the breakdown of bone associated with hormonal therapy and delay or prevent osteoporosis.

A biotechnology-derived medication called "denosumab" (brand name is "Xgeva", manufacturer's product website is www.xgeva. com) reduces the degree of osteoporosis and the risk of fractures of the spine in women receiving adjuvant hormonal therapy for breast cancer.

*Is there an additional benefit of receiving a bisphosphonate while receiving adjuvant hormonal therapy?*

Based upon large clinical studies, it appears that the bisphosphonate "zoledronic acid," when added to different forms of adjuvant hormonal therapy, further reduces the risk of breast cancer recurrence and the risk of death from breast cancer by over 30%.

## FOLLOW-UP CARE AFTER SURGERY AND ADJUVANT THERAPY

*After completing adjuvant chemotherapy or hormonal therapy, what type of follow-up care is appropriate to detect early evidence of metastatic breast cancer?*

With the current methods of treatment, early detection of the appearance of asymptomatic spread of cancer beyond the breast does not improve the chance of cure and does not appear to improve the likelihood of a longer survival. For this reason, in the absence of symptoms suggestive of recurrence, intensive follow-up with frequent blood tests and sophisticated x-rays and scans may not be necessary or recommended. This could change: as treatment of metastatic breast cancer improves, it is very possible that early diagnosis of metastatic breast cancer will lead to improved outcome. At this time, a common recommendation will be for routine check-ups every three to six months for three years, then every six to twelve months for the next two years, then annually.

If new symptoms develop, such as the appearance of nodules in the breast or chest wall area as described earlier in this chapter, prompt evaluation is essential.

At a routine check-up, a key issue will be whether the woman is experiencing any symptoms suggestive of recurrent cancer. The physical examination will focus on identification of any evidence of recurrence in the area of the surgery, in lymph nodes, in the liver, in the bones of the spine, or elsewhere. Painful bones, a new mass in the area of surgery, a painful or enlarged liver, or a weakness in the legs (which could indicate a tumor in the spine pressing on the spinal cord) will all require careful evaluation. Blood tests, x-rays, bone scans, or CT or MRI or PET scans may be useful for evaluating any areas of the body that are suspicious for recurrent disease.

Because some areas containing cancer may not be detectable by CT or MRI scan, physicians will sometimes ask a woman in whom symptoms or other findings raise a concern about the presence of metastasis, to obtain a "PET" scan. A PET scan is a sensitive test that can often detect the spread of cancer to distant organs before detection by CT scans. To do this test, an injection is made of a tiny amount of radioactive glucose into the bloodstream. Cancer cells have a greater affinity for this radioactive glucose than other cells.

The PET scanner can then find "hot spots" inside the body that contain the cancer and transmit this information to a computer for the physician to evaluate. The identification of a "hot spot" suggests, but does not prove, the presence of cancer cells in the hot spot. Although a "hot spot" may indicate the presence of cancer, areas of inflammation without cancer can also produce "hot spots". A "hot spot" indicates a suspicious area that needs evaluation, often with a biopsy, to confirm the presence or absence of local cancer.

A biopsy of an area suspected of harboring metastatic cancer could confirm the presence or absence of recurrence. If the biopsy shows recurrence, the laboratory can determine whether the area of metastatic cancer is positive for estrogen or progesterone receptors or is positive or negative for HER-2 overexpression, and whether these results are consistent with those obtained with the biopsy of the initial area of cancer as described earlier in this chapter. This could be very important for planning treatment.

## METASTATIC BREAST CANCER

### What is metastatic breast cancer?

Metastatic breast cancer means there is clear evidence of spread of the cancer beyond the breast, beyond the outside surface of the chest ("the chest wall"), and beyond the lymph nodes in the axilla. The most common areas to which metastatic breast cancer initially spreads are the bones, the lung, or the liver. Because the diagnosis of metastatic breast cancer profoundly affects the rest of a woman's life, it is critical that the diagnosis is accurate. When a suspicion of metastatic breast cancer arises because of an abnormal x-ray, CT, MRI, or bone scan finding, a biopsy of an area suspected of containing cancer can confirm the presence of cancer cells and the diagnosis of metastatic breast cancer.

## *When does metastatic cancer make its appearance?*

Metastatic cancer can occur any time from shortly after making the first diagnosis of localized breast cancer to many years from the initial diagnosis. Over half of the time, if metastatic breast cancer develops, it arises five years or more after the initial diagnosis.

## GENERAL CONSIDERATIONS THAT GUIDE METASTATIC BREAST CANCER TREATMENT

### *What general considerations guide physicians when suggesting the best form of treatment of metastatic breast cancer?*

Metastatic breast cancer generally is incurable with any treatment that is available today. Although some women with metastatic breast cancer may live for ten years or more with the disease, the treatments that are available today, however aggressively applied, are only rarely capable of curing metastatic breast cancer. The goal of treatment is, therefore, to extend healthful life as much as possible with a minimum of side effects from treatment and with a minimum of complications from the cancer itself.

### *If the treatments available for metastatic breast cancer are not curative, how effective are they?*

The available treatments of metastatic breast cancer, given sequentially, can often shrink the cancer and restrain the growth of the cancer for months and occasionally for years. This shrinkage of the cancer usually takes the form of a "partial remission", which means that the cancer has been reduced in size by 50% or more, but has not totally disappeared. Partial remissions of metastatic breast cancer induced by treatment commonly last for under a year, but if several partial remissions with different medications occur one after the other, survival can potentially be extended for several years.

## DETERMINING THE EXTENT TO WHICH BREAST CANCER HAS SPREAD

*What tests evaluate the extent of metastatic breast cancer and why is this important?*

A first step after the diagnosis of metastatic breast cancer will be to determine the extent to which the cancer has spread in the body. Physical examination, blood tests, chest x-ray and scans of the liver and bones can accurately identify areas of metastatic cancer. "Visceral metastasis" means that the cancer has spread to the liver, intestines, lungs or other body organs. Cancer that has spread to the bones is "bone metastasis". Evaluation of the areas of metastasis and of the problems these areas of metastasis may be causing is vital to making decisions about the form of treatment most likely to be beneficial.

## TREATMENT OF METASTATIC BREAST CANCER

*What types of therapy are generally available for women with metastatic breast cancer?*

Treatments available will be hormonal therapy or chemotherapy or biological therapy.

## How is the decision to treat a woman with metastatic breast cancer with hormonal therapy as opposed to chemotherapy made?

The decision regarding the choice of hormonal therapy as opposed to chemotherapy considers factors known to influence the odds of responding to hormonal therapy or chemotherapy. Hormonal therapy has fewer side effects than chemotherapy, therefore, when it is reasonable to do so, hormonal therapy is preferred.

Women whose breast cancer was estrogen receptor positive or progesterone receptor positive are likely to respond to hormonal therapy.

The "disease-free interval" is measured from the time when local therapy with surgery and radiation removed the initial cancer to the time the first evidence of metastasis appears. Women with a disease free interval of less than a year are more likely to have a rapidly growing cancer that is more responsive to chemotherapy than hormonal therapy. In addition, women whose breast cancer progressed within a year of receiving "adjuvant" hormonal treatment (see above) are less likely to respond to further hormonal treatment.

Women with areas of metastasis in the lymph nodes, the skin, or the bones, more commonly respond to hormonal therapy. Women with large areas of metastatic breast cancer in internal organs such as the liver and lungs are more likely to respond to chemotherapy.

The decision of whether to suggest hormonal therapy or chemotherapy weighs the above factors, leading a physician to prescribe hormonal therapy when hormonal therapy is likely to work and chemotherapy when hormonal therapy is not likely to work. When the considerations favoring hormonal therapy or chemotherapy can go either way, or when the risk of toxicity from chemotherapy, such as in elderly women, is a major issue, an attempt at hormonal therapy is often considered to be reasonable and best.

## SURGERY FOR METASTATIC BREAST CANCER

*Is there a role for surgery in the treatment of metastatic breast cancer?*

Occasionally, metastatic breast cancer makes its appearance as a solitary area of cancer in the lung, the brain, the liver, or on the surface of the chest. Depending on the location of this "solitary metastasis", surgical removal may be possible. Although additional areas of metastasis commonly develop after surgical removal of a solitary metastasis, recurrence of metastasis does not always occur, and many women have a prolonged "disease-free interval" after such treatment during which no additional areas of metastatic cancer develop.

## HORMONAL THERAPY OF METASTATIC BREAST CANCER

*What kind of hormonal therapy treats metastatic breast cancer?*

The most commonly used hormonal therapy of metastatic breast cancer counteracts the effect of estrogen in stimulating the growth of breast cancer cells. The beneficial effect of these anti-estrogen drugs is in women whose breast cancer cells have "estrogen receptors" on their surface, and are therefore stimulated to grow when estrogen binds to the cells.

For women who have not yet reached menopause ("pre-menopausal women") the estrogen blocking medicine used is tamoxifen. Tamoxifen treatment continues as long as the cancer stays under control. The average amount of time which tamoxifen can keep a metastatic breast cancer under control is slightly over a year. Metastatic breast cancer however, can remain under good control with tamoxifen for many years. Many physicians will advise a pre-menopausal woman to take, in addition to tamoxifen, a medicine that suppresses the functioning of the ovaries. In instances in which a woman does not want to take these ovary-suppressing medicines, a physician may suggest that a woman have her ovaries surgically removed. The medicines that suppress the functioning of the ovaries are in the family of "GnRH agonists" and include leuprolide (brand name is "Lupron", manufacturer's product website is www.lupron. com) and goserelin (brand name is "Zoladex", manufacturer's product website is www.zoladex.com).

In women who have already gone through menopause ("post-menopausal women") the most useful early form of hormonal treatment are the medicines in the family of "aromatase inhibitors". These are the same medications described earlier in this chapter: "anastrozole" (brand name is "Arimidex", manufacturer's product website is www.arimidex.com), "exemestase" (brand name is "Aromasin", manufacturer's product website is www.aromasin. com), and "letrozole" (brand name is "Femara", manufacturer's product website is www.femara.com). These medicines control metastatic breast cancer slightly more effectively than tamoxifen.

Pre-menopausal women have functioning ovaries and aromatase inhibitors stimulate their ovaries to produce estrogens. For this reason, tamoxifen is the preferred treatment for pre-menopausal women instead of aromatase inhibitors.

A recently reported clinical trial combined Arimidex, which decreases the estrogen fueling the breast cancer, with a medication called "fulvestrant" (brand name is "Faslodex", manufacturer's product website is www.faslodex.com) which blocks the receptor on the breast cancer cells that binds the estrogen. The idea behind this study was to completely shut off access of the breast cancer cells to estrogen, and, by doing so, maximize the benefit of the hormonal therapy. In this study, which involved over 700 women, the women who received the combination had, on average, a roughly six-month longer survival that the women who received Arimidex alone.

## How likely is it that a woman's metastatic breast cancer will respond to hormonal therapy?

The likelihood of a favorable response to hormonal therapy depends upon whether estrogen or progesterone receptors are present on the cancer cells. If the cancer cells have estrogen receptors only, approximately one-third of woman will respond to hormonal treatment. Approximately two-thirds of women will have a favorable response to hormonal treatment when both estrogen and progesterone receptors are present on cancer cells. If estrogen and progesterone receptors are absent, less than one woman in ten will respond. Since the side effects of the hormonal treatments are mild, it is common for cancer experts to suggest an attempt at hormonal treatment at some point during the illness of a woman with metastatic breast cancer.

### What does a "flare" mean when a woman first begins treatment with tamoxifen for metastatic breast cancer?

An additional problem that can develop when tamoxifen treatment for metastatic breast cancer begins is that of a "flare". Women with breast cancer that has spread to the bones occasionally develop a transient increase in bone pain and high levels of blood calcium (see chapter entitled "Malignant Hypercalcemia") shortly after beginning treatment with tamoxifen. Although these symptoms are very distressing, they do not mean that the tamoxifen is a bad drug or that tamoxifen will not work. The treatment of the flare will be to give medicine for pain, treat the hypercalcemia (see chapter entitled "Malignant Hypercalcemia") and continue the tamoxifen. The flare usually subsides within a month.

### What is the treatment if the initial antiestrogen medicine given is failing to control the growth of metastatic breast cancer?

Sometimes, switching from one antiestrogen medicine to another may produce another response. For example, a post-menopausal woman who is failing to respond to Femara may then respond to tamoxifen.

A very recent study evaluated women with estrogen receptor positive and HER-2 negative breast cancer whose cancer had progressed after receiving either "anastrozole" (brand name is Arimidex), or "letrozole" (brand name is "Femara"). These women were then given "exemestase" (brand name is "Aromasin") either alone or in combination with a pill called "everolimus" (brand name "Afinitor", manufacturer's product website is www.afinitor.com). The women receiving the combination of Aromasin and Afinitor clearly had the better outcome, with control of their cancer for over ten months, compared to about four months with Aromasin alone. Although this combination is not yet FDA approved, the reported results with the combination are very encouraging.

"Fulvestrant" (brand name is "Faslodex", manufacturer's product website is www.faslodex.com) blocks estrogen receptors and restrains the growth of breast cancer. Faslodex can delay progression of breast cancer and extend survival for postmenopausal women with estrogen receptor positive metastatic breast cancer whose disease has progressed after receiving tamoxifen or aromatase inhibitors. Faslodex is administered as an intramuscular injection every two weeks for the first month of treatment and every month thereafter.

Treatment with hormonal medicines such as "Megace" and "Depo Provera" which affects the "progesterone receptor" is often the next form of hormonal therapy used if antiestrogen medications are no longer controlling the breast cancer.

## HERCEPTIN IN METASTATIC BREAST CANCER

*What is the role for Herceptin in women who have metastatic breast cancer?*

Women with "HER-2 overexpression" on their breast cancer cells are "HER-2 positive".

Herceptin, given in conjunction with the hormonal treatment, can slow the growth of breast cancer in "HER-2 positive" women whose cancer cells have estrogen and progesterone receptors on their surface. The combination of hormonal therapy and Herceptin increases the chance of having shrinkage of the cancer, and improves the chance that treatment will prolong the length of time until the cancer begins to grow again.

If a women is "HER-2 positive", has progressed with hormonal treatment, and Herceptin has not yet been given, in some circumstances physicians may attempt to control the growth of the cancer with Herceptin alone.

"HER-2 positive women" whose cancer cells do not have estrogen or progesterone receptor on their surface, will commonly receive treatment with Herceptin along with chemotherapy.

### *What is done if the cancer progresses despite Herceptin treatment?*

In some circumstances, physicians may recommend continuing Herceptin treatment, since the Herceptin may be slowing, if not stopping, the growth of the cancer. Alternatively, a newer medication called "lapatinib" (brand name is "Tykerb", manufacturer's product website is www.tykerb.com) is available that also interacts with the HER-2 receptor, slowing the growth of the breast cancer, extending the period that the growth of the cancer is controlled, and extending survival. Tykerb may be given along with Herceptin, in an attempt to control the cancer by intensely inhibiting the HER-2 receptor.

### *What other HER-2 receptor targeted medications, added to Herceptin, are beneficial?*

Although Herceptin can restrain the growth of metastatic breast cancer for many months or longer, most people eventually become resistant to it, at which point the cancer begins to grow again. Researchers have found that an experimental medication, given the generic name "pertuzumab", targets the HER-2 receptor from a different angle and significantly increases the effectiveness of combination treatment with Herceptin and the chemotherapy medication "docetaxel". In a recent clinical trial involving over 800 women with metastatic breast cancer, combination treatment with pertuzumab, Herceptin, and docetaxel delayed progression of metastatic breast cancer by 18 months, compared to a 12-month delay with the combination of Herceptin and docetaxel. Although the information available is insufficient to conclude that addition of pertuzumab to treatment with Herceptin extends survival time, the early data is very encouraging and a significant survival benefit appears to be likely.

## CHEMOTHERAPY OF METASTATIC BREAST CANCER

### What is the role of chemotherapy in metastatic breast cancer?

Women with metastatic breast cancer who are unlikely to respond to hormonal therapy, or who have received hormonal therapy and have not responded or are no longer responding, can benefit from chemotherapy.

Women with metastatic breast cancer who have received hormonal therapy but have not responded, or are no longer responding, will generally not have sacrificed any of their chance of having a favorable response to chemotherapy because of having had hormonal therapy. After hormonal therapy, women are generally quite capable of having a favorable response to chemotherapy.

## What type of chemotherapy is generally administered?

A common chemotherapy treatment program for women with metastatic breast cancer is "sequential single agent therapy" which means that one drug is given at a time. Although giving combinations of chemotherapy drugs may give a higher chance of immediate shrinkage of the cancer, this benefit is associated with a higher risk of side effects and the practical problem of using up all the effective drugs too quickly so that there are no back-up medicines in case the initial treatments are failing to control the cancer.

At times, rapid growth of the cancer causes severe discomfort or dangerous complications. When this occurs, a combination of chemotherapy medicines may produce a more certain and rapid shrinkage of the cancer.

Many factors, such as estrogen, progesterone, and HER-2 receptor status, influence the choice of chemotherapy when a woman first develops metastatic breast cancer resistant to hormonal treatments.

Related medicines known as "taxanes" are common first chemotherapy treatments for metastatic breast cancer. These taxanes are "Taxol" (or its generic equivalent paclitaxel), "docetaxel" (brand name is "Taxotere") and "nab-Paclitaxel" (brand name is "Abraxane", and manufacturer's product website is www.abraxane. com). If the response to a taxane treatment is inadequate or if there is recurrence at some point despite the taxane treatment, other commonly used "second line" medicines include "doxorubicin" (brand name is "Adriamycin)", "gemcitabine" (brand name is "Gemzar", manufacturer's product website is www.gemzar.com)

and "capecitabine" (brand name is "Xeloda", manufacturer's product website is www.xeloda.com).

A new medication called "ixabepilone" (brand name is "Ixempra", manufacturer's product website is www.ixempra.com) can restrain the growth of breast cancer in women whose cancer has progressed after they have received a taxane, Adriamycin, and Xeloda. In addition, in women who have not yet received Xeloda, the combined treatment with Ixempra and Xeloda has some effectiveness.

An additional new chemotherapy medication named "eribulin" (brand name is "Halaven", manufacturer's product website is www. halaven.com) has recently been approved by the FDA for women with advanced breast cancer that has progressed despite treatment with "taxanes" and with "Adriamycin" (or related medicines called "anthracyclines"). Halaven received FDA approval based upon research indicating a slightly longer survival for women treated with Halaven compared with other treatment.

### How effective is chemotherapy?

The initial chemotherapy treatments for metastatic breast cancer produce shrinkage of the cancer about half of the time. Unfortunately, the shrinkage of the cancer and control of the cancer's growth usually lasts for less than a year. With each subsequent form of chemotherapy, there is a risk that the likelihood of tumor shrinkage and the duration of control of the cancer will be less. Although the average survival time, after chemotherapy begins, is about two years, some women, and especially women with only a few areas of the body containing evidence of cancer, can have a dramatic and very durable regression of their cancer after chemotherapy and much extended survival.

## What is the treatment if hormonal therapy or chemotherapy is failing to control the growth of the cancer?

The goal of treatment of local problems caused by treatment-refractory metastatic breast cancer will be to attempt to alleviate symptoms and prevent local complications.

An important option for a woman with metastatic breast cancer that is not responding to the hormonal therapy or chemotherapy is to seek some form of experimental treatment.

# COLORECTAL CANCER

## DEFINITIONS

### What is colorectal cancer?

Colorectal cancer is a cancer that begins in either the colon or the rectum.

### What is the colon and how are the sections of the colon named?

The colon is the "large intestine".

The colon begins in the lower right side of the abdomen (the part of the colon in the lower right side of the abdomen is the "cecum") and climbs upward to just beneath the liver. The section of the colon that ascends from the lower right side of the abdomen is the "ascending colon". The colon then crosses from the right side of the abdomen to the left. This second section of the colon is the "transverse colon". The colon then drops down from the upper left corner of the abdomen into the pelvis. This section of the colon, the "descending colon", descends into the pelvis where its final section, the "sigmoid colon" joins the rectum that ends at the anus and the outside world.

# SYMPTOMS

## *What are the symptoms of colorectal cancer?*

In its earliest stages, colorectal cancer usually produces no symptoms at all. Colorectal cancer very often is first detected when a physician does further testing after discovering a trace of blood in the stool during a routine physical examination. Routine screening colonoscopy or sigmoidoscopy, as is well publicized, can first discover a person's colon cancer.

Early symptoms of colorectal cancer, if present, can depend on where in the colon the cancer is located. Colon cancer is fragile and has a tendency to bleed into the colon. When the cancer is in the cecum or the ascending colon, an early symptom can be dark, almost black stool and a sense of general weakness. The cause of the black stool is the bowel's chemical reaction to stool with blood in it. Weakness is a result of anemia from slow and steady blood loss from the colon cancer. The closer the cancer lies to the rectum and anus, the more likely it is that the blood seen in the stool will look more red than black.

Complete blockage of the colon by cancer can occur at any part of the colon affected by the cancer. When this occurs, a person is completely constipated, the abdomen will become very bloated, and nausea and vomiting will be a prominent and distressing problem.

Occasionally, a cancer in the colon can gnaw a hole through the wall of the colon (this is called "perforation") and cause a leakage of bowel contents inside the abdomen. This will cause a severe inflammation of the inside of the abdomen called "peritonitis". Fever and severe pain and rigidity of the abdomen are the most common symptoms of peritonitis. The symptoms of perforation of the bowel by colon cancer may initially have a great deal of similarity to the symptoms of acute appendicitis. The presence of colon cancer will be evident at the time of the emergency surgery that will be necessary to treat the bowel perforation.

Rectal cancer frequently makes its presence known by frank bleeding from the rectum or by a coating of the stool with bright red blood. Partial blockage of the rectum by cancer may make the stool pencil thin. Rectal cancer may irritate the wall of the rectum and cause a continual feeling of a need to defecate.

## MAKING THE DIAGNOSIS

*How is the initial diagnosis of colorectal cancer made?*

At its earliest stages, the diagnosis of colorectal cancer is usually made by "sigmoidoscopy" or "colonoscopy".

The sigmoidoscope and the colonoscope are instruments, inserted from the anus into the colon, which allow the physician to examine the inside of the colon either directly through the instrument or through images projected onto a video monitor. The sigmoidoscope can reach up to the junction of the sigmoid colon and the descending colon. Two thirds of the time, a person's colorectal cancer is within the reach of the sigmoidoscope. The "colonoscope" can reach throughout the colon. Through the sigmoidoscope or the colonoscope, the physician can examine the inside of the colon and, if necessary, take out snips, that is, small pieces of abnormal appearing tissue for examination under the microscope. These "biopsies" can give conclusive evidence of the presence of a cancer of the colon or rectum.

## DETERMINING WHETHER COLON CANCER OR RECTAL CANCER HAS SPREAD

### What are the next steps after making a diagnosis of colon cancer?

The priority after making the diagnosis of colon cancer will be to cut the cancerous portion of the colon out. Surgical removal of the cancer provides, by far, the best chance of providing long-term control of the cancer and the possibility of a cure. Before surgery, an evaluation will determine whether the colon cancer has spread, and if it has spread, to where it has spread. Physical examination, routine blood chemistry tests, and CT or MRI scan of the abdomen and pelvis can identify obvious spread of the cancer beyond the colon. Physicians may recommend examination of the entire colon with a colonoscopy, as occasionally there may be two cancers present at the same time in different areas of the colon.

### What additional tests determine the extent of local spread of a rectal cancer?

Local spread of rectal cancer is often evident with CT or MRI scans. An additional test called a "transrectal ultrasound" provides further critical information about the local extent of the rectal cancer. To perform this test, the health professional will insert into the rectum a lubricated probe that emits sound waves that bounce off the rectum and surrounding tissues. Images transmitted from the probe to a video screen allow a physician to determine, with a high degree of accuracy, the extent to which the cancer has spread locally in the rectum and the tissues surrounding the rectum.

## SURGICAL TREATMENT IF THE CANCER APPEARS TO BE CONFINED TO THE COLON

*What treatment can cure the colon cancer if it is in the colon only and does not appear to have spread elsewhere in the body?*

If the cancer appears to involve only the colon, the goal will be to attempt a cure by surgically removing all of the cancer. The operation that accomplishes this will remove the cancerous portion of the colon and a margin of several inches of colon on both sides of the cancer. In addition, if the colon cancer has spread, it generally will have first travelled to local lymph nodes that trap cancers cells that break off from the colon cancer. The surgeon will try to remove a dozen or more of these lymph nodes for examination under the microscope. The presence or absence of cancer cells in these lymph nodes provides critical information that will guide further treatment.

The operation for colon cancer is a rather common and straightforward operation. Through an incision in the middle of the abdomen, the portion of colon with cancer in it is identified, lifted up, cut out, and the cut ends of the colon connected back together again. Because removal of only a portion of the colon has occurred, the procedure is a "hemicolectomy".

*Instead of removing the cancer through a usual operation with a large abdominal incision, can a laparoscope remove a cancerous area of the colon?*

A laparoscope is a narrow tube inserted through a small incision into the abdomen. The laparoscope can then transmit images of the inside of the abdomen via a camera on the laparoscope to a video monitor. Using these images to guide the surgery, the surgeon will insert special small instruments through small incisions in the abdomen and perform the operation to remove the area of the colon containing the cancer.

The major advantage of having "laparoscope-assisted colectomy" is a faster recovery time and a reduced risk of the complications associated with major surgery through a large abdominal incision.

Removal of the cancer and surrounding lymph nodes through the laparoscope can be quite effective, but is technically very difficult and requires that the surgeon performing this operation have very significant skill and experience in doing this. Since the surgeon, while performing the laparoscopic surgery, occasionally may run into difficulties or complications, it may become necessary to convert the laparoscopic surgery to the standard surgery involving a large abdominal incision.

*Is surgery necessary to remove cancer in the colon if the cancer has already spread from the colon to distant parts of the body?*

If the cancer is not obstructing the movement of stool through the colon, and if the cancer is not actively bleeding or causing other local problems, it does not appear that surgical removal ("resection") of the local cancer is always necessary, when the cancer has already spread to distant areas of the body. A resection not only carries some surgical risk, but also can delay initiation of chemotherapy that clearly has the potential to extend life and delay progression of the cancer both locally in the colon and in distant parts of the body.

When colon cancer, at the time of diagnosis, is in the colon and in the liver or lungs, surgical removal of all areas of cancer has the potential to cure the cancer. Before such an operation is attempted, a thorough evaluation is required to assess whether the cancer is surgically curable. Additional information about this is later in this chapter and in the chapters of the book entitled "Liver Metastasis" and "Lung Metastasis".

## STAGING OF COLON CANCER

### What are the stages of colon cancer?

The four general stages of colon cancer are named by the Roman numerals I, II, III, and IV. Stage I indicates that the cancer is at its earliest stages and is confined to the inner lining the colon. Stage II indicates that the cancer has spread through the layers of tissue in the wall of the colon and not further. Stage III indicates that the cancer has spread into local lymph nodes. Stage IV indicates that the cancer has spread to parts of the body that are distant to the colon such as the liver or the lungs.

## THE OUTLOOK FOR CURE AFTER
## COLON CANCER SURGERY

*How effective is surgery in curing colon cancer?*

The deeper the cancer has invaded into the wall of the colon, the higher the risk that the cancer will recur locally or that it will spread to other parts of the body. If the cancer has spread into the nearby lymph nodes, the risk is still higher.

Surgery cures the great majority of colon cancers that are in stage I and most colon cancers that are in stage II. If the colon cancer is removed when it is in stage III, the risk of recurrence is much higher, with the degree of this risk influenced by the size of the cancer in the colon and the extent of involvement of the local lymph nodes. When cancer has spread to other organs, such as the liver, and has been determined to be in stage IV, cure through surgery or any other form of treatment is unlikely. In some circumstances where the distant spread is very limited, such as with a single area of spread (a "metastasis") in the liver, surgical resection of the metastasis as well as of the cancer in the colon can provide a very good outcome.

## TREATMENT THAT IMPROVES THE ODDS OF A CURE
## AFTER COLON CANCER SURGERY

*What is adjuvant chemotherapy?*

Adjuvant chemotherapy is chemotherapy given after surgery to reduce the risk of return of the cancer.

## *Are there adjuvant chemotherapy treatments that improve the odds of a cure after colon cancer surgery?*

When a person's colon cancer is determined to be in stage III, chemotherapy reduces the risk of recurrence of the cancer and increases the likelihood of long-term survival. Among the chemotherapy regimens considered by many experts as "standards of care" are regimens that combine the intravenous chemotherapy medication "5-Fluorouracil" or a related oral medication "capecitabine" (brand name is "Xeloda", manufacturer's product website is www.xeloda.com) with intravenous medications called "leucovorin" and "oxaliplatin". These regimens, given the nicknames "FOLFOX" and "CapeOx" (""CapeOX" is also called "XELOX)", are, however, associated with a risk of difficult side effects including bone marrow suppression, diarrhea, and damage to the nerves in the hands and feet. Because of this, some physicians may prefer, especially in people who are elderly or in poor health, to prescribe a less toxic and slightly less effective regimen that includes the medications "5-fluorouracil" and "leucovorin" but omits the medication "oxaliplatin".

In stage II colon cancer, the evidence of benefit from adjuvant chemotherapy is not as clear-cut as it is in stage III, and there are differences of opinion as to whether or when adjuvant chemotherapy is helpful. Commonly, an expert evaluating whether to recommend chemotherapy to a person with stage II colon cancer will consider the size of the cancer found in the colon and the number of lymph nodes that a surgeon removed during the operation to remove the cancer from the colon. If the number of lymph nodes removed was low, for example, less than 12, there is a possibility that other lymph nodes not removed contain cancer, making it a stage III. These are "high-risk" factors, and may lead a physician to prescribe the same form of adjuvant chemotherapy used for stage III colon cancer.

## *What are the major side effects of the chemotherapy used in adjuvant treatment?*

Chemotherapy can suppress the ability of the bone marrow to produce white blood cells, red blood cells, and platelets, and therefore increase the risk of serious infections and serious internal bleeding (see chapter "Bone Marrow Suppression"). Because 5-Fluorouracil as well as Xeloda injures all dividing cells (including cancer cells), it also can injure normally dividing cells in the bowel and in the mouth. Sores in the mouth may occur, and an irritated bowel can produce cramping abdominal pain and diarrhea (see chapters "Severe Oral Mucositis" and "Severe Diarrhea").

Oxaliplatin commonly causes a side effect called "peripheral neuropathy" which is usually perceived as numbness, tingling, and sometimes pain and discomfort in the hands and feet. These symptoms are often mild and reversible with discontinuation of the oxaliplatin. Some people find the symptoms of peripheral neuropathy impossible to tolerate. At times, the risk of permanent nerve damage is dangerous enough to outweigh the possible benefit of continuing to include oxaliplatin in the treatment regimen.

## TREATMENT OF RECTAL CANCER THAT APPEARS TO BE CONFINED TO THE RECTUM

### *How is the diagnosis of rectal cancer made?*

The diagnosis of rectal cancer is usually made at the time of sigmoidoscopy or colonoscopy, when an abnormal growth, arising from the wall of the rectum, is plainly visible. A biopsy taken from this growth, which physicians will call a "rectal mass", will show the characteristic appearance of rectal cancer under the microscope.

## What initial steps are taken once the diagnosis of rectal cancer is made?

The critical issues, after the diagnosis of rectal cancer has been made, are to determine the exact location of the cancer, the degree, if any, to which the cancer has penetrated deep into the wall of the rectum and into surrounding tissues, and whether the cancer has spread from the rectum to distant areas of the body. This will determine the "stage" of the cancer and will provide the essential information required to plan the most effective treatment.

## What additional tests determine the extent of local spread of a rectal cancer?

A rectal examination, performed by the finger of an experienced physician, and examination with a rigid sigmoidoscope, can give vital information about the size and location of the cancer and can give evidence as to whether the cancer has spread to local tissues.

A CT or MRI scan evaluates the rectum and surrounding tissues, and looks for evidence of spread to other areas of the body, such as the liver.

As discussed earlier in this chapter, a "transrectal ultrasound" provides further critical information about the local extent of the rectal cancer.

## How can surgery treat rectal cancer?

The surgical treatment of cancer of the rectum is to remove the portion of the rectum that contains the cancer. The operation is technically more difficult than the operation for colon cancer. A major issue in the surgical treatment of rectal cancer is the risk to rectal sphincter function (the "rectal sphincter" is the muscle that gives us control over when we move our bowels).

The location of the cancer within the rectum will determine whether it is possible to both remove the cancer and preserve the rectal sphincter. When the cancer is higher in the rectum, it is more likely that the operation can completely remove the cancer and preserve the rectal sphincter. In general, it is difficult for surgery to cure rectal cancer without jeopardizing the sphincter if the cancer lies within five centimeters (approximately two inches) of the "anal verge", which is where the anus meets the outside of the body. If the rectal sphincter is not preserved, a colostomy will be necessary. To perform a "colostomy", the surgeon will attach the colon to the side of a person's abdomen and create an opening between the inside of the colon and the outside world. This will allow stool to be collected into a special plastic bag.

Depending on the size and location of the rectal cancer, radiation and chemotherapy may be given before the operation to reduce the size of the cancer. By reducing the size of the cancer, the surgery is easier to perform, has a lower risk of complications, and it is more likely that the cancer will be removed without the need for a colostomy. Also depending on the size and location of the cancer, combined treatment with radiation and chemotherapy, prior to surgery, may reduce the risk that cancer will recur months or years after the surgery. This combination of chemotherapy and radiation, given before surgery, is "neoadjuvant chemoradiotherapy".

Surgical techniques have significantly improved over the last several years and many more people with rectal cancer can have their cancer cured by surgery that does not remove the rectal sphincter and does not cause a person to require a colostomy. Surgeons who specialize in colorectal surgery are most likely to be skilled in the more recently developed procedures which spare the rectal sphincter and which give the best chance for surgical cure of the cancer.

### What is the treatment if it appears that surgical removal of the rectal cancer will be difficult or impossible?

A combination of radiation and chemotherapy can sometimes shrink the cancer to the point where surgery can remove all or most of the cancer. For this reason, and because, by far, the best chance of curing rectal cancer is through surgical removal, physicians will generally prescribe radiation and chemotherapy, followed by an attempt at total surgical removal of the cancer. Since there will be a high risk of recurrence, physicians may advise additional chemotherapy after the surgery.

### Can the radiation and chemotherapy make all evidence of the cancer disappear?

Approximately one in five people with rectal cancer treated with radiation and chemotherapy ("chemoradiotherapy") will have no evidence of their cancer with physical examination or CT or MRI scans after completion of their treatment. This absence of evidence of cancer after chemoradiotherapy is a "clinical complete remission".

## Is surgery necessary if chemoradiotherapy induces a clinical complete remission?

There have recently been studies reported in which a "wait and see" approach, involving frequent physical examinations, blood tests, and CT or MRI scans without surgery, produces comparable or better results than if a person proceeded to surgery. Surgery does have potential side effects, and if it requires a colostomy, the surgery is life changing. The great majority of people who achieve a clinical complete response after chemoradiotherapy never have had a reported recurrence of their cancer. For these reasons, avoiding surgery, if possible, is a preferred option.

## What are the complications of rectal cancer surgery?

Normal stool, which moves down the bowel into a newly repaired and stitched up rectum, contains a wide variety of bacteria. These bacteria can find the breach in the surgically injured rectal wall, slip out into the pelvis, and cause very serious infections. Vigilant medical care can spot these infections very early and cure them with antibiotics.

In order to remove the area of the rectum with cancer, the surgeon may have to cut through important nerves in the pelvis. These nerves are responsible for permitting normal urination and normal sexual function. Inability to urinate normally can occur after surgical treatment of rectal cancer, but usually returns on its own within a month or so after the operation. Inability to have an erection or inability to ejaculate normally are common problems in men after rectal cancer surgery and may be permanent. Sexual problems in women who have had rectal cancer surgery are also common, with pain during sexual intercourse a frequent problem. In addition, women commonly have urinary problems after the surgery including an urge to urinate frequently, and occasional incontinence.

## What is the likelihood that surgery with or without chemoradiotherapy can cure a person's rectal cancer?

The likelihood of cure of the rectal cancer depends upon on how deeply the cancer has invaded the wall of the rectum, and upon the skill and success of the surgeon in removing the entire area of the rectum that contains cancer. The deeper the cancer has invaded, the higher the likelihood of recurrence. When the risk of recurrence is significant, treatment given to attempt to prevent recurrence is "adjuvant treatment".

## Are there adjuvant treatments that may improve the odds of a cure after chemoradiotherapy and rectal cancer surgery?

After the chemoradiotherapy and surgery are completed, physicians may recommend "adjuvant" chemotherapy, to reduce the risk of recurrence of the cancer. Common adjuvant chemotherapy regimens for rectal cancer consist of the chemotherapy medications 5-FU or "capecitabine (brand name is "Xeloda", and manufacturer's product website is www.xeloda.com) in combination with "leucovorin", or the "FOLFOX" regimen, as described above in the discussion of adjuvant treatment of colon cancer.

## *What is the treatment if rectal cancer recurs despite the surgery, radiation and chemotherapy?*

Recurrence of the rectal cancer following initial surgery, radiation, and chemotherapy, is very hard to treat. Sometimes, depending on the size and location of the recurrence, additional surgery controls the local cancer. There will be a severe limitation on the ability to provide additional radiation treatment if radiation has already been given.

If surgery, radiation, or chemotherapy cannot control the local recurrence, there may be ways of reducing some of the pain and discomfort associated with the local recurrence. One of the most serious local complications that can develop is obstruction of the rectum by the cancer. Local measures can alleviate discomfort ("palliative treatment"), even though they do not have the potential to control the growth of the cancer. Such a measure would be the insertion of a stent, which is a rigid tube, which can prop the rectum open, and relieve the obstruction.

## WHEN COLON CANCER RECURS AFTER SURGERY

### *Where can colon cancer recur?*

Colon cancer can recur in two areas: the area near where the original cancer was originally located (this is "local recurrence") or in other body organs (this is "metastatic disease").

### *Where does the local recurrence of colon cancer appear?*

At the time of the original surgical treatment of a local colon cancer, the surgeon removes the area of the colon containing cancer and connects the cut ends of the colon together again. The area in which the cut ends of the colon were reconnected is the "anastomosis". Local recurrence is uncommon, but when it occurs, it is generally in the area adjacent to the anastomosis or in nearby lymph nodes. This local recurrence, however, may be accompanied by distant spread of the cancer.

*Why is it important to determine if the cancer has spread beyond the area of local recurrence in the colon or nearby lymph nodes?*

Localized cancer is potentially curable by surgery. If the cancer has spread to distant organs, local surgery will not cure the cancer and may be unnecessary.

*How do physicians determine if the cancer has spread beyond the area of local recurrence in the colon or nearby lymph nodes?*

A CT scan of the chest, abdomen, and pelvis can identify evidence of cancer in other body organs.

A PET scan is a sensitive test that can often detect areas of metastasis that are not visible with the CT scans. To do a PET scan, an injection is made of a tiny amount of radioactive glucose into the bloodstream. Cancer cells have a greater affinity for this radioactive glucose than other tissues, appearing as "hot spots", which, in conjunction with the CT scan, can provide vital information regarding the likely presence or absence of cancer outside the lung and liver. If cancer has spread beyond the lung and liver, surgery itself will not be able to cure the cancer.

If the CT and PET scan do not show evidence of distant spread of the cancer, a colonoscopy obtains additional information about the local area of recurrence and evaluates the entire colon for evidence of a second cancer.

### How is localized recurrence of colon cancer treated?

The treatment of a localized colon cancer recurrence is surgical removal of the area of the colon containing the cancer and some surrounding tissues.

If, in addition to the local recurrence, the cancer has recurred in distant areas of the body, and the locally recurrent cancer is not causing problems, surgical removal of the localized cancer may be deferred, and treatment of metastatic colon cancer initiated.

## TREATMENT OF METASTATIC COLORECTAL CANCER

### What is metastatic colorectal cancer?

Cancer that has spread from the colon or the rectum to distant organs is "metastatic colorectal cancer".

### Is the treatment of metastatic colon cancer and metastatic rectal cancer the same?

Metastatic colon cancer and metastatic rectal cancer respond to the same chemotherapy drugs and therefore their chemotherapy treatment is the same.

## When is surgical treatment of metastatic colorectal cancer useful?

The first organs to which colon cancer tends to spread are the liver and the lungs. If the spread, that is, if the metastasis of the cancer is truly confined to those organs, there is a possibility that the cancer, although metastatic, can be cured by surgery.

To assess the potential curability of the cancer, physicians will initially perform a CT scan, and often a PET scan as described earlier in this chapter, of the abdomen and pelvis, and sometimes, of the chest as well.

A common first area of metastasis from a colorectal cancer is in the liver. With modern surgical techniques, and with experienced surgeons, aggressive surgical removal of large areas of the liver containing cancer may be attempted, provided sufficient liver will remain after the surgery and provided blood vessels that carry blood into and out of the liver are not likely to be damaged by the surgery.

If the cancer has spread to one or both lungs, a "thoracic surgeon" will evaluate CT and PET scans to determine the likelihood that removal of the areas of metastasis can be curable. Sometimes, although the cancer has spread to both the liver and the lungs, either a cure or a significant delay in disease progression is possible, if a team of experienced surgeons remove the metastatic areas in both the lungs and the liver.

After the potentially curative surgery, physicians will often prescribe chemotherapy in an attempt to prevent the cancer from returning.

## What is "conversion therapy"?

Sometimes, a person has metastatic cancer for which surgery, although possible, is technically difficult because of either the size or location of the cancer. These cancers are "borderline resectable". In people with "borderline resectable" metastatic colorectal cancer, combination chemotherapy such as with the "FOLFOX" regimen as described below, can convert a borderline resectable cancer into a cancer that is more easily resectable and possibly curable by surgery.

## What is the treatment of metastatic colorectal cancer when surgery is not an option?

The mainstay of treatment for colorectal cancer for many years has been the marginally effective medicine 5-FU and a companion drug named "leucovorin" that slightly enhances the effectiveness of 5-FU. Over the past ten years or so, several additional medicines have become available which clearly have increased the probability that growth of the metastatic colorectal cancer is restrained and life extended. These medicines include irinotecan, oxaliplatin, Avastin, Erbitux, Vectibix, and Xeloda. With these medications, the average survival time from diagnosis of metastatic disease doubles from about 10 months to 20 months. This 20 month survival time is an average, with many people living far longer than 20 months with good control of their disease.

Medicines given initially for metastatic colorectal cancer are combinations of medicines that have nicknames related to the medicines in the combination. The most common combinations are nicknamed "FOLFOX", for 5-FU, Leucovorin and Oxaliplatin, "CapeOx" for capecitabine (Xeloda), 5-FU and Leucovorin, and

"FOLFIRI" for 5-FU, Leucovorin, and Irinotecan. FOLFOX, CapeOx, and FOLFIRI appear to produce comparable results when initially given for metastatic colorectal cancer. Some physicians and people with colorectal cancer prefer FOLFOX, since the medicines in that combination are less likely to result in the baldness that is so common in people receiving chemotherapy.

"Oxaplatin" which is the "OX" in "FOLFOX", has the very disturbing side effect of causing a form of nerve damage called "peripheral neuropathy", in which there is a loss of sensation or painful or uncomfortable sensations in the hands and feet. This toxicity accumulates, and after approximately six months of therapy can become impossible to tolerate. For this reason, physicians often limit the length of time that a person is receiving an oxaliplatin-containing regimen to six months or less, after which the oxaliplatin is removed from the regimen. This also illustrates why the choice of the best first chemotherapy treatment regimen for metastatic colorectal cancer is not "black or white", as some people may prefer to completely avoid the risk of peripheral neuropathy by receiving a combination chemotherapy that does not contain oxaliplatin, such as "FOLFORI", as mentioned above.

## When is Avastin useful?

Avastin inhibits development of blood vessels that might feed a cancer. Avastin can improve the probability that a cancer will shrink in response to chemotherapy, and may delay the time until the cancer starts to grow again. In addition, when Avastin and chemotherapy are a combined treatment, there is a further increase in average survival time.

## *Does outcome improve with direct injection of chemotherapy into liver to which cancer has spread?*

Over the past three decades, there have been many attempts to concentrate the chemotherapy in the liver by injecting the drugs directly into the artery feeding the liver. The idea makes sense: give chemotherapy directly into the liver, spare the body the side effects, and kill the cancer in the main place or the most dangerous place where it lies. There are, however, problems with the technique. Even though the cancer in the liver responds to this treatment, the catheter itself, through which medication is injected, can cause damage to the blood vessels of the liver. Chemotherapy injected directly into the liver can also cause serious damage to the cells and ducts of the liver. This technique of giving chemotherapy into the artery feeding the liver, sometimes called "intra-arterial infusions" or "hepatic artery catheterization", is not standard therapy. This is still considered experimental treatment, and has yet to prove to be of real value in extending life or improving the quality of life of people with colorectal cancer.

## *How long will the cancer generally remain under control with initial chemotherapy combined with Avastin?*

The measure of stability used in clinical trials is "progression-free survival", which means the length of time that the cancer has not grown from the point of initiation of treatment. With initial chemotherapy and Avastin, the average progression-free survival time is approximately a year. Of course, as an average, this means that some people are stable longer, some shorter, and many are stable somewhere in the middle which, in this instance, in the clinical trials evaluating Avastin with either FOLFOX or FOLFIRI, has been about a year. Most of the time, the cancer does not remain stable indefinitely.

## What treatment is given if the cancer begins to grow again?

Treatment given for recurrence is "second-line therapy". For second line therapy, physicians will usually prescribe a regimen including irinotecan for people who have had the FOLFOX or CapeOx regimens or a regimen including oxaliplatin for people who have had the FOLFIRI regimen.

## What are Erbitux and Vectibix?

Erbitux and Vectibix are biotechnology-derived medications that can find and attach themselves to a structure on the surface of cancer cells called the EGF receptor. Binding of these medications to the EGF receptor interrupts signals that cancer cells need to help them grow and spread.

Erbitux can slightly increase the effectiveness of Irinotecan when given as second-line treatment. Both Erbitux and Vectibix when given alone, if all other treatment has failed to be effective, may slightly prolong the time until the cancer progresses, but does not, yet, have a proven benefit with regard to either symptom improvement or survival.

## What options are available if all these medications have failed?

The treatment of colorectal cancer is a very active area in clinical research and many new potential treatments are under evaluation.

Large clinical trials sponsored by the National Cancer Institute and by the biotechnology and pharmaceutical industries are continually evaluating new treatments. When other treatments have failed, many people will choose to go to a major cancer center to see whether some experimental treatment is a reasonable option.

# ESOPHAGEAL CANCER

## DEFINITIONS

### What is the esophagus?

The esophagus is the tube-shaped organ through which food travels on its way from the mouth to the stomach. The esophagus begins in the back of the throat, travels downward through the chest, and ends in the stomach.

### What is esophageal cancer?

Esophageal cancer is a cancer that begins in the cells which line the inside wall of the esophagus. The growth of the cancer in the esophagus creates a lump (referred to by physicians as a "mass") that, when large enough, can block the normal passage of food to the stomach. If esophageal cancer is not controlled, it can grow into the tissues in the neck or chest that surround the esophagus and can spread to distant areas of the body such as the lung, liver, bones and brain.

# THE ANATOMY OF THE ESOPHAGUS AND ITS CRITICAL IMPORTANCE

## *What are the layers of the wall of the esophagus?*

The inner lining of the esophagus is the "esophageal mucosa". The area just beneath the mucosa is the "submucosa". Beneath the submucosa is a muscle layer that controls voluntary and involuntary contractions of the esophagus. The outermost layer of the esophagus is the "adventitia".

An understanding of the layers of the esophagus is important when considering the treatment of "superficial esophageal cancer", as described later in this chapter.

## *What is the pathway down which the esophagus travels, and what are the different portions of the esophagus called?*

The uppermost area of the esophagus begins in the back of the throat, travels downward through the neck just behind the windpipe (the "trachea"), ending inside the chest. This is the "cervical esophagus".

The middle portion of the esophagus continues downward through the chest very close to the body's main artery (the "aorta") and travels through the diaphragm into the abdomen. This is the "thoracic esophagus".

The lowest portion of the esophagus is the abdominal esophagus, and lies in a groove on the back surface of the liver. The area where it joins the stomach is the "gastroesophageal junction".

The location of the cancer in the esophagus plays a vital role in planning the type of surgery most likely to cure the cancer.

## SYMPTOMS

*What are the early symptoms of esophageal cancer?*

In its early stages, esophageal cancer usually grows without symptoms. When the cancer grows to the point where it blocks off a major space in the inside portion (the "lumen") of the esophagus, symptoms appear.

The most common early symptom of esophageal cancer is difficulty swallowing solid foods. The person with esophageal cancer may also notice a pain in their throat, chest or back when they swallow.

## MAKING THE DIAGNOSIS

*How is the diagnosis of esophageal cancer made?*

Esophageal cancer is diagnosed by having a physician (usually a gastroenterologist) look down the esophagus through a thin tube called an "endoscope" which permits thorough examination of the inside lining of the esophagus. To do this procedure, the gastroenterologist will give a person a mild sedative and have the person swallow the endoscope. The procedure is somewhat unpleasant, but is not painful and, when done properly, carries very little risk.

Looking down the endoscope, the gastroenterologist will closely examine the wall of the esophagus for abnormalities. The lesion of esophageal cancer is usually easy to identify. The gastroenterologist will scrape tissue off the surface of the lesion, take a small biopsy of the lesion, and send the scrapings and the biopsy to the laboratory for analysis by a pathologist.

If there is a cancer, the pathologist usually will have enough tissue to make the diagnosis.

The two major forms of esophageal cancer are "squamous cell carcinoma" and "adenocarcinoma". Squamous cell carcinoma can occur anywhere in the esophagus. Adenocarcinoma usually occurs very near the junction of the esophagus and the stomach (called the "gastroesophageal junction"). There are differences in the way the two forms of esophageal cancer respond to surgery, radiation, and chemotherapy. Despite this, the treatment of the two forms of esophageal cancer is similar.

Examining the tissue removed under the microscope will also allow the pathologist to assess the depth to which the cancer has invaded into or through the wall of the esophagus. This assessment is of extreme importance in planning treatment most likely to cure or control the cancer.

## DETERMINING WHETHER THE CANCER HAS SPREAD BEYOND THE ESOPHAGUS

*What further information is necessary after making the diagnosis of esophageal cancer?*

The next critical piece of information needed after making the diagnosis of esophageal cancer is whether the cancer has spread beyond the esophagus. This information is essential to planning treatment.

As with any cancer, the first priority is to determine whether the cancer is curable. In the case of esophageal cancer, the most effective way to cure the cancer, if localized, is by treatment with surgery, radiation or chemotherapy, or, very commonly, by a regimen combining all three forms of treatment. If the cancer in the esophagus initially appears to be very large and not immediately curable with surgery, treatment with radiation and chemotherapy can shrink the cancer to the point where surgical cure may later be possible. If the cancer has spread beyond the esophagus and into distant areas of the body, an initial goal of treatment will be to attempt to achieve local control of the cancer and, by doing so, prevent development of complications from locally uncontrolled cancer.

### How can physicians determine whether the esophageal cancer has spread beyond the esophagus?

A CT scan of the chest and abdomen can give useful information about spread of the cancer into other body organs such as the liver or lung. The CT scan does not always give a very clear picture of the extent, if any, to which the cancer may have spread through the wall of the esophagus into surrounding tissues. In addition, cancer cells can travel through tiny channels called "lymphatics" into local lymph nodes that normally filter material from the esophagus. These lymph nodes can retain cancer cells that multiply in the lymph node and enlarge it. The CT scan often cannot identify lymph nodes to which cancer has spread.

The test that gives the best view of the tissues surrounding the esophagus and lymph nodes into which the cancer is prone to travel is an "endoscopic ultrasound".

### What is an endoscopic ultrasound and how do physicians perform this test?

To do the endoscopic ultrasound, the healthcare professional will insert, into the esophagus, a tube that has a tiny device at its tip that can bounce sound waves off the tissues inside and surrounding the esophagus. Signals produced by these sound waves and sent to a computer, and generate images for the physicians to evaluate. Using these images, the physicians can accurately determine whether the cancer has invaded beyond the esophagus into nearby lymph nodes or other structures.

### What is a PET scan and how can it be useful?

A PET scan is a sensitive test that can often detect the spread of cancer to distant organs before it is visible with CT scans. To do this test, an injection is made of a tiny amount of radioactive glucose into the bloodstream. Cancer cells have a greater affinity for this radioactive glucose than other tissues. The PET scanner can then find "hot spots" inside the body that contain the cancer and transmit this information to a computer for the physician to evaluate. The presence of a "hot spot" suggests, but does not prove, the presence of cancer cells in the "hot spot". Although a "hot spot" may indicate the presence of cancer, areas of inflammation without cancer can also produce "hot spots". A "hot spot" indicates a suspicious area that needs evaluation, often with a biopsy to confirm the presence or absence of local cancer.

## What is bronchoscopy and why is it useful in evaluating a person with esophageal cancer?

Bronchoscopy is a medical test in which a physician looks directly into the lungs by putting a scope through the mouth, down the windpipe (the "trachea"), and into the bronchial tubes which provide air to the lungs. When esophageal cancer involves the upper portion of the esophagus, it has a tendency to grow through the wall of the esophagus and invade the trachea and very top of bronchial tubes where they divide to feed air to the left and right lungs. For this reason, depending on the region of the esophagus involved with cancer, it may be important to have a physician (usually a lung specialist) look down into the trachea and the bronchial tubes with a "bronchoscope" to see whether any evidence of tracheal or bronchial invasion by the esophageal cancer can be identified.

## What is diagnostic laparoscopy and what role does it play?

Cancers that are in the bottom portion of the esophagus can sometimes spread into the abdomen with very tiny specks of cancer that are difficult to detect with CT, PET, or endoscopic ultrasound. For this reason, physicians may suggest a diagnostic laparoscopy.

Laparoscopy is a surgical technique that allows a surgeon to examine the inside of the abdomen without performing a major operation. The instrument used, a "laparoscope", and surgical tools used to perform the operation, are inserted into the abdomen through incisions of less than an inch in length. The surgeon directs the instrument through the various parts of the inside of the abdomen and examines the abdomen through images projected to a video monitor. Abnormal tissues can be biopsied and sent to the laboratory for analysis.

## What are the next steps when the results of these tests are available?

Based upon the results of these tests, the stage of the cancer will be determined and the appropriate treatment suggested.

## What are the stages of esophageal cancer?

The common way physicians refer to the stages of esophageal cancer is through "TNM" staging.

The "T" refers to the size and invasiveness of the local cancer and ranges from $T_1$, indicating a cancer that is early and superficial to $T_4$, which is a cancer that has invaded through the wall of the esophagus and into tissues deep inside the middle of the chest (this area is the "mediastinum").

The "N" refers to the presence or absence of cancer in the lymph nodes. If the cancer has not spread to lymph nodes, it is "$N_o$" and if it has spread to lymph nodes, it is $N_1$.

The "M" refers to the presence or absence of evidence of distant spread, that is, of metastasis. If metastasis is absent, it is $M_o$. If metastasis is present, it is $M_1$.

## SUPERFICIAL ESOPHAGEAL CANCER

## What is superficial esophageal cancer?

Earlier in this chapter, the anatomy of the wall of the esophagus was described, with the innermost wall, that is, the area of the esophagus down which food slides, consisting of first, the mucosa, and second, the submucosa. Superficial esophageal cancer is a cancer that only involves the mucosa, or the mucosa and submucosa, of the esophagus.

## What is the treatment of superficial esophageal cancer?

Surgical removal of the esophagus is the treatment that is most likely to cure superficial esophageal cancer. This operation, however, carries some very significant risks, in the operating room and in the days, weeks, and months after the operation, These risks are far greater if the person's underlying health is not good, or if a person is at a very advanced age. For this reason, there is not one treatment plan that is appropriate for everyone with superficial esophageal cancer, and the unique risks, benefits, and circumstances for each person guide decisions about treatment.

If the cancer is only in the mucosa, "endoscopic mucosal resection", meaning removal of the cancer through the endoscope without removing the esophagus, can provide a cure rate, in experienced medical centers, that may approximate the cure rate achieved with total removal of the esophagus. With endoscopic mucosal resection, there is, however, a significant incidence of incomplete removal of the cancer, leading to local recurrence. For this reason, frequent examinations of the esophagus with endoscopy are essential after an endoscopic mucosal resection. The degree, if any, to which endoscopic mucosal resection compromises the chance of cure as opposed to removal of the entire esophagus has not yet been clearly determined.

If the cancer has penetrated through the mucosa, into the submucosa, and not beyond, the treatment commonly recommended will be removal of the esophagus.

## LOCALIZED ESOPHAGEAL CANCER

*What is the treatment if the esophageal cancer appears to be more than superficial but still possibly curable by surgery?*

Esophageal cancer is a highly malignant cancer that, even if apparently localized, has a high tendency to recur in the area from which it originated and to spread elsewhere in the body. For this reason, physicians employ the most aggressive treatments available in an attempt to provide an extended period of control, and possible cure, of the cancer.

With the exception of the uncommon person with a very superficial and small cancer, as described above, that is treatable by surgery alone, the treatment of localized esophageal cancer at major cancer centers usually involves "trimodality therapy", meaning three different types of treatment. The three treatments are chemotherapy, radiation therapy, and surgery.

## TREATMENT WITH THE COMBINATION OF RADIATION AND CHEMOTHERAPY AND SURGERY

*When is radiation and chemotherapy, followed by surgery administered?*

If the cancer is more than superficial, and has not spread to distant organs ($M_o$ as described above), physicians will often suggest that a person receive treatment with chemotherapy and radiation followed by surgery.

### How is radiation and chemotherapy given together?

There are many different treatment regimens. A common radiation regimen will be to have the radiation given five days a week for five weeks. The chemotherapy may consist of several different combinations of medications, but commonly includes the medicines "paclitaxel" and "cisplatin".

### What are some of the side effects of the radiation and chemotherapy treatments?

Combined treatment with radiation and chemotherapy can severely suppress the bone marrow's production of white blood cells and platelets and make a person susceptible to infections and internal bleeding (see chapter entitled "Bone Marrow Suppression").

Chemotherapy can intensify the damaging effects radiation can have on normal, non-cancer containing tissues that are irradiated. Severe sores in the throat and difficulty and pain with swallowing are common side effects.

### How is an attempt to cure esophageal cancer with surgery made?

The operation done will remove the majority of the esophagus. In order to re-establish continuity of the gastrointestinal tract, the surgeon moves the stomach into the neck and attaches the end of the stomach to the remaining portion of the esophagus.

The surgery to treat esophageal cancer is very complicated and requires that the surgeon performing the operation, and the medical professionals who will provide care after the operation, have very considerable experience in treating esophageal cancer.

## What are the problems that can result from the surgery?

After the operation, a person may develop a number of serious complications.

The junction where the esophagus is surgically re-attached to the stomach (this junction is the "anastomosis") can leak. This can cause tremendous pain and severe infections inside the chest. A leak at the anastomosis will often require a major operation to repair the leak.

Bacterial pneumonia caused by bacteria acquired in the hospital environment (see chapter entitled "Hospital-Acquired Pneumonia"), can develop, especially if a person, after the operation, requires extended treatment in an intensive care unit.

The recovery period after the operation is often prolonged. A prolonged period of bed rest and inactivity puts a person at risk for developing blood clots in the legs that can travel to the lung as a "pulmonary embolism" (see chapter entitled "Deep Vein Thrombosis and Pulmonary Embolism").

People with esophageal cancer tend to be older and commonly have other health problems such as heart failure, or COPD (see chapters discussing these diseases) which can compromise a person's chances of recovering quickly from the major operation.

*Is there general agreement among experts that surgery should follow the chemotherapy and radiation?*

Surgery after chemotherapy and radiation for esophageal cancer that has spread locally provides the best possibility for curing or controlling esophageal cancer, but can have many serious and life-threatening complications. In reviewing the various studies which have evaluated the benefit of surgery after chemotherapy and radiation for locally advanced esophageal cancer, and the risks associated with the surgery itself, there is some disagreement among experts as to whether and when surgery is necessary or appropriate. Esophageal cancer often occurs in people at an advanced age, or when other serious illnesses, such as severe heart failure or COPD, also are present. If a person's underlying health is not good and there is a significant risk that a person will not be able to tolerate the surgery, the combination treatment with chemotherapy and radiation, or with chemotherapy or radiation separately, can still provide very significant benefit, improving local control of the cancer and extending survival.

## TREATMENT WHEN CANCER RECURS OR HAS SPREAD BEYOND THE ESOPHAGUS

*What is the treatment when cancer recurs after surgery or radiation or when the cancer has spread far beyond the esophagus at the time of diagnosis?*

Esophageal cancer that has recurred after chemotherapy, radiation, and surgery is, most commonly, incurable. Similarly, cancer that has spread far beyond the esophagus at the time of diagnosis is, most commonly, incurable. Treatments administered will focus on preserving quality of life, while, to the extent possible, extending healthful life for several months, and occasionally, for much longer.

If, at the time of diagnosis, the cancer has already spread beyond the esophagus, combined treatment with radiation and chemotherapy can often relieve symptoms and provide significant local control of the growth of the cancer in the esophagus and surrounding tissues.

Cancer that has spread beyond the esophagus into distant body organs is "metastatic esophageal cancer". Chemotherapy has only a small effect in prolonging survival when metastatic esophageal cancer develops. Chemotherapy is sometimes effective in making the cancer shrink and temporarily relieving symptoms, although most of the time, growth of the cancer can only be restrained for a few months.

Chemotherapy regimens which are commonly prescribed include the medications "epirubicin", "oxaliplatin", and "capecitabine" (and may be called the "EOC regimen") or "epirubicin", "cisplatin"; and "5-Fluorouracil" (and is the "ECF regimen"). The EOC regimen may be slightly better (by about a month) as regards survival, but the average survival with chemotherapy for a person with esophageal cancer that has spread to distant parts of the body is approximately ten months.

## EXPERIMENTAL TREATMENT

### *Are there experimental treatments for esophageal cancer?*

Most experimental treatments have focused on the use of combinations of radiation, surgery and chemotherapy in the early stages of the disease before the cancer has spread.

Academic centers around the world are actively investigating new drugs for esophageal cancer.

## TREATMENT TO RELIEVE SUFFERING WHEN ESOPHAGEAL CANCER IS PROGRESSING

*What treatment can relieve some of the suffering when the esophageal cancer is progressing despite treatment?*

The key to treatment of a person who has an esophageal cancer that is relentlessly advancing will be to make the person as comfortable as possible.

Locally advanced esophageal cancer, as it grows, can obstruct the passage of food down the esophagus. When this occurs, there will be pain and severe difficulty swallowing, and associated malnutrition. There are several types of vinyl or metallic tubes called "stents" that, when placed across the area of obstruction of the esophagus, will open up the esophagus and allow food to pass through. When it is technically impossible to push the tube through the obstruction, laser beams can often create a hole large enough to allow food to pass. If all else fails, a surgeon can make a hole in the stomach and insert a tube (called a "gastrostomy tube") which will carry liquid food directly into the stomach.

Esophageal cancer can invade the trachea or bronchial tubes and create an opening (a "fistula") between the esophagus and the trachea. This fistula can allow food to leak out of the esophagus, get into the trachea, and down into the lungs. This will cause frequent severe coughing and can cause a person to choke on their food.

The same type of vinyl tube used when there is an obstruction in the esophagus, when inserted into the esophagus, can seal off the opening between the esophagus and the trachea.

Severe pain in areas to which cancer has spread is a common problem in people with advanced esophageal cancer. As with any advanced cancer, pain control with appropriate doses of narcotics will be important in maintaining a person's comfort.

# KIDNEY CANCER

## DEFINITION

### What is kidney cancer?

Kidney cancer is a cancer that begins in the kidney. Unless controlled in its earliest stages, kidney cancer will spread to major body organs including the lung, liver, and bones.

The most common type of kidney cancer in adults is "renal cell carcinoma". In children, the most common kidney cancer is a "Wilm's tumor". Renal cell carcinoma and Wilm's tumor are entirely different diseases with a completely different treatment and prognosis. The discussion in this chapter refers only to renal cell carcinoma.

## SYMPTOMS

### What are the symptoms of kidney cancer?

Kidney cancer, at the time of discovery, commonly produces no symptoms, and is discovered incidentally, when medical tests looking for other problems uncover evidence of the kidney cancer. This often happens when a CT or MRI scan of the abdomen, performed to evaluate an unrelated symptom, finds a "mass" in the kidney.

A common first symptom of kidney cancer is bloody urine. Initially, the amount of blood in the urine may be very trivial and only evident when a physician sends urine to the laboratory as part of a person's routine check-up. As the kidney cancer grows, blood in the urine may become obvious to the naked eye and the person with kidney cancer may begin to notice pain in their lower back and side.

Weight loss, loss of appetite, pain in the back just to the left or right of the spine, and fatigue are other symptoms of kidney cancer.

## MAKING THE DIAGNOSIS

### *How is the diagnosis of kidney cancer made?*

An important initial test to perform in evaluating a possible kidney cancer is the CT scan before and after injection of a "contrast" material. The CT scan permits the detailed evaluation of the kidney as well as of the "ureter", which is the tube that emanates from the kidney and travels downward, draining urine from the kidney into the bladder. The CT scan of the kidney often has a characteristic appearance when a person has kidney cancer and can give vital information as to whether the cancer has spread beyond the kidney and is curable or treatable by surgery.

A MRI scan can give further information about the size and location as well as potential curability of the cancer and help the surgeon plan the surgery with the greatest potential to cure the cancer. The MRI scan can also determine whether the cancer has invaded the main vein in the abdomen (the "inferior vena cava") or has caused the presence of a blood clot (a "thrombus") in the inferior vena cava. Invasion of the inferior vena cava by cancer, or the presence of a blood clot in the inferior vena cava, certainly does not mean that surgical cure is not possible, but, for safety reasons, it is of critical importance for the surgeon to know this before performing an operation that attempts to cure the kidney cancer.

## What is "staging" of kidney cancer?

Staging of the cancer means the determination of the size of the cancer, whether the cancer has invaded surrounding organs or tissues, and whether the cancer has spread elsewhere in the body far distant from the kidney. The determination of the stage of the cancer is essential to planning the initial treatment and can give information about the probability of cure or long-term survival.

## How is the stage of the cancer determined?

The CT and MRI scans provide vital information about the size of the cancer, whether the cancer has invaded into the ureter, and give information about involvement of other structures in the abdomen.

To determine whether the cancer has spread beyond the abdomen, a CT scan of the chest can detect evidence of cancer in the lymph nodes of the chest or in the lung, and a bone scan be done to determine whether there is evidence that the cancer has spread to the bones.

Whatever the findings of the scans and other tests, a "tissue diagnosis" is essential for making the diagnosis of kidney cancer and for deciding on the appropriate treatment.

## How do physicians make a tissue diagnosis?

If the mass is very small and localized to the kidney, there is the possibility that the mass is benign, in other words, that it is not a cancer. For that reason, it may seem reasonable for a "needle biopsy" to be done, in which using a CT scan for guidance, a needle is passed into the mass and a piece of it is taken for examination under the microscope. There is a concern, however, of a "false negative", that is, that the tiny piece of tissue obtained with a needle will falsely declare the mass benign, when it really is malignant. Small masses that are kidney cancer are very frequently curable by surgery and removing the mass as soon as possible gives the best chance of a cure. For this reason, physicians most commonly recommend removal of the portion of the kidney containing the mass without unnecessary delay.

After removal of the portion of the kidney containing the mass, the hospital pathologist will examine the removed tissue and determine whether the mass is, in fact, a cancer, and, if it is cancer, can assess the danger posed by the type of cancer cells that are within the mass.

The pathologist will examine the "margins", that is, interface between where the cancer was located and the edges of the area of the kidney from which the cancer was removed. If these "margins" do not contain cancer, it greatly improves the odds that the surgery was curative.

## <u>SURGERY</u>

### *What is the treatment of a small, incidentally discovered kidney cancer?*

Kidney cancer discovered at a time when it is still very small, may be inherently slow growing with a lower risk of spreading beyond the kidney. Many urologists will recommend, in this circumstance, a "partial nephrectomy", that is, removal of only the involved portion of the kidney and a small margin of kidney tissue surrounding the cancer.

### *How is a cancer that is localized to the kidney, but somewhat larger, treated?*

A "radical nephrectomy" is a common treatment when the cancer is relatively large and has not spread far beyond the kidney. This operation will remove the entire kidney that contains the cancer. Some surgeons will also perform a "regional lymphadenectomy" to remove lymph nodes that are in the portion of the kidney called "the renal hilum" where major arteries, veins, and the ureter, attach to the kidney.

When evaluating the treatment options for a person with newly diagnosed kidney cancer it may be discovered that, as an additional problem, the person has diminished overall kidney function such that removal of one of their kidneys may result in inadequate remaining kidney function and kidney failure. In this circumstance, an attempt to cure the cancer with a partial nephrectomy, in a person with a cancer larger than the usual threshold for partial nephrectomy, is a consideration. In making this decision, the person and their physician will have to consider the risk of recurrence of the kidney cancer compared to the risk of developing kidney failure requiring dialysis.

### How successful is the surgery at curing kidney cancer?

The success of the surgery will depend upon what the urologic surgeon finds at the time of surgery.

Cancer experts measure success of surgical treatment of kidney cancer by the percentage of people who survive five years after surgery without recurrence, since five-year survival without recurrence generally means cure.

When the pathologist confirms cancer confined to the kidney, depending on the size of the cancer and the appearance of the cells under the microscope, the cure rate can range from 75% to over 95%. If the cancer has spread into the urinary collecting system (the ureter), into the inferior vena cava (the large vein in the abdomen), or into lymph nodes, the odds of five-year survival are much lower. If cancer has spread beyond the kidney into distant organs such as the lung or bone, the odds of five-year survival are very low.

## TREATMENT TO PREVENT RECURRENCE AFTER SURGERY

### Are there treatments that can prevent recurrence of the kidney cancer after the operation?

When a surgeon has removed all visible cancer but recurrence of cancer can occur, the treatment given to a person to prevent recurrence of the cancer is "adjuvant" treatment.

At this time, there are no adjuvant treatments with a proven ability to reduce the risk of recurrence of kidney cancer after surgery. Radiation therapy or chemotherapy, given either before surgery or after surgery, does not appear to be effective in preventing or delaying recurrence.

There are some new medicines, discussed later in this chapter, which have demonstrated some benefit in very advanced kidney cancer. Clinical trials are testing these medicines as adjuvant treatments. The benefits of these medicines as adjuvant therapy are unproven, and their use outside of clinical trials is generally not encouraged.

## METASTATIC KIDNEY CANCER

*When kidney cancer has spread beyond the kidney and into major body organs at the time it is first discovered, what initial treatment is possible?*

People who have kidney cancer that has spread beyond the kidney at the time of initial diagnosis may have serious symptoms such as pain, or bleeding from the cancer in their kidney into the urine. Surgical removal of the cancerous kidney may be very useful in relieving some of the symptoms.

When it is clear that cure of kidney cancer is surgically impossible, it may be possible to perform an "angioinfarction" of the kidney. This procedure involves putting a gelatin material or another inert material into the artery feeding the cancerous kidney. This will totally block blood supply to that kidney and will cause that kidney and the cancer in it to shrivel up and die. Angioinfarction is sometimes useful in controlling the local problem with the cancerous kidney but has no effect on any cancer that is outside the kidney.

## Can surgery be helpful if the cancer has spread beyond the kidney?

Kidney cancer sometimes recurs in distant organs as a single or very small number of discrete tumors that are completely removable by surgery. It is possible for a person to have a much-extended survival after having had these isolated areas of cancer removed (see chapters entitled "Lung Metastasis", "Liver Metastasis", and "Brain Metastasis").

Sometimes, at the time of a person's kidney cancer diagnosis, there is evidence that cancer has spread far beyond the kidney to distant organs. In an attempt to make immunotherapy with interleukin-2 (discussed later in this chapter) or treatment with "targeted therapy" (also discussed later in this chapter) more effective, surgeons may suggest removal of a cancerous kidney or of other tissues in the body that are harboring cancer. This surgery (referred to by physicians as "cytoreductive or "debulking" surgery), reduces the number of cancer cells in the body and can make subsequent treatments more effective. An additional reason to remove a cancerous kidney is to relieve symptoms such as back pain and bleeding into the urine.

## IMMUNOTHERAPY

## What immunotherapy has shown some benefit in kidney cancer?

Interleukin-2, for a fortunate few people with advanced kidney cancer, can induce remarkable responses and long-lasting remissions of cancer. Having a type of kidney cancer called "clear cell carcinoma" or having had additional debulking surgery (see above) appears to improve the possibility of having a favorable response. It now appears that about 20% of people with metastatic kidney cancer who are properly selected for likelihood of response to treatment have some regression of their cancer and that about 10% of people with metastatic kidney cancer treated with interleukin-2 have complete and lasting disappearance, and sometimes a cure of their cancer. The negative side of interleukin-2 is that the treatment regimen used to obtain these remissions is quite toxic and can produce a variety of life-threatening problems affecting many different parts of the body.

## TARGETED THERAPY

*What is the targeted therapy available for advanced kidney cancer?*

Several medications "target" specific biological mechanisms that support the growth of cancer. These "targeted therapies" have proven to be effective treatments of several types of cancer, including kidney cancer.

In order to grow into large masses, cancer cells require the growth of new blood vessels to provide them with nourishment. Over the past several years, there has been a great deal of interest in "angiogenesis inhibitors", that is, in medicines that can block the growth of these blood vessels by interfering with a substance called "VEGF" that the body uses to help these blood vessels grow. Two such drugs, called "sunitinib" (brand name is "Sutent", manufacturer's product website is www.sutent.com) and "pazopanib" (brand name is "Votrient", manufacturer's product website is www.votrient.com) can be given as a pill, and can delay further growth of the cancer for many months and extend survival in people with advanced kidney cancer not previously treated with anti-cancer medications. A similar drug called "sorafenib" (brand name is "Nexavar", manufacturer's product website is www.nexavar.com) works by the same mechanism and may restrain the growth of kidney cancer that has recurred or progressed after previous treatment.

A recent clinical study compared an experimental "second-generation VEGF inhibitor", which has been given the generic name "axitinib" and the brand name "Inlyta", to sorafenib ("Nexavar") in people with advanced kidney cancer whose cancer had progressed after previous targeted therapy. Axitinib delayed further progression of the cancer approximately two months longer than with sorafenib. Based upon these results, there is optimism that axitinib will soon be available as another treatment option for people with advanced kidney cancer.

An injectable angiogenesis blocking medication called "bevacizumab", (brand name is "Avastin", manufacturer's product website is www.avastin.com) given in combination with injectable medication "interferon alfa", can shrink or stabilize the metastatic kidney cancer approximately a third of the time, delay progression of the cancer for several months, and slightly extend the average survival time for people with metastatic kidney cancer.

Another medication given by injection called "Temsirolimus", (brand name is "Torisel, manufacturer's product website is www.torisel.com) targets a protein called "mTOR" that signals cancer cells to multiply and spread. Torisel delays cancer progression and extends survival in people with advanced kidney cancer whether or not there has been previous treatment with kidney cancer medications. A related medication, a pill called "everolimus" (brand name is "Afinitor", manufacturer's product website is www.afinitor.com) has also shown some effectiveness in extending survival in people who have failed to respond to or progressed after receiving either sunitinib or sorafenib.

When one of these medications is keeping a person's cancer stable, treatment with that drug, if tolerated, continues. If it stops working, substitution of another of these medications is an option. If one angiogenesis inhibitor stops working, it is still possible that a different angiogenesis inhibitor can inhibit further cancer growth.

These new medications are generally not curative, and there is considerable research in progress developing new drugs for kidney cancer.

# LEUKEMIA

## DEFINITION

### What is leukemia?

Leukemia is a cancer of the blood and the bone marrow. Leukemia begins with the transformation of cells in the bone marrow into malignant cells that grow more rapidly and live longer than normal cells. Eventually, these malignant cells can fill up the bone marrow and interfere with its essential functions: to produce red blood cells to carry oxygen through the body, white blood cells to fight infection, and platelets to allow the blood to clot when clotting is necessary.

## THE MAJOR TYPES OF ADULT LEUKEMIA

### What are the major types of leukemia in adults?

The most common forms of adult leukemia are acute myelogenous leukemia, chronic myelogenous leukemia, and chronic lymphocytic leukemia. Acute lymphocytic leukemia, the most common form of leukemia in children, is less common in adults and not discussed in this book. Because the treatment of each type of leukemia is so different, the discussion that follows will focus on these types of leukemia separately.

## ACUTE MYELOGENOUS LEUKEMIA: AML DEFINITION

### What is acute myelogenous leukemia?

Acute myelogenous leukemia, abbreviated as "AML" is a very dangerous and rapidly progressive form of leukemia. Without treatment, acute myelogenous leukemia is generally fatal within three months. With treatment, the likelihood of a longer survival is greatly improved and cure is possible.

## SYMPTOMS

### What are the symptoms of acute myelogenous leukemia?

The symptoms of acute myelogenous leukemia can develop gradually over a period of weeks or months. In general, these symptoms reflect impaired function of the bone marrow because of the high number of malignant cells packing the marrow and crowding out the normal cells. Lack of red blood cells produces anemia that causes fatigue. Lack of white blood cells produces a high risk of infections, some of which can be serious. Lack of platelets causes small hemorrhages in the skin, or bleeding of the gums or nose.

## MAKING THE DIAGNOSIS OF ACUTE MYELOGENOUS LEUKEMIA

### What tests establish the diagnosis of acute myelogenous leukemia?

The first major indication that a person has leukemia is the finding of a very large concentration of abnormal white blood cells in the bloodstream with a routine blood test called a "CBC" ("CBC" means "complete blood count"). The CBC generally will show that the person with acute myelogenous leukemia is anemic and has a low number of platelets in their bloodstream. The diagnosis of leukemia is often apparent when an experienced physician looks at a person's blood under the microscope.

A bone marrow biopsy will make a definitive diagnosis of acute myelogenous leukemia and may give very specific information about the likelihood of responding to different forms of treatment. The bone marrow biopsy is done using a special needle that extracts a small amount of bone marrow under local anesthesia from the back of the crest of the pelvic bone.

## CONSIDERATIONS BEFORE BEGINNING TREATMENT

*Where are people with acute myelogenous leukemia treated?*

The treatment of acute myelogenous leukemia is exceedingly complicated and requires the best possible medical care right from the very beginning of treatment. Treatment in a hospital with a medical team that is highly experienced in leukemia treatment is important. The hospital must also have easy access to all blood transfusion products and to advanced antibiotic medicines.

## INITIATING TREATMENT

*What preparations are necessary for a person to receive acute myelogenous leukemia treatment?*

Acute myelogenous leukemia treatment will involve chemotherapy that will temporarily eliminate virtually all leukemia cells from the bone marrow and bloodstream. At the same time as the chemotherapy kills the leukemia cells, production of virtually all the cells in the bone marrow that produce the normal white blood cells, red blood cells, and platelets will be temporarily suppressed. This effect on normal white blood cells and platelets will leave the person with very little resistance to infection and a weakened ability to control bleeding. A number of precautionary steps are necessary before treatment begins.

Because the chemotherapy will make a person very sensitive to developing serious infections, it is important to reduce the population of dangerous microorganisms in the person's hospital environment. Specially cleaned, sterile rooms with super-clean filtered air are available at major leukemia treatment centers and can reduce the risk of infection.

Sometimes, at the time of diagnosis of acute myelogenous leukemia, a person already has some form of infection of the skin, in the mouth, in the lungs, or elsewhere. A careful examination will look for evidence of such infection. If infection is present, administration of antibiotics may precede or coincide with the beginning of chemotherapy.

Treatment of acute myelogenous leukemia involves powerful chemotherapy, many blood tests, and transfusions of different types of blood products such as red blood cells and platelets. Establishing good access to the bloodstream is critical to put medicine, blood products and antibiotics in, and to draw blood samples out. This access requires insertion of a "central venous catheter" which is a large plastic tube placed into a large vein that leads directly into the heart. Inserting this central venous catheter prevents many painful needle sticks and permits the easy administration of transfusions, chemotherapy, antibiotics, and other medications.

## "INDUCTION THERAPY"

### What is the chemotherapy that is given?

The initial course of chemotherapy for acute myelogenous leukemia is "induction therapy". The most commonly used "induction therapy" is the combined treatment with cytosine arabinoside given over a 7-day period and daunorubicin (or one of several similar drugs in the "anthracycline" family such as "idarubicin"), given for three days.

### What are the side effects of induction therapy?

The major side effects relate to the severe, but temporary, suppression of normal bone marrow. Serious infections may become a problem. (Please see chapters entitled "Febrile Neutropenia" and "Opportunistic Infections") Suppression of platelet production can cause abnormal bleeding. A person may get diarrhea or sores in the mouth because of the effect of the chemotherapy on the cells lining the mouth and the bowel. Physicians will monitor a person closely for these complications and give prompt treatment if they occur.

### What treatment can reduce the risk of serious infections?

Antibiotics in the family of medications called "fluoroquinolones" have the ability to suppress a broad range of bacteria that can cause serious infections during induction therapy, and, for this reason, are commonly given. Candida infections (see chapter entitled "Candida Infections") are common after induction therapy for acute leukemia. One of several medications that can suppress the growth of this fungal infection can diminish the risk of developing a life-threatening candida infection.

## What happens after the induction therapy?

Shortly after induction therapy begins, there will be a great reduction in the number of leukemia cells in the bloodstream and bone marrow along with a very strong suppression of the normal bone marrow. Within 2-3 weeks, the normal bone marrow should begin to recover, and the person's natural resistance to infection and bleeding should begin to return to normal.

About a week after completion of the induction therapy, physicians at many medical centers will perform another bone marrow examination looking for evidence of persistent leukemia. If there is persistent leukemia, another course of induction therapy may be given in an attempt to achieve the desired response.

## What is a complete remission?

It is critical that the person respond to treatment with a "complete remission". A "complete remission" means elimination of all leukemia cells anywhere in the body. Without a complete remission, leukemia cells not eliminated by treatment will rapidly multiply and soon cause a full relapse of the leukemia.

## "CONSOLIDATION CHEMOTHERAPY"

*Is there any treatment that can improve the odds of achieving a durable or permanent complete remission?*

After a person with acute myelogenous leukemia has had a complete remission, there still is a very high risk that the leukemia will return. The reason for this high risk of recurrence is that a small number of leukemia cells may remain alive after the induction therapy and may not be detectable. After an apparent complete remission, the number of leukemia cells in the body (if present at all) is very low and additional chemotherapy may be able to eliminate the few remaining leukemia cells and improve the odds of cure.

Cytosine arabinoside is the medicine commonly used in an attempt to prolong a complete remission and prevent relapse. A common way of giving cytosine arabinoside is to wait for the person's bone marrow to recover its ability to produce normal blood cells after induction therapy and then administer the cytosine arabinoside every other day over five days. This course of cytosine arabinoside (called "consolidation chemotherapy") will suppress the bone marrow once again and cause many of the same side effects as the induction therapy (see above). When the bone marrow recovers, which usually happens in about a month, another "cycle" of five days of cytosine arabinoside begins. In this treatment regimen, three cycles of five days of treatment complete the consolidation therapy.

## THE EFFECTIVENESS OF INDUCTION THERAPY AND CONSOLIDATION THERAPY

*How effective is induction therapy and consolidation therapy in obtaining and maintaining a complete remission?*

Approximately three out of four people with acute myelogenous leukemia who are younger than sixty years of age obtain a complete remission after induction therapy. For people over age 60, the probability of having a complete remission is somewhat lower, with approximately half achieving a complete remission. With the additional consolidation therapy, the chance of having a sustained complete remission improves still further. Overall, induction and consolidation treatment produces a complete remission lasting four years or more, and a possible cure, in slightly less than half of people with acute myelogenous leukemia under age 60. Over age 60, the likelihood of achieving a cure is lower.

"Chromosomes" consist of the genetic material well known as "DNA" coiled around protein-containing substances. Using sophisticated tests, laboratories perform "cytogenetic testing", also known as "karyotype analysis", to evaluate chromosomes inside leukemia cells for the presence of abnormalities, including "translocations" in which genetic material is shifted between chromosomes. Based upon an assessment of identified chromosomal abnormalities, a more accurate assessment is made of the likelihood that treatment can produce remission or cure of the acute myelogenous leukemia.

## Can older people respond well to treatment?

People who are over 70 years of age can very definitely have a good, although most commonly temporary, response to the intensive chemotherapy needed to get a good response to treatment.

If, however, a person is over 80 years of age, or if their kidney function is significantly impaired, or if they are severely weakened by their illness, the outcome, even with chemotherapy, is not good and survival time as a consequence of the leukemia and side effects of chemotherapy is often measured in weeks or a very few months. Older people with several of these risk factors have a very different outlook for successful treatment. For these people, low doses of chemotherapy that can relieve some symptoms but which are not likely to produce complete remission may produce the better outcome.

## What prevents some people from achieving a complete remission?

A major reason for failing to achieve a complete remission is that the person may die from an infection during the period just after the induction therapy when the bone marrow is profoundly suppressed ("the aplastic phase"). The risk of death from infection during the aplastic phase underlines the importance of receiving treatment at a top medical center with extensive expertise and experience in treating acute myelogenous leukemia. The hassles, however major, of travel to a major medical center are well worth the improved chance of surviving the aplastic phase.

Another reason a person may fail to achieve a complete remission is resistance of the person's leukemia cells to the first course of chemotherapy. If the person had a response, but not a complete remission, to initial treatment, a complete remission can sometimes be achieved with another course of the same chemotherapy. When these courses of chemotherapy fail to result in a complete remission, new forms of chemotherapy or bone marrow transplantation are considerations.

## TREATMENT OF LEUKEMIA RESISTANT TO CHEMOTHERAPY

*What is the treatment if the leukemia is resistant to chemotherapy?*

There are several treatment options available if the person's leukemia is resistant to chemotherapy. One of the first is to consider the possibility of bone marrow transplantation.

*Can the bone marrow biopsy predict resistance to standard induction and consolidation chemotherapy?*

A person's acute myelogenous leukemia cells may show, with cytogenetic testing as described earlier in this chapter, characteristics that predict that they will be resistant to the more standard treatment with induction therapy followed by consolidation therapy. In this instance, and if a bone marrow transplantation is feasible, the person may receive some initial induction therapy to reduce, as much as possible, the amount of leukemia in their bone marrow and bloodstream, followed by bone marrow transplantation.

## BONE MARROW TRANSPLANTATION AS TREATMENT OF ACUTE MYELOGENOUS LEUKEMIA

*Is bone marrow transplantation only reserved for people who are resistant to or likely to be resistant to chemotherapy?*

No. Many experts believe that the best way of increasing the odds of curing acute myelogenous leukemia is when bone marrow transplantation follows an apparent complete remission achieved with chemotherapy.

*What is "allogeneic" bone marrow transplantation?*

"Allogeneic bone marrow transplantation" is when a donor's bone marrow is transplanted into a recipient.

*How is allogeneic bone marrow transplantation done?*

The bone marrow transplant is performed by first giving massive doses of radiation and then giving the person with acute myelogenous leukemia high doses of chemotherapy. The goal of this treatment is to kill all the leukemia cells in the body. Unfortunately, the treatment will also kill the normal cells in the person's bone marrow that are necessary to form red blood cells, white blood cells, and platelets.

In order to rescue the person from the destruction of their bone marrow by chemotherapy and radiation, a healthy donor's bone marrow cells are injected intravenously after the chemotherapy and radiation treatments have been completed. These donated cells will be naturally attracted to the person's empty bone marrow and should fill their marrow up again with the normal donated cells.

## Who donates the bone marrow?

The bone marrow will come from a person whose bone marrow cells will be compatible with the immune system of the person with leukemia. Often, the donor is a sibling.

## How does the donor donate the bone marrow?

With the donor under anesthesia, large needles, inserted into both sides of the pelvic bone, will withdraw the marrow into a large syringe. The procedure does no harm at all to the donor's own bone marrow reserve. The only complaint donors commonly have after the procedure is that they feel, for a few days, as though they have taken a kick in both sides of their behind.

## What is graft versus host disease?

When a person has a transplant from a donor, white blood cells remain in the donated marrow that can have a dangerous effect. These white blood cells are part of the "graft", that is, the donated marrow, and can react with the body organs of the person who received the bone marrow transplant, that is, the "host". This can cause "graft versus host" disease, in which serious damage to body organs such as the skin, liver and intestines can occur. Initial treatment of graft versus host disease includes the administration of high doses of steroids. If steroids fail to control the symptoms, other medicines that suppress the immune system are available.

These medications include "cyclosporine" (brand names for different formulations of this are "Neoral" and "Sandimmune" (see website http://www.ncbi.nlm.nih.gov/pubmedhealth/PMH0000155), "tacrolimus" (brand name is "Prograf", manufacturer's product website is www.prograf.com) and "mycophenolate" (brand name is "CellCept", manufacturer's product website is https://www.rochetransplant.com/default.aspxl). These medications may be able to control this complication.

## What are other side effects of bone marrow transplantation?

Severe and life threatening infections may occur because of the intense suppression of the white blood cell production by the chemotherapy. Reduction of platelets in the bloodstream because of the chemotherapy can make a person susceptible to dangerous internal bleeding.

The high doses of chemotherapy can damage tiny veins in the liver and cause a very serious liver disease called "veno-occlusive disease". An experimental medicine called "defibrotide" appears to have some effectiveness in treating this and is available at some medical centers, although it is not yet FDA approved.

## Can allogeneic bone marrow transplantation cure acute myelogenous leukemia?

Successful allogeneic bone marrow transplantation can mean disease-free life for many years, and, in some circumstances, cure. Because the technology of bone marrow transplantation is rapidly improving, the odds of obtaining a cure of acute myelogenous leukemia with bone marrow transplantation are improving.

> **Is it possible to perform a bone marrow**
> **transplant when there is no compatible**
> **donor of bone marrow cells available?**

Major bone marrow transplant centers are actively investigating technologies whereby a person's own marrow can be harvested (in the same way, described above, that a donor would have their bone marrow harvested) and then cleared of leukemia cells by a variety of chemicals. This process of clearing the bone marrow of malignant cells is "purging". The "purged marrow" is then frozen, and stored. At this point, the person can be given the very high dose chemotherapy and radiation used to kill all leukemia cells, and then will have their own bone marrow cells thawed and given back to them. This process, called "autologous bone marrow transplantation", is an option when a person with acute myelogenous leukemia does not have a suitable bone marrow donor.

> **If bone marrow from donors may be difficult to obtain and**
> **may cause graft versus host disease, why is "autologous**
> **bone marrow transplantation" with a person's**
> **own cells not routinely performed?**

In addition to the leukemia killing effect of massive doses of chemotherapy given with a bone marrow transplant, the cells in a donor marrow can interact with and kill leukemia cells, causing a helpful "graft versus leukemia" effect. People who undergo a bone marrow transplant from a donated bone marrow (an "allogeneic transplant") have a better chance of a long remission and cure than people who undergo an "autologous bone marrow transplant".

## TREATMENT IF ACUTE MYELOGENOUS LEUKEMIA RELAPSES

*What treatment is helpful for people with acute myelogenous leukemia who initially achieve a complete remission with chemotherapy and then relapse?*

When leukemia recurs after induction and consolidation chemotherapy, it indicates that the leukemia is resistant to therapy. The degree of that resistance can be partially determined by the length of time between their initial complete remission and their recurrence. People who recur 12 months or more after initial complete remission are most likely to achieve another complete remission after further chemotherapy. People who recur 6 to 12 months after an initial complete remission are less likely to respond, although response is certainly possible. When someone recurs within six months of achieving a complete remission or has never achieved a complete remission, the likelihood of achieving a complete remission with another course of chemotherapy is low.

Although a second course of chemotherapy can often put the acute myelogenous leukemia back into remission, these remissions are generally shorter than the first remission.

Some large cancer centers will suggest that a person undergo bone marrow transplantation at the first sign of acute myelogenous leukemia relapse. If the person is not eligible for bone marrow transplantation, other treatment will be necessary.

## What treatment is available for people with acute myelogenous leukemia who relapse and are not eligible for bone marrow transplantation?

There is other chemotherapy, some of it not yet FDA approved, which can put the person, once again, into a complete remission. The problem is, however, that each relapse is more difficult to put into remission, these experimental treatments have many serious potential side effects, and each remission induced after the first complete remission, lasts for a shorter and shorter period.

## What treatment is possible if chemotherapy is no longer effective and bone marrow transplantation is no longer an option?

Academic medical centers are actively investigating new treatments of refractory leukemia and a person may seek enrollment in a clinical trial testing one of those new treatments.

If the options for experimental treatment do not appear to provide a realistic possibility of prolonging life and will be associated with serious toxicity, supportive care should be given, relieving symptoms and making the person as comfortable as possible.

## What type of supportive care is given?

Supportive care will treat the symptoms caused by the acute myelogenous leukemia rather than the leukemia itself. Blood transfusions will treat anemia and relieve symptoms such as severe fatigue and difficulty breathing. Bleeding caused by loss of platelets may require transfusions of platelets. Infections require treatment with antibiotics.

## CHRONIC MYELOGENOUS LEUKEMIA: CML

### What is chronic myelogenous leukemia?

Chronic myelogenous leukemia (abbreviated as "CML") is a cancer of a type of white blood cell called "a myeloid cell" that is slower growing and associated with a longer survival than acute myelogenous leukemia. Until a few years ago when new treatments became available, the natural history of this disease was that a person would begin their disease course in a chronic phase in which he or she would feel generally well aside from some discomfort from an enlarged liver or spleen and some sense of general weakness. This phase of chronic myelogenous leukemia would last, on average, for three or four years. After that, an "accelerated phase" and then a "blast crisis" would generally develop in which, the production of leukemia cells would accelerate dramatically, and leukemia cells would fill up the bone marrow and the bloodstream at an alarmingly rapid rate and usually prove fatal within several months.

The last few years have seen dramatic improvement in the treatment of chronic myelogenous leukemia. Medicine taken by mouth and generally well-tolerated can, with a high degree of likelihood, control the disease for a very long period of time and perhaps indefinitely.

### What are the early symptoms of chronic myelogenous leukemia?

As with any form of leukemia that replaces normal functioning red and white blood cells and platelets, the person may initially complain of symptoms related to anemia, frequent infections, or unusual susceptibility to bleeding. Chronic myelogenous leukemia is also associated with enlargement of the spleen and this sometimes causes a sense of fullness or a sensation of something growing in the left side of the abdomen.

### *How is the diagnosis of chronic myelogenous leukemia made?*

The diagnosis is made by examining blood and a bone marrow biopsy (see description early in the chapter in the section regarding acute myelogenous leukemia) under the microscope. The characteristic finding of a so-called "Philadelphia chromosome" in bone marrow cells of almost every person with chronic myelogenous leukemia helps make a definitive diagnosis.

## INITIAL TREATMENT OF CHRONIC MYELOGENOUS LEUKEMIA

### *How is chronic myelogenous leukemia that is still in the chronic phase treated?*

The treatment of chronic myelogenous leukemia in the chronic phase drastically changed for the better with the introduction of a class of drugs called "tyrosine kinase inhibitors". Until very recently, almost all people with newly diagnosed chronic myelogenous leukemia received a tyrosine kinase inhibitor called "imatinib", (brand name is "Gleevec", and manufacturer's product website is www.gleevec.com). With this medication, an outstanding response with complete or near complete clearance of leukemia cells from the bloodstream and improvement of symptoms will be achieved approximately 90% of the time. These responses are commonly durable, with approximately 60% of people who began receiving imatinib while in the chronic phase still taking the medicine six years later and approximately 85% still alive after eight years. New second-generation tyrosine kinase inhibitors called "dasatinib "and "nilotinib" are now available which increase this high response rate still further. Although the long-term superiority of the second-generation tyrosine kinase inhibitors to imatinib is uncertain, it appears likely that they will result in a quicker, better and more lasting responses than the first generation imatinib.

The greatest experience, including long-term follow-up for side effects, exists for imatinib. Some physicians feel, and some people with chronic myelogenous leukemia may agree, that since imatinib has an excellent track record for long term disease control and is generally a well-tolerated medicine, that imatinib should be the initial treatment of choice for chronic myelogenous leukemia with the second-line versions as a back-up in the event imatinib is no longer working. An external force, which may steer people toward imatinib, is that sometime around 2014, the drug could become generic and much less expensive than the second-generation versions. The pendulum of opinion, however, appears to be shifting toward the initial use of the dasatinib or nilotinib, because of the clear and obvious superiority of the second-generation tyrosine kinase inhibitors in head-to-head studies comparing them with imatinib over the 12 to 18 month period for which information is presently available.

## *Is bone marrow transplantation an initial treatment of chronic myelogenous leukemia?*

Although cure of chronic myelogenous leukemia with bone marrow transplantation is possible, this possibility of cure is associated with a high risk of the side effects and occasional deaths associated with bone marrow transplantation. Now that the tyrosine kinase inhibitors can control chronic myelogenous leukemia in the vast majority of people with newly diagnosed chronic myelogenous leukemia, with rare exceptions, bone marrow transplantation is not an initial therapy.

## *What is the treatment if chronic myelogenous leukemia is not responding adequately to imatinib?*

Many people with chronic myelogenous leukemia will receive initial treatment with imatinib. If it is clear that a person is taking their medicine properly and the chronic myelogenous leukemia cells remain in the bloodstream, a second-generation tyrosine kinase inhibitor often produces a better response.

If chronic myelogenous leukemia cells are still not properly cleared from the bloodstream after treatment with second generation tyrosine kinase inhibitors, consideration may be given to a bone marrow transplantation if the person is medically fit enough to have a transplant and if a suitable donor for the marrow can be found.

"Third-generation" tyrosine kinase inhibitors are in development. Very promising early results with an experimental third-generation tyrosine kinase inhibitor called "ponatinib" showed that over two-thirds of people with chronic myelogenous leukemia resistant to first and second-generation tyrosine kinase inhibitors had an excellent response to treatment. Enrolling in a clinical trial evaluating new treatments of chronic myelogenous leukemia is a very important option to consider if chronic myelogenous leukemia is not responding adequately to imatinib.

When tyrosine kinase inhibitors are not working and bone marrow transplantation is not an option, the medicines "alfa interferon" and "cytarabine" can reduce the number of chronic myelogenous leukemia cells in the bloodstream and bone marrow and occasionally be helpful in delaying the onset of life-threatening complications. Side effects of alfa interferon, such as fatigue, may be a problem, but can diminish or disappear when the interferon is taken an hour or so before bedtime. Painful sores in the mouth, diarrhea, and nausea and vomiting are other difficult side effects.

As a less effective alternative to interferon and cytarabine, an oral chemotherapy medicine called "hydroxyurea" can lower the number of chronic myelogenous leukemia cells in the bloodstream, although not to the extent that they are nearly gone.

### *What does it mean when chronic myelogenous leukemia transitions into the "accelerated phase"?*

Transition to the accelerated phase indicates that chronic myelogenous leukemia cells are more rapidly dividing and that the person's disease has become more dangerous. Among the factors that indicate the emergence of the accelerated phase are a rapidly rising number of white blood cells and a drop in the number of platelets in the bloodstream and worsening anemia. In addition, looking under the microscope, the physician would see an increased number of "blast cells" which are highly malignant and rapidly multiplying.

## *What is the treatment of the accelerated phase of chronic myelogenous leukemia?*

If the accelerated phase of chronic myelogenous leukemia develops without a person having had adequate treatment with imatinib or of other tyrosine kinase inhibitors, this medicine will be prescribed.

Since the accelerated phase indicates a dangerous transition of the disease and a higher likelihood that the disease will get completely out of control, consideration will be given as to whether a bone marrow transplant is possible.

If the accelerated phase develops despite adequate therapy with imatinib, a second-generation tyrosine kinase inhibitor may produce a good response. A key factor in this consideration will be the results of a blood test looking for a "T315I" mutation. If the person has this mutation, a response to the second-generation tyrosine kinase inhibitors is unlikely.

If tyrosine kinase inhibitors and bone marrow transplantation are not options, enrollment in a clinical trial evaluating a new treatment is an important option.

## CHRONIC MYELOGENOUS LEUKEMIA IN BLAST CRISIS

### *What is blast crisis?*

Blast crisis is the most dangerous phase of chronic myelogenous leukemia in which the blood and the bone marrow is filling up rapidly with the highly malignant leukemia cells.

## What is the treatment if blast crisis develops?

As with the accelerated phase, the first consideration will be whether the person has had adequate treatment with the tyrosine kinase inhibitors and whether bone marrow transplantation is an option. Although the results of either treatment are not as good as in earlier stages of CML, a good response to treatment with tyrosine kinase or with bone marrow transplant is still possible.

The other options for treatment of blast crisis are not good. Although chemotherapy can reduce the white blood cell count, leukemia cells usually begin to grow back again and rapidly fill up the bone marrow.

A person with blast crisis who wants an aggressive attempt to control their disease may want to consider seeking experimental treatment at a major medical center with experience in the investigation of new treatments of leukemia.

# CHRONIC LYMPHOCYTIC LEUKEMIA: CLL DEFINITION

## What is chronic lymphocytic leukemia?

Chronic lymphocytic leukemia, generally abbreviated as "CLL", is a slowly progressive form of leukemia that primarily affects people over 50 years of age. The slow multiplication of leukemia cells in most people with chronic lymphocytic leukemia allows many people to survive ten or more years from the time a person first receives their diagnosis. With treatments that have recently become available, the survival time of people with chronic lymphocytic leukemia is likely to extend still further.

# SYMPTOMS

## *What are the symptoms of chronic lymphocytic leukemia?*

A person with chronic lymphocytic leukemia will commonly notice enlarged lymph nodes( "called "lymphadenopathy"), particularly in the neck area ("cervical lymphadenopathy"), and in the armpit ("axillary lymphadenopathy"). Sometimes, there is a general sense of fatigue. An enlarged spleen may cause pain in the left side of the abdomen.

In the early stages of the illness, a person may have no symptoms and suspicion of chronic lymphocytic leukemia only arises when a high level of a type of white blood cell called a "lymphocyte" appears on a routine blood test. "Lymphocytosis" reported by the laboratory means that a high number of lymphocytes are present in the blood stream.

People with chronic lymphocytic leukemia are unusually susceptible to infections. These infections may require medical attention and may lead to the discovery of the diagnosis of chronic lymphocytic leukemia.

# STAGES OF CHRONIC LYMPHOCYTIC LEUKEMIA

## *What are the stages of chronic lymphocytic leukemia and why are they important?*

The stage of chronic lymphocytic leukemia is indicative of how far the disease has progressed and gives vital information about the person's outlook and about the appropriate treatment to administer.

There are several different ways physicians can consider the stage of chronic lymphocytic leukemia, but one of the most common methods will classify someone as having low risk, intermediate risk, or high risk chronic lymphocytic leukemia.

People with low risk chronic lymphocytic leukemia only have lymphocytosis (see above), and no other symptoms: their average survival time from diagnosis is over ten years. With intermediate risk chronic lymphocytic leukemia, there is enlargement of lymph nodes and there may be enlargement of the liver or the spleen; this is associated with an average survival time of approximately seven years. With high-risk chronic lymphocytic leukemia, anemia or low platelet counts give evidence of a reduction of the bone marrow's ability to make blood cells. High-risk chronic lymphocytic leukemia is associated with an average survival time of approximately a year and a half. Extension of these survival times is likely with new treatments that have recently become available.

## **TREATMENT**

### *Is chronic lymphocytic leukemia curable?*

No currently available treatment can safely cure chronic lymphocytic leukemia. There are medicines, however, which can induce a "complete remission", which, although not permanent, can eliminate all evident leukemia cells from the body for an extended period.

## What is the treatment of chronic lymphocytic leukemia at its earliest stages when a person does not have troubling symptoms?

When chronic lymphocytic leukemia is not producing significant symptoms, it is not certain that immediate intensive treatment with all its dangerous side effects will improve a person's outlook. Many physicians will suggest that a person with low risk chronic lymphocytic leukemia not have any treatment at all.

During the period when no treatment is given, examinations of the blood every few months will determine the extent, if at all, that the number of lymphocytes in the blood stream is increasing. Based upon this assessment of the lymphocytes, and based upon whether there is emergence of worrisome new symptoms suggesting significant progression, physicians will suggest either further delay or initiation of therapy.

As the disease progresses, symptoms related to impairment of bone marrow function and enlargement of the lymph nodes and spleen can become a problem. When this occurs, treatment with one of several forms of chemotherapy will be helpful to relieve symptoms and extend survival.

## What form of chemotherapy is used?

The most effective chemotherapy medications used to treat chronic lymphocytic leukemia have the highest degree of side effects. For this reason, at the time a person needs treatment to relieve symptoms and extend survival, the person's underlying health and willingness to tolerate the side effects of treatment are important considerations. For example, the treatment given to a frail 80-year-old person with many other medical problems will differ from that given to an otherwise healthy 50-year-old person.

The older standard first-line treatment is the combination of two medicines, chlorambucil and prednisone. These medicines have fewer side effects than the more effective new combination treatments, but can reduce the number of leukemia cells in the bloodstream, relieve symptoms, and have some modest benefit in extending survival. They generally do not induce complete remissions in which all evidence of the chronic lymphocytic leukemia disappears, and for this reason, this older form of treatment is less effective than more recently developed treatments.

A medication, called "fludarabine", is far more effective than chlorambucil and prednisone in reducing and sometimes entirely clearing leukemia cells in the bloodstream. Fludarabine is a component of initial treatment for people with chronic lymphocytic leukemia whose underlying health is good. For people who, because of poor health, initially received treatment with chlorambucil and prednisone and had progression of their disease, fludarabine may be a second line treatment. A new form of fludarabine is now available as a pill, which makes administration of this medication simpler and safer.

Recently, the FDA approved a chemotherapy medication called "bendamustine" (brand name is "Treanda", manufacturer's product website is www.treanda.com) as an initial treatment of chronic lymphocytic leukemia. Although bendamustine is clearly more effective than chlorambucil in inducing remissions of chronic lymphocytic leukemia and in delaying its progression, it is not yet clear how bendamustine measures up to fludarabine-containing regimens as regards response rate, longer term outlook or survival. The relative effectiveness of bendamustine as opposed to fludarabine is under evaluation by a clinical study in progress comparing a treatment regimen containing bendamustine with a treatment regimen containing fludarabine.

## Which medicines, administered along with fludarabine, enhance the responses still further?

If a person is able to tolerate more intense treatment with a somewhat higher likelihood of side effects, a combination of medications appears to be the most effective way to suppress chronic lymphocytic leukemia. A medication in the family of "monoclonal antibodies" called "Rituximab" given along with the chemotherapy medication "cyclophosphamide" increases the response rate of fludarabine and decreases the likelihood that the disease will progress or prove lethal for a period of three years or longer. This combination of fludarabine and Rituximab and cyclophosphamide significantly reduces the number of chronic lymphocytic leukemia cells in the bloodstream approximately 90% of the time, and clears the bloodstream of evidence of chronic lymphocytic leukemia approximately half of the time.

## What are the side effects of the chemotherapy of chronic lymphocytic leukemia?

For chlorambucil and for fludarabine and for bendamustine, the major side effects are suppression of the white blood cells called "neutrophils" which help a person fight bacterial infections.

This drop in the number of neutrophils in the bloodstream, called "neutropenia", is far more common with fludarabine than it is with chlorambucil. For a detailed discussion of neutropenia, please see the chapter "Bone Marrow Suppression".

With the combination of fludarabine and Rituximab, there is a much higher risk of neutropenia than with fludarabine alone. In addition, during the intravenous injection of the Rituximab, a person may develop severe shaking chills along with low blood pressure. For a detailed discussion of these side effects of Rituximab, please see the chapter "Infusion Reactions".

### How long is the chemotherapy given?

Chemotherapy is generally administered in cycles in which the drugs are given for several consecutive days every month or so. Chemotherapy treatments continue either until a person has a complete clearing of chronic lymphocytic leukemia cells from the bloodstream or until reaching a point at which no further reductions of chronic lymphocytic leukemia cells in the bloodstream is occurring with continued treatment.

### What is the treatment if a person is not responding to initial treatment?

If the initial treatment is not having the desired effect on the chronic lymphocytic leukemia, alternate treatment regimens are available. Fludarabine, Rituximab, and bendamustine are the three drugs that are most effective in destroying chronic lymphocytic leukemia cells. If one of these drugs has not administered earlier, it is likely that a physician will recommend that it be given.

## What is the treatment if the disease recurs after a previous remission?

If chronic lymphocytic leukemia remained in remission for six months or longer, physicians may attempt to regain control of the disease by administering the same medications as given before to get the original remission. Before doing so, physicians may test a person's leukemia cells for an abnormality called a "17-p deletion". If present, a "17-p deletion" is a sign that a response to the previous chemotherapy is unlikely, and that alternative therapy could be more appropriate.

The chemotherapy medication called "bendamustine" which was mentioned earlier in this chapter can produce very good remissions, especially when given in combination with Rituximab, when chronic lymphocytic leukemia has relapsed or progressed after other therapy.

People who are failing to respond to fludarabine or Rituximab or bendamustine have a difficult outlook, since treatment options that remain may not be as effective. A monoclonal antibody known by the brand name of "Campath" (manufacturer's product website is www.campath.com) can significantly reduce the number of chronic lymphocytic leukemia cells in the bloodstream in approximately a third of people refractory to fludarabine and may be an important treatment option if the "17-p deletion", mentioned above, is present. Campath causes a very potent suppression of the immune system, and is associated with a high risk of developing serious and life-threatening infections.

A new monoclonal antibody called "Arzerra" has shown some effectiveness in people who are refractory to treatment with fludarabine and Campath. With Arzerra treatment, approximately 40% of people have some clearing, which is not complete, of chronic lymphocytic leukemia cells from their bloodstream. Favorable responses to treatment last, on average, for approximately six months. Like Campath, this treatment is associated with serious suppression of the immune system and a high risk of developing serious and life-threatening infections.

Clinical trials evaluating new treatments of refractory chronic lymphocytic leukemia are in progress at major medical centers and enrollment in one of these trials may be another option.

## VACCINES TO PREVENT INFECTION

*Which vaccines can prevent serious infections in people with chronic lymphocytic leukemia?*

Vaccination against influenza, given every year, and against "pneumococcus", given every five years, is a common recommendation. Because of the suppressed immune system associated with chronic lymphocytic leukemia, live virus vaccines, such as the vaccine against herpes zoster, are not given.

## TREATMENT OF RECURRENT INFECTIONS IN PEOPLE WITH CHRONIC LYMPHOCYTIC LEUKEMIA

*How are recurrent infections in a person with chronic lymphocytic leukemia treated?*

The person with chronic lymphocytic leukemia, their families, and their physicians, must be vigilant about early symptoms of infection. Fever, cough, pain in the sinuses, skin infections, and any other early sign of infection are important warning signals. Prompt evaluation, and, if appropriate, prompt initiation of antibiotics, are essential to preventing serious, life-threatening infections.

Some people with chronic lymphocytic leukemia who have recurrent infections may be better able to fight off infections after beginning treatment with intravenous immunoglobulin injections given every three or four weeks.

Herpes zoster, a virus infection known by many as "shingles", causes a painful blistering skin rash and can be a recurrent difficult problem in people with chronic lymphocytic leukemia. For additional information about "shingles", please see the discussion in the chapter "Opportunistic Infections".

# LUNG CANCER

## DEFINITION

### What is lung cancer?

Lung cancer is a cancer that arises in the lung. Unless controlled in its earliest stages, lung cancer will usually spread from the lung to other areas of the body.

It is important to distinguish between "lung cancer" and "metastasis of cancer to the lung". "Lung cancer" means the cancer started in the lung. "Metastasis of cancer to the lung" means that the cancer began somewhere outside the lung and spread to the lung. The treatment of cancer that has spread to the lung is completely different from treatment of cancer that started in the lung. This chapter only discusses lung cancer. A review of the treatment of cancer that has spread to the lung is in the chapter entitled "Lung Metastasis", and in the chapters of this book that discuss the individual cancers that can spread to the lung.

## SYMPTOMS

### What are the symptoms of lung cancer?

The most common first symptom of lung cancer is a new, persistent cough. As time goes on, the coughing worsens and bloody sputum may come up with the cough. Shortness of breath, pain in the chest, fever, weight loss and a general feeling of unremitting weakness are among the many symptoms that may reflect the presence of a growing lung cancer.

## MAKING THE DIAGNOSIS

*How is the diagnosis of lung cancer made?*

Specific abnormalities seen on a plain chest x-ray can lead to a tentative diagnosis of lung cancer. A "mass lesion", "coin lesion", or "pulmonary nodule" are words for the same thing, which is something new or abnormal on the chest x-ray in the form of a somewhat round or oval white spot that should not be there. Spread of the cancer beyond the lung to lymph nodes in the center of the chest or to the bones of the rib cage may be evident on the chest x-ray.

Although a chest x-ray alone may strongly suggest a diagnosis of lung cancer, further testing is necessary. Benign tumors of the lung certainly do occur. A wide variety of infections, including tuberculosis, can have similarities to lung cancer's x-ray appearance. Before a diagnosis of lung cancer is made with certainty, it is important to confirm the diagnosis of lung cancer and determine the exact type of lung cancer the person has by having a pathologist examine a piece of the lesion under the microscope (called "making a tissue diagnosis").

*How does the physician make a tissue diagnosis?*

In the early stages of lung cancer, there usually is a mass of fragile cancer sitting inside a bronchial tube somewhere in the lung. When a person gives a strong cough, cells can be broken off the cancer and caught up in sputum. A pathologist examining this sputum under a microscope may find cancer cells.

Bronchoscopy is usually necessary to make a more precise diagnosis. The device used to perform this test (called a "bronchoscope") is a flexible long tube that projects images from inside the bronchial tubes in the lungs to a video monitor. To perform the bronchoscopy, a lung specialist will administer mild sedation, spray the throat with a light anesthetic, and then advance the bronchoscope down the windpipe into the bronchial tree. Based upon the location of the mass found with the x-ray or CT scan, the physician finds the tumor with the bronchoscope and the appearance, size, and location of the tumor will be determined. The bronchoscope itself has a space inside of it that allows the physician performing the bronchoscopy to put an instrument down the scope that can snip off a piece of the lesion for the pathologist to examine under the microscope.

## What happens if bronchoscopy is unable to make a tissue diagnosis?

There are other ways of getting a tissue diagnosis aside from bronchoscopy. When the lesion is close to the outer surface of the lung close to the rib cage (this is a "peripheral lesion" or "peripheral nodule"), it may be possible, guided by a CT scan or ultrasound machine, to put a long, fine biopsy needle through the chest wall and into the lung mass. This procedure is a "needle biopsy". The risk of a needle biopsy is that the lung punctured by a biopsy needle may release air into the chest cavity and cause a "pneumothorax" (see chapter entitled "Pneumothorax"). A needle biopsy may serve as a tremendous shortcut to a diagnosis by preventing the need for performing a major operation on the lung to make the diagnosis.

Sometimes lung cancer has already spread far beyond the lung at the time the person first develops symptoms of their cancer. In these cases, the cancer may be in the bones, in lymph nodes, in the liver or other organs of the body. If such a spread or "metastasis" has occurred, it may be easiest to biopsy the metastasis itself. Biopsy of the metastasis can confirm the diagnosis of cancer and make a biopsy of the tumor in the lung unnecessary.

A tissue diagnosis is essential for making the diagnosis of lung cancer and for deciding on the appropriate treatment. If a piece of the tumor is unavailable by any other method, it may be necessary to perform a major operation to remove the portion of the lung that contains the mass. The hospital pathologist examines the removed mass.

### How does the tissue diagnosis guide treatment?

A tissue diagnosis will confirm whether cancer is present or not. If the diagnosis is cancer, the biopsy will give precise information as to the type of lung cancer that the person has.

Lung cancers belong to two broad categories– "non-small cell lung cancer" and "small cell lung cancer". Among people with lung cancer, those with non-small cell lung cancer outnumber those with small cell lung cancer by about four to one.

Because there is a vast difference between the treatment of non-small cell lung cancer and small cell lung cancer, it is necessary to split the discussion about the treatment of lung cancer into two separate sections.

## NON-SMALL CELL LUNG CANCER DEFINITION

### *What does non-small cell lung cancer mean?*

There are four major types of lung cancer: "squamous cell" lung cancer, "large cell" lung cancer, "adenocarcinoma" and "small cell" lung cancer. In practical terms, the first three cancers–the "non-small cell lung cancers"–respond in a similar way to therapy and have a similar outlook. Because of this, the non-small cell lung cancers, with some exceptions, are one disease when therapy is planned or evaluated.

## DETERMINING WHETHER NON-SMALL CELL LUNG CANCER HAS SPREAD BEYOND THE LUNG

### *How is the extent of spread, if any, of the non-small cell lung cancer determined?*

The most effective way to cure lung cancer is, when possible, to cut it all out. Successful surgical cure of lung cancer is, however, highly unlikely if the cancer has spread from the lung and neighboring lymph nodes to distant areas of the body. Therefore, an essential first step after the tissue diagnosis confirms non-small cell lung cancer is to evaluate the areas of the body to which lung cancer tends to spread and to determine whether the cancer is surgically curable.

When non-small cell lung cancer spreads, it tends to spread first to the lymph nodes that are near the lung, and then to the pleura (the pleura is the inner lining of the rib cage), and to the bones of the rib cage. Spread of the cancer inside the chest may be evident with a plain chest x-ray and by a CT scan of the chest. When non-small cell lung cancer spreads beyond the chest, it can spread to almost any major organ, but spreads most commonly to the liver, the bones and the brain. Evidence of spread of the cancer to liver, bones or brain is detectable by simple blood tests, by physical examination, by CT scans, or by a bone scan.

## STAGING THE CANCER

### What is the significance of the stage of the cancer?

The stage of the cancer is designated as stage I, stage II, stage III, or stage IV with the letter "a" or "b" after a designated stage of I, II, or III. A higher Roman numeral means that the cancer is more advanced and that treatment has a lower likelihood of curing the cancer. Similarly, the letter "b" after a numeral means that the cancer has advanced more than, if it had the letter "a". These numerals and letters reflect the size of the cancer, location in the chest, involvement of lymph nodes, and evidence of invasion of adjacent or distant structures. Determination of the stage of the cancer at the time of diagnosis is essential to planning the treatment with the highest likelihood of curing the disease, or, failing that, extending survival and relieving symptoms.

### How is the stage of the cancer determined?

A CT scan of the chest and abdomen is a crucial test that provides detailed information about the location and size of the cancer, and involvement of nearby or distant structures or organs in the chest or the abdomen.

Because some areas involved with cancer may not be detectable by the CT scan, physicians will sometimes ask a person to obtain a "PET" scan. A PET scan is a sensitive test that can often detect the spread of cancer to distant organs before detection by CT scans. To do this test, an injection is made of a tiny amount of radioactive glucose into the bloodstream. Cancer cells have a greater affinity for this radioactive glucose than other tissues. The PET scanner can then find "hot spots" inside the body that contain the cancer and transmit this information to a computer for the physician to evaluate. The identification of a "hot spot" suggests, but does not prove, the presence of cancer cells in the hot spot. Although a "hot spot" may indicate the presence of cancer, areas of inflammation without cancer can also produce "hot spots". A "hot spot" indicates a suspicious area that needs evaluation, often with a biopsy to confirm the presence or absence of local cancer.

If there are new symptoms of impaired brain function or headaches, a physician may advise a CT or MRI of the brain. It is uncommon for non-small cell lung cancer to have spread to the brain at the time of first diagnosis.

## ASSESSING LUNG FUNCTION

*Why is it important to assess lung function?*

The most effective way of curing lung cancer is to remove the portion of the lung that contains the cancer. If this is not possible, intense radiation focused on a localized cancer can stop its local growth and can occasionally cure it. Since surgery removes functioning lung and intense radiation causes some collateral damage to surrounding uninvolved lung, it is important to assess a person's lung function to make sure that they can tolerate this treatment. Since smoking is the most common cause of lung cancer, it is common for the cancer to develop against a background of pre-existing severe lung disease such as COPD (see the chapter).

## What tests evaluate lung function?

One of the most important tests done is "spirometry" which will measure the maximum volume of air a person can forcefully exhale in one second. This test is an "FEV1 ", which stands for "forced expiratory volume, one second". The measurement of FEV1 before and after the person inhales a medicine that widens or "dilates" the bronchial tubes (a "bronchodilator") gives very important information about the presence and severity of COPD, which is common in smokers.

Another important spirometry measure is the "FVC" or "forced vital capacity". This measures the amount of air that a person can expel from their lungs after taking a full deep breath. The relationship between the FEV1 and the FVC in a ratio called the "FEV1/FVC ratio" provides important information about the severity of the person's COPD and helps to provide guidance with regard to a person's ability to tolerate lung cancer treatments such as surgery or radiation.

In addition to pulmonary function tests, the physician may advise tests to determine pulmonary and cardiac function during exercise.

# THE MEDIASTINUM

## What is the mediastinum?

The mediastinum is the area in the chest that is between the lungs. The mediastinum contains the heart, the esophagus, and the major arteries and veins leading to and from the heart. The mediastinum also contains lymph nodes to which the cancer can travel.

## How are lymph nodes in the mediastinum evaluated?

A CT or MRI scan can show evidence of enlargement of lymph nodes in the mediastinum, which is suggestive of, but not proof of, presence of cancer in these lymph nodes. To determine whether these lymph nodes are involved, a surgeon can perform a "mediastinoscopy". To do this, a surgeon will make a small incision in the very top of the chest between the collarbones. Through this incision, the physician will put a scope inside the chest and look around. Suspicious lymph nodes will be biopsied, and then sent to a pathologist to determine whether they contain cancer cells.

A newer and very effective way of evaluating lymph nodes in the mediastinum is with "endosonography" which involves putting separate tube-like instruments inside the esophagus and inside the bronchial tubes in the lung, and, using sound waves bounced off internal organs, generating images transmitted to a video screen. The images generated by endosonography can identify enlarged lymph nodes in the mediastinum and can identify other areas inside the chest that may contain cancer. Guided by endosonography, these areas can be biopsied and the presence or absence of cancer determined.

## *What is the significance of cancer in lymph nodes in the mediastinum?*

When cancer is in lymph nodes in the mediastinum, there is a much lower possibility that surgery will be able to cure the cancer. Depending on which lymph nodes in the mediastinum are involved, and particularly depending on whether this involvement is extensive or on both the left and right side of the chest, very different surgical, radiation, and chemotherapy treatments could be required.

## SURGERY

## *What type of surgery is most effective in removing a cancer from the lung?*

The lungs divide into "lobes" with the left lung having two lobes and the right lung having three. When the cancer has not spread beyond a lobe, the surgeon can perform a "lobectomy", which effectively removes the cancerous portion of the lung. When it does not appear that a lobectomy is likely to remove the entire cancer while removing the entire lung might, a "pneumonectomy", that is, removal of the entire lung, has the potential to remove all of the cancer.

## *What is stage I non-small cell lung cancer and what is its common treatment?*

Stage I non-small cell lung cancer means that the cancer is relatively small and confined to the lung, without spread to nearby lymph nodes or any other near or distant structures. This cancer is potentially curable with surgery and the standard treatment would be either a lobectomy or a pneumonectomy.

## What is stage II non-small cell lung cancer and what is its common treatment?

Stage II non-small cell lung cancer means that the cancer appears to be confined to the lung with the exception of some cancer that has spread to lymph nodes that are within the lung or lymph nodes that are very close to the involved lung. These lymph nodes are "peribronchial" and "hilar" lymph nodes. Lymph nodes on the same side as the involved lung are "ipsilateral lymph nodes". Lymph nodes surrounding the opposite lung are "contralateral lymph nodes". When the cancer is relatively small, localized to the lung and only involves ipsilateral peribronchial and/or hilar and/or lymph nodes in the lung, it is stage II non-small cell lung cancer.

Stage II non-small cell lung cancer is also potentially curable with surgery and the standard treatment would either be a lobectomy or a pneumonectomy.

## What is the difference in outlook between stage I and stage II non-small cell lung cancer?

Non-small cell lung cancer is a very dangerous form of cancer that has a high risk of recurring even after an apparent surgical removal of all cancer. For stage I, depending on the size of the lung cancer and the surgical or radiation treatments administered, cure of the lung cancer is very possible. For stage II, the risk of recurring is much higher.

## What can reduce the odds of recurrence after surgery?

For people with stage I non-small cell lung cancer and a very small cancer (technically speaking this is a cancer that is less than 3 centimeters in diameter and is called "Stage $I_a$"), that is completely removed by surgery, it is not clear that any treatment reduces the risk of recurrence. If the stage I cancer lesion is somewhat larger (more than 3 centimeters and considered "stage $I_b$"), or if the cancer is considered to be in stage II, chemotherapy containing the medicine "cisplatin", along with one other chemotherapy medication, can add several percentage points to the likelihood that the cancer will be cured by the surgery.

## Is radiation therapy helpful in reducing the risk of recurrence after surgery for stage I or II non-small cell lung cancer?

After surgery, the pathologist will examine the lobe of the lung from which the cancer was removed. The pathologist will examine the "margins", that is, the interface between where the cancer was located and the edges of the area of the lung from which the cancer was removed. If these "margins" are negative, radiation therapy does not reduce the risk of recurrence and may actually have a negative effect on likelihood of long-term survival. In this setting, that is, given to prevent recurrence after surgery, it appears to be more harmful than helpful.

If the "margins" are positive, it implies that cancer cells remain in the lung and there may be some benefit to radiation therapy.

*Can chemotherapy, given before surgery, improve the odds of the surgeon removing all of the cancer and curing it?*

This is an area of ongoing research, but, despite many attempts at this in large clinical trials, giving chemotherapy before the attempt at surgical cure does not appear to improve outcome.

*When is it not a good idea to attempt a surgical cure of a localized lung cancer?*

Long-time cigarette smokers often have many medical problems. Severe COPD is very common in middle-aged and elderly smokers. Removal of large amounts of lung tissue from a person with limited functioning lung may be medically impossible. People with a history of serious heart disease may also not be able to withstand the major surgery.

*What is the treatment if the person, because of poor health, would not be able to tolerate a lobectomy or pneumonectomy?*

Depending on the size and location of the tumor, surgeons may attempt to remove only the segment of the lung ("a segmentectomy") or a wedge of the lung ("a wedge resection") thereby sparing the remainder of the lung. These are difficult operations to do, especially in people with non-small cell lung cancer with poor underlying health, and have a lower cure rate than lobectomy or pneumonectomy.

There are some new surgical techniques by which, using a very small incision and special instruments including a scope and video device (called "video assisted thoracoscopic surgery"), small cancers can be removed in people with severe COPD without causing unacceptable lung damage or the trauma of a major operation. Such surgical techniques are available at centers of excellence with very experienced "thoracic surgeons".

When these limited operations are not feasible for reasons related to the person's underlying health or the size and location of the cancer, a treatment regimen of high doses of radiation has the potential to cure the cancer in about one in five people with stage I or II non-small cell lung cancer. If the radiation fails to cure the cancer, it often is able to slow or stop its continued growth in the lung and the surrounding structures in the chest. This radiation commonly causes inflammation in the esophagus that can make swallowing difficult. In addition, the radiation can damage nearby lung and somewhat worsen a person's lung function, although not nearly as much as by removing a lobe of a lung or an entire lung.

## Can elderly people withstand the surgery?

People over age 70 are definitely candidates for surgery so long as their heart, lungs, and general health are in reasonably good shape. With increasing age, complications of surgery are somewhat more common, but there is no doubt that lung cancer is curable in elderly people with surgery.

# WHEN MEDIASTINAL LYMPH NODES HAVE CANCER IN THEM

*What is a common treatment plan if the
lymph nodes in the mediastinum contain cancer?*

When the lymph nodes in the mediastinum contain cancer, it generally is a sign that surgery is less likely to cure the cancer. There are differences of opinion regarding the best treatment if the lymph nodes in the mediastinum contain cancer. Despite these different opinions, there is general agreement that the greatest risk that a person with lung cancer in lymph nodes in the mediastinum faces is the risk of spread of the cancer beyond the lung to distant areas of the body. Because of this, treatment regimens prescribed usually include chemotherapy.

A common approach is to first assess whether the degree of cancer in the lymph nodes in the mediastinum is extensive and whether the cancer involves lymph nodes on both the right and left sides of the chest.

If the degree of involvement of the lymph nodes in the mediastinum is minimal, and the surgeon believes the entire cancer can be surgically removed, a treatment plan could include chemotherapy, followed by potentially curative surgery, followed by radiation therapy given to the chest.

If the surgeon and other physicians believe that surgery will not be able to cure the cancer, a treatment approach would be a combination of radiation treatment along with chemotherapy.

*What is the treatment if the pathology laboratory discovers cancer in lymph nodes in the mediastinum after a surgeon has removed a lobe of a lung or an entire lung in an attempt to cure the lung cancer?*

It is not uncommon for a person's cancer to be "upstaged" after surgery, that is, that a cancer that appeared to be at an earlier stage is found, by microscopic examination of tissue removed during surgery, to have spread to lymph nodes in the mediastinum. In this circumstance, it is generally recommended that a person receive chemotherapy which could somewhat reduce the risk of cancer recurrence.

## TREATMENT WHEN SURGERY CANNOT CURE THE CANCER

*What is the treatment for people who are not surgical candidates, that is, who would clearly have cancer left after an attempt at curative surgery?*

Over half of people with non-small cell lung cancer have a cancer that is incurable by surgery at the time of initial diagnosis. Many other people with lung cancer have a heavy smoking history and COPD (see chapter) or heart failure (see chapter) and would not be able to withstand the surgery required to cure the lung cancer. The goal of therapy when non-small cell lung cancer is not surgically curable will be to restrain, as much as possible, the growth of cancer in the chest and elsewhere in the body, and to prevent disabling symptoms and complications of the disease.

# RADIATION THERAPY

## Can radiation prevent complications of lung cancer?

Radiation therapy is a potent method of shrinking a non-small cell lung cancer. By shrinking the cancer in or surrounding the lung, radiation can prevent local complications of cancer such as collapse of portions of the lung or recurring pneumonia.

## What are the side effects of the radiation therapy?

While under the radiation therapy machine, the zap of the radiation is painless. There are, however, several potentially serious side effects of the radiation therapy.

Radiation therapy will not only zap the lung cancer, but will zap any tissues that are in the path of the radiation. Radiation can cause inflammation and scarring of the lung, leading to significant, chronic shortness of breath. A radiated esophagus may become inflamed and swallowing may become painful and difficult. The inflammation of the esophagus usually heals up on its own when the radiation therapy is finished.

During radiation therapy, people usually complain of feeling weak and tired. This ill feeling will usually pass when the radiation therapy is completed.

## How effective is radiation therapy for surgically incurable non-small cell lung cancer?

The non-small cell lung cancer that is surgically incurable because of its size and location or involvement of lymph nodes in the mediastinum, usually spreads either within or beyond the chest despite the radiation therapy. Although radiation therapy prevents some problems in the chest, the distant spread of the cancer remains the most serious impending problem. About one in twenty people with locally advanced, surgically incurable non-small cell lung cancer are curable by radiation therapy. The average survival time after radiation therapy is less than one year.

## TREATMENT WITH BOTH RADIATION THERAPY AND CHEMOTHERAPY

*Does combined treatment with chemotherapy and radiation control inoperable non-small cell lung cancer only evident in the chest?*

The combined use of radiation and chemotherapy appears to be somewhat more effective than radiation alone in extending survival of people with non-small cell lung cancer. Combining radiation therapy with the chemotherapy drug "cisplatin" and one other chemotherapy drug (such as "Gemcitabine" or "Paclitaxel") may have some modest effect in prolonging survival when given to people with inoperable non-small cell lung cancer which is only evident in the chest.

## TREATMENT OF METASTATIC NON-SMALL CELL LUNG CANCER

*What is metastatic non-small cell lung cancer?*

Non-small cell lung cancer that has spread outside the chest is "metastatic non-small cell lung cancer".

## What chemotherapy treatment is helpful for
## metastatic non-small cell lung cancer?

Chemotherapy can delay progression of the cancer for several months, and, by doing so, extend survival.

The standard treatment for metastatic non-small cell lung cancer involves the use of chemotherapy. The most common chemotherapy treatment involves the use of two drugs (a "doublet" treatment). One component of this "doublet" is most commonly either "cisplatin" or "carboplatin". The other medication for people with non-small cell lung cancer is generally one of seven or eight chemotherapy drugs that make approximately the same contribution to the effectiveness of the cisplatin or carboplatin. When the cancer is a type of non-small cell lung cancer called an "adenocarcinoma" the chemotherapy medication called "pemetrexed" (brand name is "Alimta" and manufacturers product website is www.alimta.com), when given in combination with cisplatin, may be a slightly more effective treatment than another two commonly used two drug regimen (gemcitabine + cisplatin), although this has not been firmly established. On the other hand, if the non-small cell lung cancer is a "squamous cell carcinoma", Alimta is less effective and therefore not used.

The choice of the second component of the doublet chemotherapy regimen will take into consideration the side effects of the different medications and the probability, based upon a person's medical history, of tolerating these side effects. The decision may reflect, to some extent, the cost and availability of the different medications as well the physician's experience and judgment.

## Which other medications, given along with chemotherapy, can delay progression and extend survival?

The biotechnology medication "bevacizumab" (brand name is "Avastin", and the manufacturer's product website is www.avastin. com) may slow the growth of the non-small cell lung cancer by preventing formation of blood vessels feeding the cancer. When given in combination with the chemotherapy medicines carboplatin and paclitaxel, Avastin slightly increases the likelihood of longer survival.

An oral medication called "erlotinib", (brand name is "Tarceva" and manufacturer's product website is www.tarceva. com), when given after a response to chemotherapy, may slightly increase the odds of longer survival in people with non-small cell lung cancer. There is some controversy, however, as to the benefit, in that the increase of average survival is about a month, Tarceva is expensive, and there is a potential for troubling side effects.

## Is chemotherapy always the best first treatment?

In the past several years, many important discoveries have revealed the unique chemical structure of components of cancer cells. With this knowledge, researchers have been creating potential medications that can bind to these structures or "molecular characteristics" and, disrupt whatever they do to make cancers cells grow and spread. These forms of treatment are "targeted treatments" and have clear benefit for some people with non-small cell lung cancer.

At experienced hospitals or clinics treating lung cancer, physicians may test a sample of a person's cancer (taken at the time of surgery or of a biopsy) to see whether the cancer cells contain something called an "EGF receptor mutation". If this is present, physicians may initially prescribe "Tarceva" which can initially slow the growth of cancers that carry this "EGF receptor mutation". If the cancer begins to grow despite Tarceva, physicians may then suggest beginning chemotherapy.

A second test that has now become important evaluates the non-small cell lung cancer cells for an abnormality (technically called a "rearrangement") of the "ALK gene". Rearrangement of the ALK gene is present in approximately one in twenty people with non-small cell lung cancer. If ALK gene rearrangement is present, it is likely that a person's cancer will reduce in size or stabilize with an oral medication called "crizotinib" (brand name is "Xalkori" and manufacturer's product website is www.xalkori.com). Xalkori is a very new medication, approved by the FDA in August of 2011.

*Are there ways of improving the odds that the chemotherapy or targeted therapy chosen will be effective in stopping the growth or spread of the cancer?*

One of the most active areas of research in cancer treatment is in identifying characteristics of cancer cells (called "biomarkers") that can predict whether an individual's cancer will respond to the different available forms of treatment. There is some recent evidence that this is possible with non-small cell lung cancer and can improve the odds of identifying a medicine with a better chance of controlling the person's cancer and extending survival. This is an important early step. Unfortunately, the medications that are currently available generally have only a limited ability to control non-small cell lung cancer.

## How long is chemotherapy given?

If a person has shrinkage of their cancer, or stabilization of the growth of their cancer, with chemotherapy, the chemotherapy is often given as four cycles of treatment, with each cycle consisting of two chemotherapy drugs given at approximately 3-4 week intervals. Although administration of additional cycles of the same chemotherapy in people who respond or remain stable does not appear to provide significant additional benefit, there is some evidence that, for people whose cancer has regressed or stabilized with four cycles of treatment, switching to a different single chemotherapy medication may delay disease progression and, perhaps, extend survival. Alternatively, some physicians may recommend a break from chemotherapy and resume chemotherapy if the cancer recurs. The relative success of these two treatment strategies, that is, an immediate switch to another chemotherapy medication as opposed to delaying further treatment until recurrence, is under evaluation.

If the cancer is progressing despite chemotherapy, or, if after four cycles of chemotherapy the cancer does not appear to have responded to treatment, the chemotherapy is unlikely to be beneficial.

For people with metastatic non-squamous cell lung cancer who have responded to combination chemotherapy that does not contain Alimta, Alimta, given intravenously every three weeks, appears to delay progression of the cancer and extend survival by, on average, roughly three months.

If Avastin was prescribed along with the chemotherapy, some physicians will advise continuing Avastin treatment indefinitely, or until there is evidence, the cancer is progressing.

> **What is the treatment if the cancer begins to grow again despite the initial chemotherapy?**

Metastatic non-small cell lung cancer that recurs or progresses despite initial chemotherapy has a difficult outlook with an average survival, depending on the characteristics of the recurrence, in the 6-9 month range.

Additional chemotherapy, called "second-line treatment" does add some additional possibility of a slightly longer (in the range, on average, of two months or so) of increased survival, with the occasional person having a much longer duration of cancer control. The most common medications used as "second line" are "Taxotere" and "Alimta". In addition, in some circumstances, physicians may suggest using "Tarceva", which occasionally is able to control the cancer.

Because the second line treatment of non-small cell lung cancer has such a low rate of long-term control of the cancer, seeking some form of experimental treatment at a major cancer hospital or a community affiliate is an important option to consider.

## SMALL CELL LUNG CANCER
## DEFINITIONS

### *What is small cell lung cancer?*

Small cell lung cancer is one of the most highly malignant, rapidly growing and rapidly spreading cancers. Because this cancer grows and spreads so quickly, it usually has spread beyond the lung at the time of diagnosis. Without treatment, death usually occurs within four months. Small cell lung cancer, is, however, very sensitive to the effects of radiation and chemotherapy and excellent, though usually transient, responses can be often be obtained with treatment.

## CONFIRMING THE DIAGNOSIS
## BEFORE INITIATING TREATMENT

### *How is the accuracy of the diagnosis of small cell lung cancer reviewed?*

The accuracy of the diagnosis of small cell lung cancer is extremely critical. Small cell lung cancer, under the microscope, can be somewhat difficult or misleading to diagnose. Because of this, physicians commonly send microscopic slides of the lung biopsy to an academic medical center or another expert for a second opinion.

## DETERMINING THE EXTENT
## OF SPREAD OF THE CANCER

### *How is the extent of the cancer determined?*

The areas of the body to which small cell lung cancer frequently spreads are the bone, the liver, the bone marrow, the adrenal glands and the brain. A person's symptoms, physical examination and blood chemistry profile can provide important information as to where the cancer has spread. A bone scan can identify areas of bone metastasis. CT scan of the liver and abdomen and CT or MRI scan of the brain can show whether cancer has spread to the areas scanned.

At times, a physician may suggest a test called a "bone marrow aspiration and biopsy" that can indicate whether the cancer has spread into the bone marrow. To perform this test, a physician will put local anesthesia into the area around the back of the crest of the pelvic bone, insert a needle into the bone and take out a tiny bit of bone marrow tissue. The test is a bit uncomfortable, takes about ten minutes to perform, and leaves a mild feeling of soreness that lasts for a few days.

## What do physicians do with the information about the extent of the cancer?

When considering the extent of the spread of the cancer, people with small cell lung cancer fit into one of two broad categories. The first category includes people with "limited stage disease" which means that after the staging work-up the cancer that can be identified with x-rays or other tests can only be found on one side of the chest. The second category includes people with "extensive stage disease" which means that cancer is evident both in the chest and in areas outside of the chest, or on both sides of the chest. At the time of diagnosis, about a third of people with small cell lung cancer have limited stage disease and about two-thirds of people have extensive stage disease.

# TREATMENT OF LIMITED STAGE SMALL CELL LUNG CANCER

## What is the treatment of limited stage small cell lung cancer?

The goal of treatment of limited stage small cell lung cancer is to clear all cancer cells out of the chest and to eradicate any cancer cells which may be present elsewhere in the body. The treatments used to accomplish this are radiation and chemotherapy.

## Is surgery an option in small cell lung cancer?

Small cell lung cancer, most commonly, is incurable by surgery. There are, however, uncommon circumstances when the cancer presents itself as a very small round spot ("a solitary pulmonary nodule") without evidence of cancer anywhere else. In this circumstance, some centers may remove the portion of the lung containing the cancer and follow this surgery with radiation and chemotherapy.

## How is radiation therapy given?

Radiation therapy begins as soon as possible concurrently with chemotherapy. The radiation is commonly given as two doses of radiation daily over a three-week period. If the twice-daily zaps are difficult from a practical point of view, an alternative is for a person to have one zap of radiation per day over a five to six week period.

## How is chemotherapy given?

The most common way that physicians treat limited stage small cell lung cancer is to give the chemotherapy medications called "cisplatin" and "etoposide". These two medications, when given concurrently with radiation therapy, will shrink the cancer over 80% of the time. Approximately half of the time, this treatment will result in complete disappearance of the visible cancer. If this clear shrinkage or disappearance of the cancer occurs, the treatment is commonly continued for somewhere between three and six months.

## How long do the responses last?

Most people who have an initial response of small cell lung cancer develop recurrence of the cancer. The average time it takes until the cancer returns is in the range of nine months. There is quite a bit of variation, however, with regard to time to recurrence, with some people having brief remissions and some having very long-lasting remissions. Approximately, a third of people with limited stage small cell lung cancer survive two years after diagnosis and approximately, one out of ten people with limited stage small cell lung cancer survive five years or longer.

## What are the side effects of the chemotherapy and radiation therapy treatments?

The chemotherapy that is given is quite toxic to the bone marrow. After intense chemotherapy, blood cells produced by the bone marrow will not form normally for about two weeks. During this time, an abnormally low number of white blood cells in the bloodstream can put a person at risk for developing serious and life threatening infections. In addition, a low number of platelets in the bloodstream after chemotherapy will put a person at risk for developing serious internal bleeding. For a further discussion of this side effect, please see the chapter entitled "Bone Marrow Suppression".

Combining radiation therapy with chemotherapy will increase the incidence and severity of side effects. Radiation therapy to the chest will zap bone marrow in the ribs and spine and will somewhat worsen the suppressive effect which chemotherapy has on bone marrow. Radiation therapy can cause painful irritation and damage to the lungs and esophagus.

## What is "prophylactic cranial irradiation"?

Because the chemotherapy hardly penetrates into the brain, and because small cell lung cancer tends to travel to the brain, the brain can serve as a sanctuary where cancer cells can grow. If the cancer recurs in the brain (please see chapter entitled "Brain Metastasis"), it is very difficult to treat and is associated with a very short survival. To prevent the brain from serving as such a sanctuary, people who have an excellent response to chest radiation and chemotherapy may be advised to have brain irradiation in an attempt to obliterate small deposits of cancer in the brain that may be present. This treatment, called "prophylactic cranial irradiation", does carry some risk of inducing memory loss and confusion. Without prophylactic cranial irradiation, a person with small cell lung cancer who survives 2-3 years after chest radiation and chemotherapy has an approximately 60% chance of having recurrence of the cancer appear in the brain. Prophylactic cranial irradiation appears to cut this risk in half. The decision for or against the "prophylactic cranial irradiation" must be made after careful consideration of the potential risks and benefits of having this treatment.

# TREATMENT OF EXTENSIVE STAGE SMALL CELL LUNG CANCER

### What is the treatment of extensive stage small cell lung cancer?

When small cell lung cancer is both in the chest and outside the chest, or on both sides of the chest, the treatment of choice is usually to treat with chemotherapy alone. The chemotherapy drugs initially used are similar to those used for limited stage small cell lung cancer, with some physicians preferring to use etoposide in combination with "carboplatin" instead of cisplatin. These medicines commonly are given in 21-day "cycles", with etoposide given on the first three days of the cycle, and carboplatin or cisplatin on the first day of the cycle.

After two cycles of chemotherapy, the physician will examine x-rays or other tests to see whether the cancer has responded to treatment. If the cancer has responded, an additional two cycles are often given, followed by another two cycles if a person's cancer has continued to respond.

### How is the outlook with extensive stage small cell lung cancer different from that of people with limited stage?

With extensive stage small cell lung cancer the response rate, meaning significant shrinking of the cancer with treatment, remains very high, in the 60-80% range, however only approximately one person in five has a complete disappearance of their cancer. People with extensive stage small cell lung cancer generally have progression of their cancer much sooner than with limited stage small cell lung cancer. The average survival of a person with extensive stage small cell lung cancer is approximately a year.

## WHEN SMALL CELL LUNG CANCER RECURS AFTER INITIAL CHEMOTHERAPY

*What can be done if the cancer grows back again after chemotherapy?*

The cancer that returns despite chemotherapy is generally resistant to further chemotherapy. Although additional chemotherapy may make the cancer shrink temporarily, the responses usually last for only weeks or a few months. Commonly used "second line" chemotherapy medication for people with extensive stage small cell lung cancer includes "topotecan" and "irinotecan". Only one in four people with recurring small cell lung cancer have shrinkage of their cancer with this, and most of the time, this shrinkage is temporary, lasting in the range of three months. Enrollment in a clinical trial testing an experimental cancer treatment is an important option to consider, when a person has recurrent small cell lung cancer.

# LYMPHOMA

## DEFINITION

### *What is lymphoma?*

Lymphoma is a malignancy of a type of white blood cell called a "lymphocyte". When a person has malignant lymphoma, the lymphocytes tend to grow in clumps or clusters and can form tumor masses in various parts of the body.

The two major forms of malignancy of lymphocytes in which tumor masses form are "Hodgkin's Disease" and "non-Hodgkin's lymphoma". These diseases have very different behavior and respond in very different ways to treatment. This chapter only discusses non-Hodgkin's lymphoma.

## SYMPTOMS

### *What are the early symptoms of lymphoma?*

The most common early symptom is a painless enlargement of lymph nodes in the neck, the armpit, or the groin. Lymph nodes containing lymphoma usually are somewhat round in shape and feel to the fingers like tiny firm rubber balls.

Some people with lymphoma may first notice an involuntary loss of weight. Slight fevers (around 100 degrees Fahrenheit) and sweating in the middle of the night are occasional early symptoms of lymphoma. The symptoms of fever, weight loss and night sweats, in the context of lymphoma, are referred to as "B symptoms".

Lymphoma masses that grow in the chest or abdomen can interfere with the function of major organs that are located in their vicinity. Symptoms related to the presence of lymphoma in the lungs, liver, bowels, or any other area of the body can bring a person to the attention of a physician.

## MAKING THE DIAGNOSIS

### *How is the diagnosis of lymphoma made?*

Most people with lymphoma have enlarged lymph nodes ("lymphadenopathy") in the groin ("inguinal lymphadenopathy"), armpit (axillary lymphadenopathy") or neck ("cervical lymphadenopathy"). These lymph nodes are just under the skin and it is very easy to make a small incision and remove ("excise") a lymph node for examination by a pathologist under the microscope. The removal of a lymph node for examination under the microscope is a "lymph node biopsy" and is the most common way of making the diagnosis of lymphoma.

### *In addition to making the diagnosis of lymphoma, what information can the pathologist determine from examining the lymph node biopsy?*

There are over 20 different types of lymphoma, each with its own pattern of behavior and ability to respond to treatment. By examining the lymph node under the microscope and through other specialized examinations of the lymph node biopsy, the pathologist can provide vital information about the exact type of lymphoma that the person has and the likelihood that it will respond to the many available forms of treatment.

A critical test the pathologist performs examines the surface of the lymphoma cells in the lymph node biopsy. The technique used to do this is "immunophenotyping".

## What is immunophenotyping?

The genetic material of lymphoma cells gives cells instructions regarding the manufacture of complex proteins that end up on the cell's surface. These proteins are "antigens" and bind tightly to "monoclonal antibodies" that are designed to identify and bind specific proteins.

To identify specific proteins on the surface of lymphoma cells, a liquid solution containing a variety of "monoclonal antibodies" are poured over the lymphoma cells. The ability of the different "monoclonal antibodies" to stick to lymphoma cells will allow the pathologist to determine whether critical proteins are on the surface of the lymphoma cells, and will provide important information about the likelihood that a person's lymphoma will respond to available forms of therapy.

The two major types of lymphocytes are "T cells" and "B cells", which, if they turn malignant, cause "T cell lymphoma" and "B cell lymphoma". "B cell lymphoma" is the more common of the two. This chapter discusses the most common B cell lymphomas, "follicular lymphoma" and "diffuse large B-cell lymphoma". A critical item revealed by immunophenotyping is whether a protein called "CD20" is on the surface of the lymphoma cells. If CD20 is present, it indicates that the lymphoma is a B cell lymphoma and will be vulnerable to the lymphoma-killing effects of recently developed treatments and, possibly, of treatments that are currently being developed.

### What behaviors do lymphomas exhibit?

There are over twenty different types of lymphoma. Some grow very slowly and are "indolent" or "low grade" lymphomas. Others grow more rapidly and are "aggressive" or "high grade lymphoma". The pattern of growth and susceptibility to different forms of treatment, largely predicted by immunophenotyping, is extremely important in determining the type of treatment most likely to control or cure the disease.

## DETERMINING THE EXTENT TO WHICH THE LYMPHOMA HAS SPREAD

### How is the extent to which lymphoma has spread determined?

A history and physical examination can give important clues regarding the areas of the body to which lymphoma has spread. Simple blood tests evaluating the number of red blood cells, white blood cells, and platelets in the bloodstream, and evaluating liver and kidney function can provide evidence as to whether the lymphoma has spread to bone marrow, or is affecting the functioning of the liver or the kidneys. A chest x-ray and a CT scan of the abdomen evaluate whether lymphoma is forming tumor masses inside the chest or abdomen. A biopsy of the bone marrow (in which a needle withdraws a small sample of bone marrow from the back of the pelvic bone) can give important information about the presence or absence of lymphoma in the bone marrow.

## How do physicians use this information about the extent of disease?

With information about the extent of a person's disease a person's disease can be "staged", with the Roman numeral "I" being the earliest stage with the smallest amount of lymphoma in the body and the Roman numeral "IV" the most advanced stage with either the greatest amount of lymphoma in the body or spread of the lymphoma to body organs.

Stage I, the earliest stage, indicates that the lymphoma involves only a single area of lymph nodes or a single cluster of malignant lymphocytes in a single organ.

With stage II lymphoma, two or more lymph nodes areas are involved on the same side of the diaphragm. To lymphoma doctors, the diaphragm, which is at the level of the lower part of the chest, is a type of dividing line between the top half of the body above the chest and the bottom half of the body from the abdomen downward.

Stage III means lymph nodes are involved above and below the diaphragm.

Stage IV means that whether lymph nodes are involved or not, major organs such as the bone marrow, liver, or lung are involved.

If "B symptoms" as described earlier in this chapter are present, the letter "b" is used after the Roman numeral.

The stage of the disease is important in planning therapy and predicting outcome. The stage, however, is less important than the appearance and characteristics of the lymphoma, as determined by the pathologist, in determining the behavior of a person's disease and the treatment most likely to extend survival or possibly cure the disease.

## TREATMENT

### What is the treatment of lymphoma?

The treatment of lymphoma is very different depending on whether the lymphoma is "indolent" or "aggressive". "Indolent lymphomas" grow slowly, but are difficult to cure with treatment. "Aggressive lymphomas" grow rapidly, and, although highly lethal without treatment, are often curable with current treatments.

Although there are many different types of lymphoma, the two most common are the indolent lymphoma called "follicular lymphoma" and the aggressive lymphoma called "diffuse large B-cell lymphoma". The remainder of this chapter will focus only on those two forms of lymphoma.

## TREATMENT OF THE MOST COMMON INDOLENT LYMPHOMA: FOLLICULAR LYMPHOMA

### How indolent are indolent lymphomas?

Although indolent lymphomas are usually very slow growing, without treatment and with the passage of sufficient time, life-threatening complications commonly develop. Even without treatment, some people with indolent lymphoma can remain in good health for many years after receiving a diagnosis of an indolent lymphoma. The most common indolent lymphoma is "follicular lymphoma".

### What are the symptoms of follicular lymphoma?

Most commonly, follicular lymphoma makes its appearance with painless enlarged lymph nodes in the armpit, the neck, or in the groin area. These lymph nodes commonly undergo some fluctuation up and down in their size. Other symptoms such as the "B symptoms" described earlier in this chapter or symptoms related to compression of nearby organs can occur, but are not common in the early stages of follicular lymphoma.

## TREATMENT OF LOCALIZED FOLLICULAR LYMPHOMA

### What is "localized follicular lymphoma"?

Localized lymphoma means that the lymphoma only involves a small region of lymph nodes. At the time of diagnosis, about one in ten people with follicular lymphoma have only a small area of localized disease.

### What is the treatment of localized follicular lymphoma?

Radiation of the localized area of follicular lymphoma can be curative. Follicular lymphoma is very slow growing and, if localized, may produce very few symptoms. Observation alone is sometimes recommended in people who are elderly, have other significant medical conditions, or if the radiation needed to potentially cure the lymphoma would pose too much of a danger to parts of the body that are within the region that would have to be radiated.

## TREATMENT OF ADVANCED FOLLICULAR LYMPHOMA

### What is "advanced follicular lymphoma"?

Lymphoma found above and below the diaphragm or in major body organs outside of lymph nodes is "advanced follicular lymphoma". The great majority of people with follicular lymphoma have advanced disease at the time of diagnosis.

### What is Rituxan?

Follicular lymphoma, as well as diffuse large B cell lymphoma and some other types of lymphoma, is composed of malignant "B cells". "Rituxan", (manufacturer's product website is www.rituxan.com) is a "monoclonal antibody" that binds to a substance on the surface of malignant B cells called the "CD20 antigen". By binding to the CD20 antigen, Rituxan can destroy the malignant cells or limit their growth. It is one of the most important medications used in the treatment of lymphoma.

### What general considerations guide physicians when suggesting the best form of treatment of follicular lymphoma?

Advanced follicular lymphoma generally is incurable with any treatment that is available today. Although people with follicular lymphoma commonly survive for ten years or more with the disease, the treatments that are available today, however aggressively applied, are only rarely capable of curing the disease. The goal of treatment is, therefore, to extend healthful life as much as possible with a minimum of side effects from treatment and with a minimum of complications from the follicular lymphoma itself.

**If the treatments available for follicular lymphoma are not curative, how effective are they?**

The available treatments of follicular lymphoma, given sequentially, usually shrink the size of the lymphoma and restrain its growth for months or years. This shrinkage of the lymphoma can take the form of a "complete remission", which means evidence of the disease disappears, or "partial remission", which means that the cancer has reduced in size by 50% or more, but has not totally disappeared. The remissions induced by treatment are usually not permanent, although with several complete and partial remissions induced with different medications occurring one after the other, treatment can extend survival for many years.

**What is the treatment of advanced follicular lymphoma when a person does not have troubling symptoms?**

When follicular lymphoma is not producing significant symptoms, immediate treatment does not clearly appear to improve a person's outlook. Many physicians will suggest that a person without significant symptoms of their follicular lymphoma not have any treatment at all until troublesome symptoms appear. During the period of no treatment, physical examination, blood tests, and CT scans can determine the extent, if any, that the disease is progressing.

The treatment of follicular lymphoma that is not yet producing symptoms is controversial. A clinical trial demonstrated that Rituxan delays the time until symptoms requiring chemotherapy appear, but did not demonstrate an effect of Rituxan on improvement of survival time. There are different opinions about the significance of this clinical trial. Rituxan treatment for people with advanced follicular lymphoma without symptoms has an effect that some consider very promising, but until demonstration of a survival benefit, many experts believe that it is best to delay Rituxan treatment until symptoms appear that indicate a need for treatment.

As the disease progresses, symptoms related to bone marrow failure and enlargement of the lymph nodes and spleen can become a problem. When this occurs, treatment with one of several forms of chemotherapy will be helpful to relieve symptoms and extend survival.

*What is the treatment of advanced follicular lymphoma when symptoms develop, or if the growth of the lymphoma appears to be accelerating?*

The chemotherapy given often consists of the medications "cyclophosphamide", "vincristine" and "prednisone". This regimen is the "CVP" regimen. Rituxan, when given with the CVP regimen, is the "R-CVP" regimen. R-CVP increases the likelihood of having shrinkage of the lymphoma and prolongs, by approximately an additional year, the time until the disease progresses.

The great majority of people with follicular lymphoma have a significant shrinkage of their lymphoma when treated with the CVP in conjunction with Rituxan. This combined treatment delays the time until the tumor progresses, on average, to approximately 2 ½ years, and by doing so, extends survival.

Based upon recent information, a regimen combining the newly available chemotherapy medication "bendamustine" (brand name is "Treanda", manufacturer's product website is www.treanda.com) with Rituxan appears to be another effective treatment regimen that can restrain the growth of follicular lymphoma. Because Treanda has only recently become available, the long-term experience with this medication in people with previously untreated follicular lymphoma is limited.

### How is the R-CVP administered?

The four medicines comprising the R-CVP regimen are administered in 21-day cycles, with Cyclophosphamide, Vincristine, and Rituxan given intravenously on the first day of the cycle and Prednisone, as a pill on the first five days of the cycle.

After 4 cycles, physicians will commonly make a determination as to whether it appears that the lymphoma has had a "partial response", meaning 50% or more reduction in size, or a "complete response", meaning complete disappearance of visible tumor. If there has been a partial or complete response to treatment, an additional 4 cycles of R-CVP are administered.

### What treatment provides further benefit after the 8 cycles of R-CVP are completed?

If, after 8 cycles of R-CVP therapy, a person has had a partial or complete response, continued treatment called "maintenance therapy" can further restrain the growth of the follicular lymphoma. With maintenance therapy, Rituxan is given every two months for two years. Maintenance therapy roughly doubles the chance that the disease will not worsen during the two years of additional Rituxan treatment.

Please see the chapter "Cancer Therapy Complications: Infusion Reactions" for a discussion of an important side effect of Rituxan.

## WHEN FOLLICULAR LYMPHOMA RECURS AFTER CHEMOTHERAPY

*What happens if the initial regimen of chemotherapy fails to control the follicular lymphoma?*

When the initial regimen of chemotherapy fails to control the follicular lymphoma, decisions regarding the immediate need for treatment consider a person's symptoms, with the realization that treatment administered, whether immediate or delayed, is unlikely to cure the person's follicular lymphoma. If very few symptoms are present, it may be prudent to delay additional chemotherapy until symptoms appear.

The most effective treatment when follicular lymphoma is progressing is under evaluation in many ongoing clinical trials. Outside of a clinical trial, and depending on how well the person responded to the initial treatment, physicians may suggest re-treatment with either Rituxan alone, chemotherapy alone (perhaps with different medications), or the combination of Rituxan with chemotherapy. Because the initial treatment regimen is often the

"R-CVP regimen discussed earlier in this chapter, "bendamustine" (brand name is "Treanda", manufacturer's product website is www. treanda.com) is often prescribed, sometimes as a single treatment, and often in combination with Rituxan.

Although these treatments can induce another very good response, these "second-line" treatments tend to be less effective when follicular lymphoma relapses after the first regimen.

There are biotechnology medications available that use a monoclonal antibody to guide a radioactive material directly to the follicular lymphoma cell. The available medications in this category have the brand names "Zevalin" (manufacturer's product website is www.zevalin.com) and "Bexxar" (manufacturer's product website is www.bexxar.com). Because of the serious side effects (see chapters "Bone Marrow Suppression" and "Infusion Reactions"), and because of the many complexities associated with administering these radioactive medications, many physicians prefer to reserve the use of these medications to people with follicular lymphoma refractory to chemotherapy and Rituxan.

There have been several reports of excellent responses and apparent cures after bone marrow transplantation in people with follicular lymphoma resistant to chemotherapy. This is very intensive treatment with a great deal of risk of life-threatening toxicity and is only appropriate for the person whose underlying health would permit them to undergo this treatment. The odds of achieving a cure of follicular lymphoma after bone marrow transplantation have not yet been clearly determined.

# EXPERIMENTAL TREATMENTS OF FOLLICULAR LYMPHOMA

## Are there other experimental treatments for follicular lymphoma?

A number of biotechnology products are under evaluation as treatment of follicular lymphoma. New monoclonal antibodies carrying potent toxins are in development that specifically binds to molecules on the surface of lymphoma cell, delivering these toxins to the lymphoma cells and destroying them. Enrolling in a clinical trial evaluating new treatments of follicular lymphoma is an important option to consider if the disease is progressing despite initial treatment.

## TREATMENT OF AGGRESSIVE LYMPHOMA

### How aggressive is aggressive lymphoma?

Aggressive lymphoma is a very rapidly growing malignant tumor. Without therapy, aggressive lymphoma is usually fatal within months of diagnosis. Aggressive lymphoma can respond very well to treatment and is potentially curable.

This chapter will only discuss the most common form of aggressive lymphoma: "diffuse large B-cell lymphoma".

### What is the initial treatment of diffuse large B-cell lymphoma?

The foundation upon which the treatment of diffuse large B-cell lymphoma is built is a four-drug combination treatment, nicknamed

"CHOP", that combines the medicines "Cytoxan", "Adriamycin", "Vincristine", + "Prednisone". "CHOP" appears to be more effective when combined with the monoclonal antibody "Rituximab" (brand name is "Rituxan", and manufacturer's product website is www. rituxan.com). How this is given depends upon the stage of a person's disease at the time of diagnosis.

The treatment of diffuse large B-cell lymphoma is evolving and there are different views regarding the most effective and safe treatment regimens. The discussion that follows outlines a common treatment plan for early stage and late stage diffuse large B-cell lymphoma.

## CHEMOTHERAPY OF LOCALIZED DIFFUSE LARGE B-CELL LYMPHOMA

*What is the treatment for early stage and localized diffuse large B-cell lymphoma?*

Diffuse large B-cell lymphoma in an early stage and located on only one side of the diaphragm is potentially curable with a combination of chemotherapy, Rituxan, and radiation therapy. Initially, this treatment involves three courses of chemotherapy with CHOP in conjunction with Rituxan at three-week intervals. Following this initial treatment, radiation therapy is given to the localized area of the body that contained the lymphoma.

With this treatment, almost 80% of people with localized diffuse large B-cell lymphoma are free from progression of their disease for five years or longer.

# CHEMOTHERAPY OF ADVANCED DIFFUSE LARGE B-CELL LYMPHOMA

## *What is the common treatment if the diffuse large B-cell lymphoma is advanced?*

Advanced diffuse large B-cell lymphoma means that the disease is located both above and below the diaphragm, or it involves body organs such as the stomach, liver, or bone marrow. The treatment required must eradicate the cancer throughout the body and will require chemotherapy that is more intensive. This intensive treatment consists of eight courses of chemotherapy with CHOP in conjunction with Rituxan at three-week intervals. There are variations on this regimen that are being studied that have the same goal of providing intensive chemotherapy with the intention of destroying lymphoma cells wherever they may be in the body, and curing the disease.

The chemotherapy with CHOP and Rituxan is most effective when full intensive doses of the chemotherapy medicines are administered. Reductions of the dosage of the individual chemotherapy drugs in the regimen may compromise the chances of achieving a complete remission and obtaining a cure. For this reason, it is best for the person with aggressive lymphoma to have their treatment coordinated and managed by medical professionals with extensive experience in treating this aggressive lymphoma. This will improve the chances of receiving the doses of chemotherapy needed to achieve a maximal response and a possible cure

### How effective is CHOP plus Rituxan as a treatment of diffuse large B-cell lymphoma?

Approximately two-thirds of people with diffuse large B-cell lymphoma achieve a complete remission with therapy and are without evidence of lymphoma four years after treatment. Since most relapses occur soon after treatment, most people who have not had recurrence within four years will remain free of recurrence of their disease.

Approximately one-third of people with diffuse large B-cell lymphoma do not respond adequately to CHOP plus Rituxan or relapse after the treatment.

## WHEN DIFFUSE LARGE B-CELL LYMPHOMA RECURS AFTER CHEMOTHERAPY

### What happens if the diffuse large B-cell lymphoma progresses or recurs after chemotherapy?

Chemotherapy given after diffuse large B-cell lymphoma progresses or recurs is far less effective than the initial chemotherapy. Although additional chemotherapy can induce regression of the lymphoma, it very commonly begins to grow again after several months. The treatment with the best chance of producing a long-lasting remission appears to be an "autologous hematopoietic cell transplant", abbreviated as "autologous HCT".

### What is an autologous HCT?

When a person has relapsed diffuse large B-cell lymphoma, very high doses of chemotherapy are necessary to destroy all lymphoma cells and induce a complete remission. These high doses will also destroy the normal cells in the bone marrow, and would ordinarily be lethal. To permit the bone marrow to recover, physicians will harvest "hematopoietic stem cells" from either the person's own blood or bone marrow and inject them after the high dose chemotherapy is completed. The hematopoietic stem cells find their way to the bone marrow and permit its recovery. This is an autologous HCT.

## Who is a candidate for autologous HCT?

The chemotherapy administered is very intense and produces many serious side effects. A person's underlying health must be sufficient to withstand these side effects.

## How effective is autologous HCT?

Autologous HCT can produce long-lasting remissions, especially in people with diffuse large B-cell lymphoma that relapsed after a previous response to chemotherapy. As experience grows with autologous HCT and treatments given after the autologous HCT to maintain the remission, the effectiveness of this treatment is likely to improve.

## What treatment options are available if autologous HCT is not possible?

Chemotherapy medications currently available have a very limited ability to control the growth of recurrent or refractory diffuse large B-cell lymphoma.

Focused radiation, applied directly to the area of the body containing a lymphoma mass, can relieve localized pain and discomfort.

A critical option when a person's disease is refractory to standard treatments is to seek a promising experimental therapy.

## EXPERIMENTAL TREATMENT OF AGGRESSIVE LYMPHOMA

*What forms of experimental treatment are available for recurrent aggressive lymphoma?*

A large number of experimental medications are under evaluation for the treatment of the various forms of this lymphoma. Many of these medications are monoclonal antibodies that specifically attach to proteins on the surface of lymphoma cells, and by a variety of mechanisms, can destroy them.

The development of new treatments of lymphoma is one of the most active areas of cancer research and there is a general optimism that new medications for treating lymphoma will improve outlook further over the next several years.

# MELANOMA

## DEFINITION

### What is melanoma?

Melanoma is a cancer of the pigment-producing cells in the skin. Unless found and treated, melanoma can extend deeply into the skin, spread to local lymph nodes, then spread throughout the body. If found and treated in its earliest stages, it is usually curable.

## SYMPTOMS

### What are the symptoms of melanoma?

The person who develops a melanoma usually comes to medical attention after noticing a new spot on their skin or a change in the size, color, or consistency of a spot on their skin that had previously existed. A melanoma is usually brownish black or black, somewhat raised, and may have a jagged or irregular border. The occasional melanoma has a cover of broken or ulcerated skin.

## MAKING THE DIAGNOSIS

### When there is a suspicion that a spot on the skin is a melanoma, how is the diagnosis of melanoma made?

An "excisional biopsy" makes the diagnosis of melanoma. With an "excisional biopsy", the physician removes the entire lesion along with a narrow margin of skin around the lesion and sends it to a pathologist for examination under the microscope.

## What information will the pathologist provide?

The pathologist will determine whether the lesion is a melanoma. If the lesion is a melanoma, the pathologist will determine the depth to which the melanoma has penetrated downward (the "depth of invasion") into the skin, whether the layer of tissue on top of the melanoma is intact (if it is not, it is "ulcerated"), and will estimate the "mitotic rate", meaning how rapidly the cancer cells are dividing. If the mitotic rate is high, the melanoma is more likely to grow and spread. These three factors guide decisions regarding the next step in treatment. Depending on the depth of invasion, the melanoma will be assigned a designation of $T_1$ (indicating the lowest risk), $T_2$, $T_3$, or $T_4$ (indicating the highest risk). If there is no ulceration or a low mitotic rate, it is also assigned the letter "a" (indicating a lower risk) or and if there is ulceration or a high mitotic rate it is also assigned the letter "b" (indicating a higher risk).

## INITIAL TREATMENT

### What are the next steps after the making the diagnosis of a melanoma?

The pathologist's report will indicate the "thickness", (also referred to as the "depth") of the melanoma that has been removed. Based upon the thickness of the melanoma, the dermatologist may remove an additional margin of one or two centimeters of skin and tissue surrounding the area from which the original melanoma was removed.

An immediate key issue with regard to treatment planning is determining whether lymph nodes to which melanoma can travel need evaluation. Occasionally, based upon a person noticing or the physician feeling hard lymph nodes, there may be a suspicion that the melanoma has already spread in an obvious way to local lymph nodes.

If the melanoma is less than ¾ of a millimeter thick, and does not have ulceration or a high mitotic rate, and if the lymph nodes that are nearby do not appear enlarged, it is unlikely that lymph nodes will be involved. In this situation, removal of the melanoma (if not already done with the excisional biopsy) with a one centimeter margin of skin around the edges of the melanoma is generally curative. If the tumor is deeper than one millimeter, or if it is more than ¾ of a millimeter thick and there is ulceration, a high mitotic rate, or a person is under the age of 40, the physicians may recommend further evaluation of the lymph nodes with sophisticated tests.

## EVALUATING LYMPH NODES FOR EVIDENCE OF SPREAD

### To which lymph nodes do melanomas spread?

The first place to which melanoma usually spreads is to lymph nodes close to the area of the body involved by the melanoma. Melanoma of the legs can travel to lymph nodes in the groin (groin lymph nodes are "inguinal nodes"). Melanomas of the arm travel to lymph nodes in the armpit (the technical term for the armpit is the "axilla"; nodes in the axilla are "axillary nodes"). Melanomas of the head or neck travel to lymph nodes in the neck (neck nodes are "cervical nodes").

### How can it be determined whether the cancer has spread to these lymph nodes?

In the past, lymph node evaluation required an "elective lymph node dissection" in which a surgeon removed all the lymph nodes surrounding the melanoma as well as lymph nodes in the region to which it was suspected the melanoma could travel. Now, there is a newer technique called "sentinel node biopsy" that can determine, without major surgery and with good precision, whether the cancer has spread to lymph nodes.

### How is the sentinel node biopsy done?

To do a sentinel node biopsy, the physician will put a special blue dye, or a weakly radioactive material (called a "radioisotope"), or both, into the tissue directly adjacent to the melanoma or the excisional biopsy margin. This dye will then travel through channels called "lymphatics" to "sentinel lymph nodes" where the melanoma, if it has travelled, is most likely to be. If these few lymph nodes are removed, examined under the microscope, and do not contain melanoma, it is very unlikely that cancer will be found in other lymph nodes and further lymph node dissection can be avoided. If the sentinel node does contain melanoma cells, the physicians may recommend a "lymph node dissection" which removes the sentinel lymph nodes and other nearby lymph nodes.

## *What is the treatment if the sentinel node biopsy shows evidence of melanoma?*

If the sentinel node biopsy shows evidence of melanoma, a common recommendation will be to have the regional lymph nodes surgically removed with an operation called a "therapeutic lymphadenectomy".

## *If the sentinel lymph node biopsy shows evidence of melanoma, should a person have a thorough work-up to see whether the melanoma has spread elsewhere before the therapeutic lymphadenectomy is done?*

It is very uncommon that a thorough work-up will find melanoma beyond the sentinel lymph node. Because of this, extensive tests such as CT, MRI, or PET scans of the chest or abdomen are not always recommended.

If the melanoma that was removed was very thick (over 4 millimeters) or ulcerated, or if the sentinel lymph nodes removed had a lot of melanoma in it, physicians may recommend additional tests, including a CT or MRI scan, to see whether the melanoma has spread elsewhere. If the melanoma has spread to areas of the body far distant from where the melanoma began, it may not be appropriate to attempt to remove all the local lymph nodes since the cancer will have already spread beyond them.

Because some areas involved with melanoma may not be detectable by the CT or MRI scan, physicians will sometimes ask a person to obtain a "PET" scan. A PET scan is a sensitive test that can often detect the spread of melanoma to distant organs before detection by CT scans. To do this test, an injection is made of a tiny amount of radioactive glucose into the bloodstream. Melanoma cells have a greater affinity for this radioactive glucose than other tissues. The PET scanner can then find "hot spots" inside the body that contain the cancer and transmit this information to a computer for the physician to evaluate. The identification of a "hot spot" suggests, but does not prove, the presence of melanoma cells in the hot spot. Although a "hot spot" may indicate the presence of melanoma, areas of inflammation without melanoma can also produce "hot spots". A "hot spot" indicates a suspicious area that needs evaluation, often with a biopsy to confirm the presence or absence of melanoma.

## What are the complications of therapeutic lymphadenectomy?

Complications of therapeutic lymphadenectomy depend upon the area from which the lymph nodes are removed.

Removal of inguinal nodes can cause a serious problem with swelling of the leg (called "lymphedema") on the side of the lymph node dissection. A person having a therapeutic lymphadenectomy can somewhat reduce their risk of developing leg swelling by wearing elastic stockings on the leg on the side of the surgery and by regularly performing leg exercises.

Removal of axillary nodes can occasionally damage the nerves in the armpit that control arm function. Swelling or infection in the area of the surgical incision can occasionally be a problem.

Years ago, removal of cervical nodes involved a radical neck dissection with removal of muscles and nerves in the neck. Many surgeons now believe that a modified neck dissection that spares muscles and nerves in the neck is the correct procedure. Even this modified elective node dissection in the neck can damage nerves which control the ability to raise the shoulders. Persistent neck pain is another occasional problem after removal of cervical lymph nodes.

## TREATMENT TO REDUCE THE RISK OF RECURRENCE OF MELANOMA

*Are there any medications such as chemotherapy or immunotherapy that can reduce the risk of developing recurrence of the melanoma?*

Alfa interferon, in trials sponsored by the United States National Cancer Institute has demonstrated some modest, but significant effectiveness in reducing the risk of recurrence of melanoma. Alfa interferon, given by injection five days a week for a month, followed by three times a week for eleven months, appears to reduce the risk of recurrence by approximately 25%, along with a very slight improvement in the odds of long survival and cure.

At this time, there is no chemotherapy with the proven ability to reduce the risk of developing recurrent melanoma.

Reduction of risk of recurrence of melanoma is an active area of research and many experimental medications are under evaluation that could prove to be more effective with fewer side effects than alfa interferon. Participation in a clinical trial coordinated by a major cancer center is a very important option to consider.

## What are the most common side effects of recombinant alfa interferon?

The most common side effects of recombinant alfa interferon are fevers, chills, and an overall sense of fatigue, headache and depression. These side effects vary greatly from person to person and tend to lessen with continuing treatment. Some people, however, find these side effects impossible to live with and decide to discontinue treatment.

## LOCAL OR REGIONAL RECURRENCE

### What is meant by local recurrence?

Local recurrence means that, after surgery to remove the melanoma and the margin of normal appearing skin around it, the melanoma has reappeared within two centimeters of the edges of the area from which the melanoma was initially removed.

### What is meant by in-transit metastasis?

In order for melanoma cells to travel to lymph nodes, they move through "lymphatic channels". Along the way to the regional lymph nodes, they can leave deposits of melanoma cells that grow into little malignant nodules. These are "in transit metastasis".

### How is local recurrence or in-transit metastasis treated?

Both local recurrence and in-transit metastasis indicate that a person is at a far higher risk of developing distant spread ("distant metastasis") of their cancer. Depending on the size and location of the recurrence, physicians may recommend an evaluation to determine whether the cancer has spread into the chest, abdomen or elsewhere. This could have an influence on the type of treatment given for the local recurrence since cure of melanoma by a local treatment is not possible if there is distant metastasis.

Surgery can remove small locally recurrent lesions. Because this local recurrence may have spread to local lymph nodes, sentinel lymph node biopsy, even if done before, may be recommended. If spread to local lymph nodes is identified, surgical removal of local lymph nodes may be recommended.

At times, the recurrence is on an arm or leg and is very large and difficult to remove surgically. In this circumstance, physicians may suggest a complicated procedure in which the circulation of blood in and out of the arm or the leg is isolated and a very large dose of chemotherapy is circulated for a brief period through the limb (called "isolated limb perfusion"). Most people treated with isolated limb perfusion have a shrinkage of their melanoma and about half of the time all evidence of the local melanoma disappears (this is referred to as a "complete remission"). People who have a complete remission of their melanoma after isolated limb perfusion have a higher likelihood of long survival and possible cure of their melanoma.

Another treatment option for people with locally recurrent melanoma with lesions too large for surgical removal is to have local radiation. Radiation can often produce excellent tumor shrinkage and is usually well tolerated. Unfortunately, radiation probably adds little to improving the probability of long survival.

## *Is interferon helpful after the surgery or isolated limb perfusion?*

Based upon the extensive research showing a reduction in the risk of melanoma recurrence in people at high risk of recurrence, many physicians will recommend alfa interferon for people who have not received it previously or who have recurred a significant period of time after having previous treatment with interferon.

## METASTATIC MELANOMA

### *What is done when melanoma recurs in body organs?*

Melanoma that recurs in body organs such as lung, liver, bone, brain or kidney, is "metastatic melanoma". Metastatic melanoma is rarely curable. The occasional person with a single metastasis or several small and discrete areas of metastasis can have the metastasis surgically removed and can have a very long survival and, occasionally, never have another melanoma recurrence. It is common, however, to develop multiple areas of metastatic disease shortly after the appearance of the first area of metastasis in a body organ.

### *Is there any non-surgical therapy that can cure metastatic melanoma?*

There is a "biological" or "immunotherapy" medication called "interleukin-2", which, if given in very high doses, can induce a very good shrinkage of the melanoma roughly 20% of the time. Complete disappearance of all melanoma in the body (a "complete remission") occurs in about 5% of people with metastatic melanoma treated with interleukin-2. Most of these complete remissions are long lasting and may indicate a cure. The treatment, however, is extremely toxic to multiple body organs. Because of this serious toxicity and the requirement of good health to withstand the toxicity, interleukin-2 therapy is most effective for people with underlying good health and then, only in medical centers with physicians and support personnel that are experienced in taking care of people undergoing this rigorous and toxic therapy.

*What treatment is available for people with metastatic melanoma who are not candidates for interleukin-2?*

The three available forms of treatment are "immunotherapy", "targeted therapy" and "chemotherapy".

## IMMUNOTHERAPY OF METASTATIC MELANOMA

*What form of immunotherapy is available for people with metastatic melanoma?*

The FDA, in March 2011, approved a new medicine called "Ipilimumab", as a treatment of metastatic melanoma. Ipilimumab, which, has been given the brand name "Yervoy" (manufacturer's product website is www.yervoy.com), is an antibody that binds to a molecule on a type of white blood cell called a "T-cell", that helps regulate a person's natural immune responses. Ipilimumab blocks the activity of a molecule that inhibits this immune response, thereby promoting an active immune attack on cancer cells. Ipilimumab extends the life of people with metastatic melanoma, on average, for several months, with some people having stability of their disease for two years or longer. Approximately one person in eight treated with Ipilimumab in clinical trials evaluating its safety and effectiveness developed serious or life-threatening side effects related to inflammation of the intestines, liver, skin, or other body organs.

## TARGETED THERAPY

### What targeted therapy is available for metastatic melanoma?

Cancer researchers discovered that approximately half of people with melanoma have a type of "mutation" in their melanoma cells called a "BRAF" mutation, which makes the melanoma cells susceptible to destruction by a medicine called "vemurafenib" (brand name is "Zelboraf, manufacturer's product website is www.zelboraf.com). Over half of people with this BRAF mutation treated with vemurafenib have shrinkage of their melanoma, with most people having stabilization of their melanoma for six months or longer. Vemurafenib was approved by the FDA in August of 2011, therefore extensive long-term outcome results, as well as information about its benefit as compared to, or combined with, Ipilimumab, are not yet available.

## CHEMOTHERAPY

### How effective is chemotherapy for metastatic melanoma?

The most commonly used chemotherapy medication for metastatic melanoma, DTIC, only shrinks a person's cancer about 15% of the time. Responses usually last for a very few months and are associated with many side effects (especially nausea and immune system depression) from the medication. Combining DTIC with other forms of chemotherapy or biologic or immunologic therapy has not convincingly added any benefit with regard to control of the melanoma or extending survival.

# OVARIAN CANCER

## DEFINITION

### What is ovarian cancer?

Ovarian cancer is a cancer that starts in the ovary. Unless controlled by treatment, cancer of the ovary can spread into other areas of the abdomen and pelvis, into the chest, and potentially to other areas in the body.

## SYMPTOMS

### What are the symptoms of cancer of the ovary?

The initial symptoms of cancer of the ovary are usually very slight and difficult to attribute to any particular medical condition. A woman with cancer of the ovary may first notice discomfort in the abdomen associated with a loss of appetite or a change in bowel habits. Because vague discomfort in the abdomen is so common, this symptom may have been present for weeks or months. Some women with cancer of the ovary may have the sensation of a need to urinate more frequently. There may be changes in a woman's menstrual pattern. At some point, these symptoms may lead the women to see her physician.

## <u>MAKING THE DIAGNOSIS</u>

### *How does the first suspicion of cancer of the ovary usually arise?*

The first suspicion of cancer of the ovary usually arises when a physician (usually a gynecologist) discovers that an ovary feels enlarged during a pelvic examination. In the context of the other symptoms, and particularly in women who have gone through menopause, further evaluation for the possibility of cancer of the ovary will begin.

### *What steps are taken when there is a suspicion of cancer of the ovary?*

An initial step in evaluating the possibility of ovarian cancer will be to perform an "ultrasound" examination in which harmless sound waves, bounced off the abdomen and organs inside the abdomen, transmit images to a video display terminal.

The ultrasound can show, with good accuracy, the size of the ovaries and whether they are solid or whether the ovaries contain fluid-containing areas (called "cysts") and whether cysts identified are large or small or contain solid components within them. Based upon suspicions raised by the results of the ultrasound examination, the physician may recommend additional evaluation.

If the ultrasound shows an abnormal enlargement of the ovary that is suspicious of being an ovarian cancer, an operation that obtains tissue from the ovary for examination under the microscope is generally required. Nevertheless, prior to performing an operation, the gynecologist may want to perform a CT or MRI scan of the abdomen and pelvis that can provide evidence as to whether or not ovarian cancer is present and if so, the extent, if any, to which the cancer has spread beyond the ovary. The CT or MRI scans can help guide the surgeon in planning initial treatment.

Simple blood tests are usually not helpful in the initial diagnosis of cancer of the ovary or in the initial determination of the extent to which cancer of the ovary has spread. A blood test called "CA-125" will often be abnormal in women with ovarian cancer, but can also be abnormal because of many health problems that are completely unrelated to ovarian cancer.

The definitive evaluation of a suspected cancer of the ovary requires an operation.

### Who performs the operation to evaluate and initially treat cancer of the ovary?

A physician called a "gynecologic oncologist" who specializes in the surgical treatment of gynecological cancers most effectively does the operation. Gynecologic oncologists are surgeons or gynecologists who have had additional training in the treatment of cancer of the ovary. Because of this training, and because much of their professional time is spent treating ovarian cancer, they are more likely to do a thorough and competent job of performing the technically difficult operation required to treat ovarian cancer than a physician without this level of training and experience.

# SURGERY TO MAKE THE DIAGNOSIS AND DETERMINE THE EXTENT TO WHICH THE CANCER HAS SPREAD

## What kind of operation makes the diagnosis of cancer of the ovary?

In the operating room, the physician performing the operation will first examine the enlarged ovary and determine by visual inspection and a biopsy whether the mass in the ovary is a cancer of the ovary.

If the diagnosis of cancer of the ovary is confirmed in the operating room, the standard surgical procedure (except in some women with stage I cancer as described later in this chapter) will include removal of the uterus, both ovaries and the fallopian tubes. The gynecologic surgeon will carefully inspect the liver, the undersurface of the diaphragm, and the sidewalls of the inside of the abdomen, the bowel, and other structures inside the abdomen and will take biopsies from areas that appear suspicious for containing cancer.

If cancer is present, the gynecologic oncologist will attempt to remove as much of the cancer as is possible. This type of surgery, called "debulking" or "cytoreductive" surgery, removes the great majority or all of the visible cancer, and will help make subsequent chemotherapy more effective.

## **ATTEMPTING TO PREVENT RECURRENCE AFTER THE OPERATION**

*How do physicians make decisions regarding further treatment after the operation?*

The operation will provide two critical pieces of information: the exact type of cancer of the ovary and the extent to which the cancer has spread.

There are several different types of cancer of the ovary. Approximately 90% of the time, a woman's ovarian cancer is an "epithelial" cancer of the ovary. This chapter will only discuss the treatment of epithelial cancer of the ovary.

The extent to which the tumor has spread will be determined by the gynecologic surgeon's visual inspection and by evaluation of the biopsies taken during the operation. This information will produce a "stage" for the woman's cancer of the ovary that will provide important guidance regarding the appropriate next steps in treatment.

*What are the stages of ovarian cancer?*

Stage I ovarian cancer means the cancer involves one ovary (Stage $I_a$) or both ovaries (Stage $I_b$) and does not extend beyond the ovaries. Approximately, a quarter of women have stage I cancer of the ovary at the time of the initial operation.

When a woman has Stage II ovarian cancer, it means that the cancer involves one or both ovaries as well as some other tissues inside the pelvis. Approximately, one in ten women has stage II cancer of the ovary at the time of the initial operation.

Stage III ovarian cancer means that the cancer has spread beyond the pelvis and into other portions of the abdominal cavity. Approximately, half of women have stage III cancer of the ovary at the time of the initial operation.

When a woman has Stage IV ovarian cancer, it means that the cancer involves organs and tissues that are both inside and outside of the abdomen. Approximately, one woman in eight has stage IV cancer of the ovary at the time of the initial operation.

## TREATMENT
## TREATMENT OF EARLY OVARIAN CANCER: SURGERY

### *How is stage I cancer of the ovary treated?*

Removal of the left and right ovaries and fallopian tubes as well as the uterus is usually adequate to cure stage I cancer of the ovary. At the time of surgery, a careful exploration of all structures inside the abdomen will also occur to identify and remove suspected tiny deposits of cancer.

Some women with stage I cancer of the ovary may be pre-menopausal and may still want to have children. If the cancer of the ovary has not extended beyond one ovary, removal of that ovary alone could be a reasonable option. If the tumor has spread to the opposite ovary or if malignant cells are in the tissues or other material obtained at the time of the operation, removal of both ovaries, the fallopian tubes and the uterus will give the better odds of obtaining a cure.

After the operation, pathologists will carefully examine all the tissues removed to be sure that cancer cells are not present beyond the ovaries. In addition, the pathologist determines if the cancer cells look almost normal (called "well differentiated", which is good) and will see if the cancer has a type of cell called a "clear cell" which is not good. The pathologist will also examine the ovary or ovaries to see if cancer cells have penetrated though to the outer surface of the ovary, which, if present, would make the cancer a "stage $I_c$". With surgical treatment alone, about 90% of women with well-differentiated stage $I_a$ or $I_b$ cancer of the ovary are cured of their cancer. If the cancer is confined to the inside of the ovary and is well differentiated, it is considered "low risk stage I". Chemotherapy is not usually recommended for women with low risk stage I cancer of the ovary.

If the cancer has penetrated to the outer surface of the ovary and is considered stage $I_c$, or if the cancer cells are not well-differentiated, or the cancer cells are considered to be "clear cell", the woman is generally considered to have "high risk stage I ovarian cancer" and chemotherapy is commonly recommended.

### What is adjuvant chemotherapy?

Chemotherapy given to reduce the risk of cancer recurrence after surgery has removed all visible evidence of cancer is "adjuvant chemotherapy".

### What is a common adjuvant chemotherapy regimen for women with high-risk stage I ovarian cancer?

A common adjuvant treatment regimen combines the chemotherapy medicines called "carboplatin" and "paclitaxel". These medicines are given intravenously on the first day of a 21-day cycle of treatment. To some extent, a physician's recommendation on the appropriate number of cycles of treatment may reflect the woman's underlying health, tolerance of the chemotherapy, and the appearance of her ovarian cancer cells, as reported by the pathologist. Most experts believe that a minimum of three treatment cycles and a maximum of six treatment cycles are appropriate. Six treatment cycles are more likely to cause severe bone marrow suppression with anemia as well as a low white blood cell count and increased susceptibility to developing serious infections (see chapter "Bone Marrow Suppression"). Because the treatment can cause severe nausea and vomiting as well as "infusion reactions", medicines to prevent this are necessary (see chapters "Nausea and Vomiting" and "Infusion Reactions").

Surgery and adjuvant chemotherapy cure most women with stage I high-risk ovarian cancer.

### How is stage II cancer of the ovary treated?

The risk of recurrence following surgical removal of all visible cancer is higher with stage II ovarian cancer than it is with stage I. Because of this, treatment with six cycles rather then three, of the same adjuvant treatment with carboplatin and paclitaxel described above is advocated by many physicians as the preferred way of reducing the risk of recurrence for women with stage II ovarian cancer.

# SURGERY

## How is stage III and IV cancer of the ovary surgically treated?

The initial treatment of stage III or IV cancer of the ovary is to have a gynecologic surgeon perform an operation to remove as much of the cancer as is possible.

At the time of diagnosis, the cancer may have spread very widely in many areas inside the abdomen. Sometimes the cancer has grown so that tentacles of the cancer have spread deeply into tissues, making surgical removal of the visible cancer difficult. The surgical difficulties associated with removing as much cancer as possible serve to emphasize the importance of having the initial surgery performed by a physician with extensive training and experience in the surgical treatment of cancer of the ovary.

## Why is it important to remove as much cancer as possible at the time of initial surgical treatment?

There is a direct correlation between the amount of cancer that remains after surgery and the probability of long survival and cure. Women with a significant amount of visible cancer remaining after the surgery have a much lower chance of having a long survival or of ultimately being cured of their ovarian cancer.

## CHEMOTHERAPY

*Why is it important to give chemotherapy after removal of all visible cancer in women with stage III or IV ovarian cancer?*

Despite the removal of all visible cancer, ovarian cancer generally recurs after an operation for stage III or IV ovarian cancer. Chemotherapy can delay, and possibly prevent this recurrence.

*Is chemotherapy ever given before the debulking surgery?*

If a woman has cancer deposits in her abdomen that are larger than three-quarters of an inch across, or if the cancer has spread to the lungs or the liver or other organs outside of the abdomen, some physicians may suggest "neoadjuvant" therapy prior to the operation. "Neoadjuvant therapy" would consist of three courses of chemotherapy to shrink the cancer, followed by surgery to remove any remaining cancer, followed by three or more courses of chemotherapy.

*Is it more effective to do debulking surgery immediately followed by chemotherapy or to have the neoadjuvant therapy just described before the surgery?*

The effectiveness of these two treatment strategies with regard to survival and freedom from progression appears to be very similar. The more common approach and the general standard of care, is to have an experienced gynecologic surgeon begin treatment by performing debulking surgery and, following the surgery, begin treatment with chemotherapy. If, however, the cancer is so extensive as to make optimal surgical debulking difficult or impossible, chemotherapy followed by surgery is a common recommendation.

Surgical removal of all visible cancer, whether done before or after chemotherapy, is of critical importance in delaying or preventing recurrence of ovarian cancer.

## What is the chemotherapy treatment after an operation for advanced ovarian cancer?

Whether the surgeon removes all visible tumor or not, women with advanced (stage III or IV) cancer of the ovary will be advised to receive chemotherapy within weeks of their operation.

The most important chemotherapy medication for cancer of the ovary is "cisplatin" or its close relative "carboplatin". The addition of the chemotherapy medication "paclitaxel" to cisplatin can increase the probability of achieving complete disappearance of the cancer. These two medications are given together, in a "cycle" which repeats every three weeks for six cycles. It does not appear that giving more than six consecutive cycles adds further benefit. The six treatment cycles can cause severe bone marrow suppression with anemia as well as a low white blood cell count and increased susceptibility to developing serious infections (see chapter "Bone Marrow Suppression"). Because the treatment can cause severe nausea and vomiting as well as "infusion reactions", medicines to prevent these complications are necessary (see chapters "Nausea and Vomiting" and "Infusion Reactions").

## What is "intraperitoneal chemotherapy" and when is it given?

If it appears that the gynecologic surgeon has removed all visible cancer, it is still likely that very tiny deposits of cancer are present on the surface of the organs and tissues inside the abdomen. By placing a catheter directly into the inside of the abdomen, the chemotherapy medicines cisplatin and paclitaxel can be delivered directly to these tissues. This direct therapy into the abdomen, called "intraperitoneal chemotherapy", appears to enhance the effectiveness of chemotherapy when given in conjunction with intravenous chemotherapy for women with no visible cancer after their initial surgery.

When cancer remains visible after surgery, most physicians will administer "intravenous" chemotherapy with either cisplatin or carboplatin in conjunction with paclitaxel. Intraperitoneal chemotherapy is less effective when visible tumor remains after surgery, since directly applied chemotherapy does not penetrate well into any area of cancer more than a few millimeters in size or thickness.

## Does intraperitoneal chemotherapy have drawbacks?

Intraperitoneal chemotherapy has many serious potential side effects including serious suppression of the bone marrow, injury to the intestines, nausea, vomiting, severe fatigue, and serious infections. This is not an easy therapy to administer, and should be done only by physicians and medical centers with the proper level of experience, and with a full understanding of the potential for serious side effects.

227

## Which is more effective: cisplatin or carboplatin?

The two medicines appear to be equally effective. There is a difference in the toxicities of the two medicines. Cisplatin appears to have a higher chance of causing kidney damage and damage to the hearing than carboplatin. For this reason, many physicians prefer carboplatin.

The major side effect of carboplatin is nausea and vomiting. The nausea is transient and usually controlled with new anti-nausea medicines (see chapter "Nausea and Vomiting"). The other major side effect, suppression of the bone marrow, usually does not produce problems that greatly curtail therapy or jeopardize life.

## How effective is the chemotherapy of advanced cancer of the ovary?

About three out of four women with advanced cancer of the ovary will have significant shrinkage of their cancer of the ovary with chemotherapy. About half will have complete disappearance of all evidence of their disease. Women who respond well to chemotherapy clearly have a better outlook with regard to control of the symptoms of their disease, survival, and the possibility of lasting remission or cure.

The effectiveness of the chemotherapy will depend, largely, upon the amount of cancer that remains after the initial operation. It is for this reason that it is critically important to have the initial operation performed by a physician experienced in gynecologic oncology surgery.

Despite the best available therapy, over half of women with stage III or IV ovarian cancer will eventually have a recurrence of their ovarian cancer.

*Is there any medication that, when added to chemotherapy, improves outlook?*

The biotechnology medication "bevacizumab" (brand name is "Avastin", manufacturer's product website is www.avastin.com) inhibits the growth of blood vessels that feed cancers and sustain their growth. When Avastin is added to chemotherapy of women with ovarian cancer, there appears to be a small but real increase in the length of time until progression of the ovarian cancer occurs. This increase in "time to progression" is likely, although not certain, to translate into a longer average survival time. Additional information from ongoing clinical trials of Avastin in ovarian cancer will provide critical guidance as to the contribution Avastin can make to the treatment of ovarian cancer.

## IF OVARIAN CANCER RECURS OR PROGRESSES AFTER CHEMOTHERAPY

*Can early identification of recurrence improve the likelihood of long-term survival?*

Although it is logical to assume that early diagnosis of recurrence can improve outlook, this does not appear to be the case. A recent study evaluated women who had a very early diagnosis of recurrence, based upon rising blood levels of the ovarian cancer marker "CA-125", to see whether early intervention to treat the recurrence improved outcome. It did not. For this reason, some physicians are now recommending that women with rising levels of CA-125 delay resuming chemotherapy until problems or symptoms related to the recurrence appear.

There still is controversy around this, but the key to improved outlook with early diagnosis of recurrence will be improvement of the medications available for treatment.

## What is the treatment if advanced cancer of the ovary recurs or progresses after chemotherapy?

Most women with stage III or IV ovarian cancer will, at some point, and perhaps years after initial treatment, have recurrence of their cancer despite having had a response to chemotherapy. Recurrent ovarian cancer is incurable with treatments that are currently available. The goal of treatment for women with recurrent ovarian cancer will be to extend life as much as possible and to delay the onset of symptoms that are painful and harmful to quality of life.

The physician evaluating a woman with recurrent or progressive advanced cancer of the ovary will evaluate the type of treatment the woman previously received and her response to that treatment. In the uncommon circumstance where a woman has never received either cisplatin or carboplatin, the woman will usually receive one of those medications.

Women who received cisplatin, carboplatin, or paclitaxel in the past and who responded well, meaning that the tumor shrank and that shrinkage lasted for six months or longer, if treated again with the same medicines, will often respond again with shrinkage of their cancer. The longer the period of time between the previous chemotherapy and recurrence, the better the chance of responding.

*What additional medicines are available for women with advanced cancer of the ovary that is no longer responding to chemotherapy with cisplatin or carboplatin?*

There are several chemotherapy medications, including Doxil, Gemcitabine, and Topotecan, which have approximately the same minor degree of effectiveness, with approximately one in five women having significant shrinkage of their cancer and a slight increase of survival time with treatment.

## EXPERIMENTAL TREATMENT

*Are experimental treatments available?*

An important option for a woman who develops recurrent ovarian cancer is to seek some form of experimental treatment. Ovarian cancer is a very active area of research, and many experimental drugs are currently under evaluation.

## WHEN OVARIAN CANCER CANNOT BE CONTROLLED WITH CHEMOTHERAPY

*What treatment is possible for a woman who is failing to respond to all chemotherapy?*

When a woman is no longer responding to chemotherapy or any other form of therapy, severe problems related to uncontrolled cancer of the ovary can develop.

Women with uncontrolled advanced cancer of the ovary very commonly develop a large and uncomfortable collection of fluid in the abdomen (this fluid is called "ascites"; please see chapter entitled "Ascites"). Ascites caused by ovarian cancer that is no longer responding to chemotherapy does not respond very well to diuretics or other medical treatments. By putting a needle into the abdomen with local anesthesia, a quart or more of fluid can be removed, giving immediate relief from some of the discomfort of the ascites.

Women with advanced ovarian cancer can develop mechanical intestinal obstruction (see chapter entitled "Mechanical Intestinal Obstruction"). Most of the time, intestinal obstruction in women with ovarian cancer is treatable with an operation that will unblock the intestine and restore intestinal function. This is, however, a major operation, and may not be an appropriate treatment for a woman with far advanced ovarian cancer and a life expectancy of days or very few weeks. Supportive measures such as draining fluid from the stomach with a "nasogastric tube" that is passed through the nose down into the stomach and generous use of pain medications may, in the very advanced stages of ovarian cancer, be the most appropriate treatment of intestinal obstruction.

# PANCREATIC CANCER

## DEFINITION

### What is pancreatic cancer?

Pancreatic cancer is a highly malignant cancer that begins in the pancreas and spreads quickly to other vital parts of the body. It is among the most dangerous of all the cancers.

## THE SYMPTOMS

### What are the symptoms of pancreatic cancer?

Major symptoms of pancreatic cancer are pain and weight loss. The pain creeps up on a person over a period of weeks. At first, the pain feels like indigestion or just a vague bellyache. As time goes on, the pain localizes in the upper part of the abdomen and feels as though it is gnawing its way into the center of the back. Appetite for food gets less, and weight may begin to drop off at a startlingly rapid rate.

A very common and dramatic early symptom of pancreatic cancer is the sudden appearance of the yellow eyes and yellow skin that are characteristics of jaundice.

## *Why do people with pancreatic cancer get jaundice?*

The thick and somewhat round right side of the pancreas, called "the head of the pancreas", contains the duct that carries bile from the liver into the duodenum (the "duodenum" is the first part of the small intestine). As the cancer grows, it compresses the tissues surrounding the duct and can completely obstruct the flow of bile through the duct. When this happens, bile cannot flow, as it should, from the liver into the duodenum. The system backs up, bile leaks into the bloodstream and turns the skin, and eyes yellow. This is "obstructive jaundice".

## **MAKING THE DIAGNOSIS**

## *What tests confirm the diagnosis of pancreatic cancer?*

When a person sees a physician because of symptoms suggestive of pancreatic cancer, the physician will perform a thorough physical examination. If the cancer is advanced, it may be possible for the physician to feel an abnormal hard mass in the abdomen just below the breastbone. If the cancer has spread into the liver, the physician may feel an enlarged, bumpy edge of the liver just below the right rib cage. An experienced physician can also detect signs of an abnormal collection of fluid inside the abdomen (called "ascites") which may be associated with pancreatic cancer. Regardless of the findings of the physical examination, if there is a suspicion of pancreatic cancer, further evaluation is necessary.

A type of x-ray called a "CT scan of the abdomen" is the gold standard for making the diagnosis of pancreatic cancer.

## How does a CT scan help make a diagnosis of pancreatic cancer?

A very high quality CT scan called a "spiral" CT (also called a "helical CT"), along with the intravenous injection of "contrast material", (which is a radiologist's dye that makes organs, blood vessels, and other structures more visible) is a very effective way of providing vital information about the cancer. In the majority of people with pancreatic cancer the CT scan will show an abnormal area of enlarged tissue (sometimes called a "mass lesion") wherever it is located in the pancreas. The CT scan can also show evidence of spread of cancer to the liver or elsewhere inside the abdomen.

The injection of contrast material during the scan enables physicians reviewing the CT scan to evaluate major arteries and veins affected by the cancer. Since these arteries and veins are essential for supplying blood to internal organs, their preservation is essential during any operation that would attempt to cure the cancer. If cancer surrounds important blood vessels, it may be impossible for the surgeon to remove the cancer. The information provided by the CT is critical in making a decision as to whether surgical cure of the pancreatic cancer is possible.

## What is endoscopic ultrasound?

An ultrasound device uses sound waves that bounce off organs inside the body and transmit images to a screen for evaluation. In endoscopic ultrasound, the ultrasound device is put on the end of a thin tube with a light on its end and is passed down the mouth, then down the esophagus, then down the stomach, and then into the duodenum. As the scope is advanced, the physician will examine the inside of the esophagus, stomach and duodenum. With the tip of the ultrasound device inside the duodenum and directly next to the pancreas, the ultrasound device will transmit images to a screen for the physician to evaluate. These images can provide critical details about the size, location, and density of the abnormal area in the pancreas. The endoscopic ultrasound can also evaluate the lymph nodes to which pancreatic cancer tends to travel, and give information regarding the extent to which the cancer may have invaded or wrapped itself around critical blood vessels.

### What is "endoscopic ultrasound-guided celiac plexus neurolysis" and when is it useful?

Pancreatic cancer, especially when it is locally advanced and inoperable, irritates and damages a group of nerves called the "celiac plexus". This can cause very severe pain in the upper part of the abdomen that radiates to the back. The pain of locally advanced pancreatic cancer can be very disabling, and often requires high doses of morphine to keep it under control.

During endoscopic ultrasound, a physician, using the ultrasound for guidance, can inject these nerves with 99% pure ethanol ("absolute alcohol") which can eliminate or reduce the ability of these nerves to transmit the sensation of pain. This can greatly reduce the pain from locally advanced and inoperable pancreatic cancer and reduce the requirement for morphine to control the pain. This procedure, called endoscopic ultrasound-guided celiac plexus neurolysis, can be helpful when it is clear that an attempt at surgical cure of the pancreatic cancer is not possible.

## What is an ERCP?

An ERCP is a type of x-ray test that can be useful in making a diagnosis of pancreatic cancer. An ERCP evaluates the ducts which drain fluid from the pancreas and which drain bile from the liver and gall bladder. The full technical name for the test is "endoscopic retrograde cholangiopancreatography".

## How is an ERCP done?

In order to do an ERCP, a physician will give a person a mild sedative and advance a tube from the mouth to the stomach to the duodenum. The duct of the pancreas (the pancreatic duct") as well as the bile duct empty digestive juices into the duodenum through a small opening. The physician finds this opening (the opening is called "the Ampulla of Vater") and injects into it a dye which will light up the pancreatic duct when an x-ray picture is taken.

## What information does the ERCP provide?

When the ERCP shows that the pancreatic duct is narrow or obliterated, physicians will have a very high level of concern that the person may have pancreatic cancer. At the time of the ERCP, the physician may be able to gently scrape or suck out malignant cells for a pathologist to look at under the microscope. The identification of these malignant cells under the microscope would confirm a diagnosis of pancreatic cancer.

## *What is a therapeutic ERCP?*

With ERCP, it is possible to relieve an obstruction of the bile duct that is causing jaundice.

To understand how the obstruction is relieved, it is important to understand the anatomy of what is causing the problem. Bile produced by the left and right side of the liver travels down ducts that join to form the "common hepatic duct". This duct continues downward, joins the duct from the gall bladder, and forms the "common bile duct". The common bile duct travels through the pancreas and empties its bile into the duodenum through the small hole called "the Ampulla of Vater". In the duodenum, the bile helps us digest our food.

When a bulky cancer develops in the head of the pancreas, the bile duct is compressed and blocked, backing up the bile that then leaks into the blood stream.

With an ERCP, the physician will put the scope down into the duodenum, find the Ampulla of Vater, and, through it, can advance a tube-like structure called a "stent" up into the common bile duct that props open the duct and allows bile to flow again. This is a "therapeutic ERCP".

Therapeutic ERCP is useful in relieving obstruction when it appears that the pancreatic cancer is inoperable. When the pancreatic cancer appears to be operable, therapeutic ERCP is associated with a higher risk of complications without clear benefit, and many physicians will prefer to proceed immediately to the operating room. Surgery is a more definitive way of bypassing the obstruction and permits an attempt at curing the pancreatic cancer without additional delay.

### How is a definite diagnosis of pancreatic cancer made?

Although the CT scan or endoscopic ultrasound or an ERCP can raise a high level of suspicion of the diagnosis of pancreatic cancer, a "biopsy" of the tumor is essential in order to make a definite diagnosis.

### Why is the biopsy so essential?

Occasionally, inflammation of the pancreas (please see chapter entitled "Acute Pancreatitis") can give the same appearance on CT scan as pancreatic cancer. In addition, less common tumors, such as lymphoma, can look like a pancreatic cancer on CT scan. Because the treatment of these other conditions is so vastly different from the treatment of pancreatic cancer, it is essential to make a definite diagnosis with a biopsy before proceeding with treatment.

### When is the biopsy done?

If, based upon the testing described above, it is likely that the diagnosis is pancreatic cancer, and if these tests suggest that a surgical cure is possible, a biopsy is done in the operating room, at the time surgeons attempt to cure the pancreatic cancer.

If it is evident that surgical cure would be impossible, a biopsy without major surgery can confirm the diagnosis. Using an endoscopic ultrasound as a guide, a physician can advance a very thin needle into the area most suspicious for containing cancer, and pull out a small piece of tissue for the pathologist to examine under the microscope. If cancer is present, this biopsy will generally make the diagnosis.

## LAPAROSCOPY TO DETERMINE WHETHER THE CANCER HAS SPREAD

### What is laparoscopy?

Laparoscopy is a surgical technique that allows a surgeon to examine the inside of the abdomen without performing a major operation. The instrument used is a "laparoscope", and, through incisions of less than an inch in length, surgical tools used to perform the operation, are passed into the abdomen. The surgeon directs the instrument through the various parts of the inside of the abdomen and examines the abdomen through images projected to a video monitor. Tissues that are abnormal can be biopsied and sent to the laboratory for analysis.

### How useful is laparoscopy in evaluating people with pancreatic cancer?

Pancreatic cancer commonly spreads to the "peritoneum", which is the tissue that lines the inside of the abdomen. Small cancer deposits in the peritoneum (called "peritoneal seeding") or tiny spots of cancer on the surface of the liver may be impossible to identify with a CT scan or with an endoscopic ultrasound but may be obvious to the surgeon examining images projected by the laparoscope from the inside of the abdomen onto a video monitor. Identification of obvious spread of the cancer can lead to the conclusion that the cancer is surgically incurable and can save the person from having an unnecessary major operation. With laparoscopy, approximately a third of people thought to have a potential for a cure by surgery are determined to be surgically incurable.

## Is laparoscopy always necessary prior to major surgery?

There are differences of opinion as to whether or when laparoscopy should precede surgery. On the one hand, if the cancer has already spread, it can prevent a major operation. On the other hand, it can delay definitive surgery. When the CT scan and the endoscopic ultrasound show no evidence of spread beyond the pancreas, and when the cancer is relatively small and located in the head of the pancreas, many physicians feel strongly that a person should proceed directly to surgery.

## How often will evaluation with a CT scan, endoscopic ultrasound, laparoscopy, and other tests lead to the conclusion that the cancer is potentially curable?

Less than one in five people with pancreatic cancer who undergo this thorough evaluation have no evidence of spread of their cancers, and can potentially be cured by surgery.

## ATTEMPTING SURGICAL CURE

### What kind of an operation attempts to cure a pancreatic cancer?

This is a major operation usually performed through a large incision in the upper abdomen. As a first step, the surgeon will search around the inside of the abdomen for any evidence that the cancer has spread beyond the pancreas. Biopsies of areas suspicious for containing cancer are sent to the pathologist for immediate examination under the microscope. If visual inspection or a pathologist's review indicates that cancer has spread beyond the pancreas, an attempt at surgical cure would be dangerous and unnecessary and will not be made.

If it appears that the cancer is restricted to the head of the pancreas and that cure is possible, the surgeon will usually do an operation removing the head of the pancreas, the duodenum, the gall bladder, the bile duct, and parts of the stomach and small intestine. This operation is called a "Whipple's procedure" and takes about six hours or so to perform.

Some major cancer centers with extensive experience treating pancreatic cancer have begun performing the Whipple's procedure using robotic surgical technology. With robotic surgery, the surgeons use a computer to guide the movement of multiple robot arms that actually perform the surgery. Robotic surgery may allow smaller incisions, improve the safety, and shorten the recovery time from the Whipple's procedure.

### What is the success rate of the Whipple's procedure in curing pancreatic cancer?

Even under the most favorable circumstances, the majority of pancreatic cancers recur after surgery. In top medical centers with surgeons experienced in performing the Whipple's procedure, about one in five people with an apparently small, localized pancreatic cancer who undergo the Whipple's procedure are cured by surgery.

The odds of cure reflect the findings of the pathologist examining the tissues removed by the surgeon. If the cancer does not involve lymph nodes that are near the pancreas, and the cancer does not appear to have spread beyond the pancreas, approximately a third of people survive five years, which, with pancreatic cancer, generally means a cure. If the cancer does involve lymph nodes, the odds of five-year survival are approximately one in ten.

## Is it helpful to give chemotherapy before the Whipple's procedure?

If it appears that surgery has the potential to cure a person's pancreatic cancer, it is not clear that giving chemotherapy prior to the surgery has benefit. Having said this, some major cancer centers are investigating the role chemotherapy, given before surgery, may have in improving the outcome after surgery with regard to local control of the cancer and prevention of distant spread.

There are circumstances where it appears that surgical removal of the cancer is possible, but difficult. Specifically, pancreas cancer has a tendency to grow around major blood vessels in the abdomen such as the "portal vein" that must be preserved in any operation. In this situation, in which a person has a "borderline resectable" pancreatic cancer, a combination of radiation and chemotherapy can sometimes shrink the cancer to the point where subsequent surgery can remove all visible or detectable areas of cancer. This type of treatment is "neoadjuvant therapy".

### *Is there any treatment after a Whipple's procedure to reduce the risk of recurrence?*

There is general agreement among experts, based upon recent clinical trial results, that chemotherapy with the medication "gemcitabine", given for several months after Whipple's surgery, is beneficial. For people who eventually have a relapse of their cancer, gemcitabine more than doubled the average time until the cancer relapsed. Gemcitabine also more than doubled the odds of not having the cancer come back for five years or more, which may equate with a cure.

Some experts also suggest giving radiation to the area from which the pancreatic cancer was removed along with the chemotherapy medication called "5-FU" to reduce the risk of cancer recurring in that local area. The usefulness of this combination of chemotherapy and radiation ("chemoradiotherapy") is controversial and is a subject of ongoing clinical trials.

## WHEN SURGICAL CURE IS NOT POSSIBLE

### *What is the treatment if surgical cure of the pancreatic cancer is not possible?*

If the cancer is not curable with surgery, the goal of treatment will be to attempt to prolong life as much as possible and prevent painful or life-threatening complications of the pancreatic cancer.

## SURGERY TO RELIEVE SYMPTOMS OR PREVENT COMPLICATIONS

*Can a surgical operation prevent
complications of the pancreatic cancer?*

The pancreas is located immediately next to the stomach, the duodenum and the bile duct. As the cancer grows, it can invade any of these organs and cause serious problems. To prevent this, an operation can be done in which the gastrointestinal plumbing and biliary duct drainage can be re-routed so that it bypasses the vicinity of the pancreas. This can prevent a great deal of pain and suffering.

As described earlier in this chapter, pancreatic cancer, especially when it is locally advanced and inoperable, irritates and damages a group of nerves called the "celiac plexus", causing severe pain in the upper part of the abdomen that radiates to the back. During an operation, the celiac plexus can be injected with 99% pure ethanol ("absolute alcohol") which can eliminate or reduce the ability of these nerves to transmit the sensation of pain.

## RADIATION THERAPY AND CHEMOTHERAPY

*Is there any way to cure pancreatic
cancer other than by surgery?*

Aside from surgery, there no available or known treatment is capable of curing pancreatic cancer.

## What is the role of radiation therapy?

The two major issues associated with pancreatic cancer that is incurable by surgery are local growth and distant spread of the cancer. Radiation can be quite helpful in controlling local growth of the cancer and associated pain, and may prevent distant spread ("metastasis"), but has no effect on controlling areas of metastasis that are already present.

In many cancer centers, radiation for locally advanced pancreatic cancer is given over a period of several weeks along with chemotherapy. A chemotherapy medication commonly used is "gemcitabine". This combination of treatment, called "chemoradiotherapy" is not curative, but can delay the growth of the cancer and slightly increase the likelihood of a longer survival.

Some cancer centers are evaluating a highly focused form of radiation therapy called "stereotactic body radiation treatment", abbreviated as "SBRT", which may deliver a comparably effective course of radiation in one to three days. SBRT, though somewhat more convenient, appears to have more side effects related to the intense dose of radiation to which neighboring organs, such as the intestines, are subjected. With a higher level of side effects, and no demonstrated benefit over more standard radiation, in either disease control or survival, many experts, regard SBRT as an experimental and unproven treatment of locally advanced pancreatic cancer.

## What type of chemotherapy is given and how effective is the chemotherapy?

The most commonly used chemotherapy is the medication "gemcitabine", and can produce a beneficial effect in about one in four people. This beneficial effect primarily means a reduction of symptoms associated with the pancreatic cancer. The beneficial effect on survival time is very small, measured in only a few months. The medication "erlotinib" (brand name is "Tarceva", manufacturer's product website is www.tarceva.com), given with gemcitabine, can add, on average, a few additional weeks to survival time, and is associated with troublesome side effects such as skin rash and diarrhea.

A recently developed combination of the chemotherapy medications "5 FU", "leucovorin", "irinotecan" and "oxaliplatin" given together in a regimen that has been given the nickname "FOLFIRINOX" appears to be more effective than gemcitabine. With this regimen, about a third of people with metastatic pancreatic cancer will have a significant shrinkage of their cancer, and average survival extended by several months from approximately six months with gemcitabine to approximately eleven months with FOLFIRINOX. The side effects of this treatment are very significant, and include bone marrow suppression, a higher risk of infections and severe fatigue. These side effects are so severe that, in the context of pancreatic cancer as an incurable disease, many physicians and people with pancreatic cancer believe this treatment is too toxic. "Neulasta" may be given to reduce the risks associated with white blood cell suppression; a detailed discussion of this is in the chapter "Bone Marrow Suppression". FOLFIRINOX appears to be most appropriate when given to people with previous good health who are willing to trade severe side effects for an opportunity for several additional months of survival.

Early results of a clinical study evaluating the combination of the chemotherapy medications "Gemcitabine" and "Abraxane" suggest that this regimen has approximately the same level of effectiveness as the FOLFIRINOX regimen.

There was a good deal of enthusiasm regarding the possibility that the biotechnology medications "cetuximab" (brand name is "Erbitux", manufacturer's product website is www.erbitux.com) and bevacizumab ("Avastin", manufacturer's product website is www.avastin.com) might be helpful for people with advanced pancreatic cancer. These medications, tested in large clinical trials, did not show any benefit when added to gemcitabine for people with advanced pancreatic cancer.

When cancer is progressing despite initial treatment with Gemcitabine or FOLFIRINOX, additional treatment options are largely experimental.

New medications are necessary. Many experts believe that the best hope for prolonged survival for a person with advanced pancreatic cancer is to receive and respond to some new form of experimental treatment.

## OUTLOOK

*What is the outlook for a person with pancreatic cancer?*

The great majority of people diagnosed with pancreatic cancer are not curable by surgery. Those not cured by surgery have a difficult outlook. The average survival time for a person with pancreatic cancer that is surgically incurable is under a year, although with some recent advances in chemotherapy it is probable that this average survival time will be lengthened. These statistics encourage many people to seek out experimental treatment as soon as possible after receiving a diagnosis of pancreatic cancer.

# PROSTATE CANCER: METASTATIC

## DEFINITION

### What is metastatic prostate cancer?

Metastatic prostate cancer is a cancer that began in the prostate gland and has spread beyond the prostate gland in a way that makes it incurable by surgery, radiation, or any other locally directed therapy. Most commonly, prostate cancer which has become surgically incurable or incurable with radiation initially spreads to the nearby lymph nodes and other tissues adjacent to the prostate, and then into the bones of the pelvis and the spine. Once prostate cancer has spread either to the bones or to major body organs, it is incurable with treatments currently available.

## GENERAL CONSIDERATIONS THAT GUIDE METASTATIC PROSTATE CANCER TREATMENT

### What general considerations guide physicians when suggesting the best form of treatment of metastatic prostate cancer?

Current treatments of metastatic prostate cancer, however aggressively applied, are not capable of curing the disease. The goal of treatment is, therefore, to extend healthful life as much as possible with a minimum of side effects from treatment and with a minimum of complications from the cancer itself.

The most effective initial treatment for metastatic prostate cancer suppresses and neutralizes the male hormones that fuel the growth of prostate cancer. This treatment, which can clearly, although not permanently stop the progression of a man's prostate cancer, has very bothersome side effects. Almost all men become impotent, that is, will lose the ability to get an erection, while receiving treatment. Loss of male hormones causes muscles in the body to weaken and become smaller and body fat to increase. Bones become thinner and may break more easily. Hot flashes, similar to those women get around the time of menopause, can be extremely uncomfortable and can cause sleep problems. The most common type of medication used, the "GnRH agonists" slightly increase the risk of heart attacks, strokes, diabetes and sudden death.

*If the treatments available for metastatic prostate cancer are not curative and have such difficult side effects, why are they useful?*

The available treatments of metastatic prostate cancer can shrink the cancer and restrain the growth of the cancer for months or years. The benefit of this shrinkage of the cancer usually manifests itself as relief of bone pain and prevention of complications related to spread of the cancer in the bones. The remissions induced with different medications can occur one after the other, while delaying progression of the prostate cancer for several years.

## *When is it best for a man with metastatic prostate cancer to begin treatment?*

There is considerable disagreement among experts regarding the best time to begin treatment. Some feel that treating soon after first identifying the presence of metastatic cancer will delay growth of the cancer at its earliest stages and, by doing so, delay the onset of the painful symptoms and complications of bone metastasis. Others believe that the side effects of the treatment are so unpleasant, that it is best to delay treatment until bone pain or other symptoms of metastasis are severe and require treatment. Clinical studies are in progress evaluating the benefits and risks of immediate, as opposed to delayed, treatment of metastatic prostate cancer. Weighing all the information available today, and all the information likely to become available, a man will have to make the choice of whether, and when, to begin treatment.

## INITIAL CONSIDERATIONS IN THE TREATMENT OF METASTATIC PROSTATE CANCER

### *What are potential short-term dangers with metastatic prostate cancer?*

The most common danger is that of developing a "pathologic bone fracture", which means that a bone weakened by cancer can fracture far more easily than any bone should. Radiation therapy can radiate the local area of cancer, shrink the cancer in the bone, relieve pain, and reduce the risk that the local cancer will cause a pathologic fracture.

Because the pelvis and the femur, which is the bone in the upper leg, bear the full weight of the body when walking, these bones, if weakened, may be especially susceptible to pathologic fractures. When an x-ray of a bone shows a seriously weakened bone, it sometimes helps to have an orthopedic surgeon strengthen the bone with surgical cement or other surgical material in order to prevent a disabling fracture.

The uppermost portion of the femur contains the "femoral head" that fits into a socket in the pelvis, and the "femoral neck" that connects to the remainder of the femur at the "intertrochanteric region". Extensive involvement of this area by metastasis can seriously weaken the femur and expose a person to a high risk of fracture. The most practical way of immediately strengthening this area and relieving the risk of a dangerous fracture may be a partial hip replacement with a device that replaces the damaged area of the femur.

Prostate cancer can spread to the bones in the spine and occasionally press on the spinal cord. This is a medical emergency, and is discussed in the chapter entitled "Malignant Spinal Cord Compression".

## INITIAL HORMONAL THERAPY

### What is the initial hormonal treatment of metastatic prostate cancer?

Male sex hormones accelerate the growth of prostate cancer. When these male hormones disappear, growth of prostate cancer slows down. Initial therapy of metastatic prostate cancer suppresses and neutralizes male hormones. Male hormones are "androgens" and treatment that suppresses androgens is "androgen deprivation therapy".

### How are male sex hormones, that is, androgens, suppressed or neutralized?

Two types of treatment can neutralize male hormones and extend the life of men with metastatic prostate cancer. Each has major drawbacks.

Surgical removal of the testicles ("orchiectomy" or "surgical castration") certainly diminishes the production of male hormones. Many men, however, view orchiectomy as an unpleasant, irreversible, and unacceptable form of treatment. It is, however, an option, which some may wish to take after considering the other options.

Medicines are available that have the same effect as orchiectomy in stopping the production of male hormones. The most common medications initially used to stop production of male hormones are the "GnRH agonists".

### What are GnRH agonists and how do they work?

GnRH agonists are medicines given by injection that block the body's ability to produce testosterone.

The pituitary gland, which is a pea-sized structure that is located on the bottom of the brain, controls the function of the key glands of the body. The pituitary gland produces a hormone called "LH", which drives the testicles to produce testosterone.

253

GnRH agonists cause an overstimulation of pituitary gland production of LH to the extent that the pituitary gland runs out of this hormone and can no longer drive the testicles to produce testosterone.

## Can initial overstimulation of the pituitary gland cause problems?

Initially, stimulation of the pituitary can cause a transient increase of testosterone production and cause a worsening of the symptoms of prostate cancer. Because of this, physicians commonly prescribe a second medication, called an "anti-androgen", which can block the effect of the testosterone. "Flutamide" and "Casodex" are commonly used anti-androgens. A month or so of anti-androgen medication is generally sufficient, by which time the hormones from the pituitary gland that were stimulating testosterone should have shut down.

## How are GnRH agonists given?

Two major brands of GnRH agonists that are available are "Lupron" and "Zoladex". These medications are given by injection, and, depending on the way the medication is formulated, can be given once monthly or once every three or four months.

## What is "intermittent androgen deprivation"?

Intermittent androgen deprivation is an experimental way of treating prostate cancer with the GnRH agonist for several months then, if the cancer appears to be under control, discontinuing the

GnRH agonist for several months. GnRH agonist treatment resumes sooner, if symptoms of the cancer return, or blood tests (see below) suggest the cancer is growing. Intermittent androgen deprivation has the advantage of reducing the side effects of GnRH agonists and the possible disadvantage of allowing the prostate cancer to grow when treatment with the medication temporarily discontinues. The benefits and risks of intermittent androgen deprivation are still under investigation.

### How effective are the GnRH agonists in treating metastatic prostate cancer?

The GnRH agonists successfully restrain the growth of the prostate cancer and relieve, or delay, development of symptoms most of the time. This benefit is, however, not permanent. Metastatic prostate cancer is very likely, eventually, to become resistant to the effect of GnRH agonists at which point other treatment will be needed to control the cancer.

### What effect does androgen deprivation therapy have on bones?

Androgen deprivation therapy decreases the amount of minerals in the bone and, by doing so, weakens them. The loss of bone minerals and resulting loss of the structural strength of bone is "osteoporosis". Osteoporosis associated with androgen deprivation therapy may become evident as early as six months after androgen deprivation therapy has begun, and increases the risk of developing bone fractures after only minor trauma. Because of this, many physicians will recommend a simple and painless "bone mineral density test" at the beginning of androgen deprivation therapy, and at regular intervals, so that the effect of the treatment on the strength of the bones can be followed closely.

## What can prevent osteoporosis during androgen deprivation therapy?

Dietary supplementation with calcium and Vitamin $D_3$, to some extent, can be helpful. The medications called "bisphosphonates", which are discussed in the chapter entitled "Bone Metastasis", may also inhibit the breakdown of bone associated with androgen deprivation therapy, and delay or prevent osteoporosis.

A biotechnology-derived medication called "denosumab" (brand name is "Xgeva" manufacturer's product website is www.xgeva.com) appears to have effectiveness in reducing the degree of osteoporosis, and the risk of fractures of the spine in people receiving androgen deprivation therapy for prostate cancer that has not yet spread to the bone. Xgeva also reduces the risk of "skeletal related events", defined as a broken bone, pain in a bone needing radiation, or malignant spinal cord compression (see chapter entitled "Malignant Spinal Cord Compression") in men who have bone metastasis from prostate cancer. Xgeva works by inhibiting the development of bone damaging cells called "osteoclasts". Xgeva is given by an injection under the skin (a "subcutaneous injection") in the arm, abdomen, or thigh, every 4 weeks.

Comparing the effectiveness of the bisphosphonate "Zometa" with Xgeva, Xgeva appears to be more effective in preventing or delaying "skeletal related events" in people who have bone metastasis.

## EVALUATING RESPONSE TO TREATMENT

### *How is the response to treatment evaluated?*

Most of the time, prostate cancer cells release a substance called "prostate specific antigen" (abbreviated "PSA") into the bloodstream when a man has metastatic prostate cancer. As the cancer responds to treatment, the elevated PSA level in the blood generally drops, and as the cancer stops responding, the PSA level generally increases. The PSA level is not, however, a perfect indicator of response and does not always correlate with a good or bad outlook.

Imaging studies, such as CT scans or MRI scans are generally not helpful in assessing response, since the metastatic cancer predominantly involves the bones, which CT and MRI scans are not good at evaluating. Other forms of imaging bone metastasis from prostate cancer are still under development.

Cancer in the bones can produce bone pain and pathologic fractures and compress nerves exiting the spinal column. Worsening symptoms, primarily related to bone pain, are often a reflection of progression of disease.

## SECOND LINE HORMONAL THERAPY

### *What is the treatment if the cancer stops responding to the initial hormonal therapy?*

Despite the continued use of Lupron or Zoladex, the growth of metastatic prostate cancer generally resumes at some point in time.

Part of the reason for this is that male hormones ("androgens") produced by the adrenal gland, are not adequately suppressed by Lupron or Zoladex. By binding to the "androgen receptor" on the surface of prostate cancer cells, these adrenal-produced male hormones can stimulate prostate cancer growth. The medicines "Casodex" and "Flutamide" block binding of androgens to androgen receptors and by doing so can often regain control of the prostate cancer growth. Casodex and Flutamide are most effective if the person keeps taking Lupron or Zoladex. The combined treatment with a GnRH agonist and an androgen receptor blocking medicine is "complete androgen blockade"

### Is complete androgen blockade a more effective initial treatment of metastatic prostate cancer as well?

Although complete androgen blockade may more effectively control the prostate cancer, it is associated with more side effects, and it is not clear that giving both hormonal treatments initially gives a better outcome, as regards symptom control and survival, than GnRH initially given alone. There is controversy here, but physicians commonly give Lupron or Zoladex alone and reserve complete androgen blockade for the point in time when a person is becoming inadequately responsive to the single therapy.

### What is the treatment if the cancer begins to grow again with complete androgen blockade?

It is not uncommon, for reasons that are obscure, that discontinuation of the anti-androgen drug, that is, of Casodex or Flutamide, with continued treatment with Lupron or Zoladex, will trigger another regression of the cancer.

Another medication with hormonal effects is a pill called "Ketoconazole", which will temporarily regain control of prostate cancer growth approximately half of the time.

When the hormone treatment is no longer working, the person's cancer is "hormone refractory prostate cancer".

The steroid medicine "prednisone" can reduce the production of androgens by the adrenal glands and appears to have some direct effect on inhibiting the growth of prostate cancer. Approximately a third of men who receive prednisone have a temporary reduction of bone pain, which generally lasts for a very few months.

## PROVENGE

### *What is Provenge?*

Provenge is a newly FDA approved form of immune therapy. To give the treatment, a man's immune cells are separated from his own blood by a process called "leukapheresis". The immune cells collected are sent to a special laboratory where they are exposed to a protein called "prostatic acid phosphatase". Because of this exposure, the immune cells develop the ability to recognize prostate cancer cells containing "prostatic acid phosphatase" on their surface. This slows prostate cancer cell growth. These immune cells are injected by vein every two weeks for three injections. Side effects of the immune therapy are generally very mild and transient, and consist of chills, fever, and fatigue.

## How effective is Provenge?

Without exposing men to significant side effects, Provenge can extend survival for several months. In the largest study done, the average survival of men with hormone refractory prostate cancer receiving Provenge was 25 months, as opposed to 21 months for the men not receiving Provenge. These survival times are averages, and it is possible that some men had an excellent response to Provenge and lived significantly longer because of treatment.

## CHEMOTHERAPY

### What happens if the metastatic prostate cancer begins to grow again despite hormonal therapy?

When prostate cancer is progressing despite hormonal therapy and, if available, immune therapy with Provenge, chemotherapy can, at times, restrain the growth of the cancer.

A chemotherapy regimen considered effective in treating hormone-refractory prostate cancer combines the medicine "Taxotere" with oral prednisone. Several years ago, it was reported that with this treatment, approximately half of men have a reduction in their bone pain, and an average survival of a bit over 1½ years, with an approximately one in five chance of survival for three years or more. The possibility of longer survival may have improved somewhat with the recent approval of a new "second line treatment" (see below) for men who are no longer responding to Taxotere. The Taxotere is given every three weeks and does have significant side effects, including nausea, vomiting, fatigue, and a risk of developing serious infections.

If prostate cancer progresses despite treatment with Taxotere, a medicine called "abiraterone" (brand name is "Zytiga" and manufacturer's product website is www.zytiga.com), given with the steroid medication "prednisone", can slow progression of the cancer. Zytiga is an oral, once-a-day medicine that blocks the product of androgens by the testicles, the adrenal glands, and by the tumor itself. This more complete suppression of androgens extends the average survival of men with prostate cancer that has progressed after Taxotere by approximately four months. The delay in tumor progression and increased survival with Zytiga treatment is associated with a lower risk of serious side effects than with chemotherapy treatments for advanced prostate cancer. Clinical trials are in progress evaluating the effectiveness of abiraterone before treatment with chemotherapy.

A new medication related to Taxotere, "cabazitaxel" (brand name is "Jevtana", manufacturer's product website is www.jevtana.com) has been approved by the FDA as a "second line treatment" in men with prostate cancer who are no longer responding to Taxotere. Men treated with Jevtana in combination with the oral steroid medicine "prednisone" appear to have an approximately three-month improvement in average survival compared to previously available "second-line" treatment, with some men surviving much longer with extended periods of disease stability. Jevtana can cause serious side effects, such as severe bone marrow suppression and "neutropenic sepsis" (see chapters entitled "Bone Marrow Suppression" and "Febrile Neutropenia and Neutropenic Sepsis"), as well as nerve, kidney, and liver damage. Before prescribing this medication, physicians assess whether the person with advanced metastatic prostate cancer will be physically able to tolerate this potentially toxic medication.

When metastatic prostate cancer grows despite Taxotere, Zytiga, and Jevtana, further treatment options, aside from medications to relieve symptoms, are primarily experimental.

# STOMACH CANCER

## DEFINITION

### *What is stomach cancer?*

Stomach cancer is a cancer that begins in the wall of the stomach. As the cancer grows larger, it can penetrate through the wall of the stomach, shed cancer cells into the abdominal cavity, and spread throughout the body. Stomach cancer, also known as "gastric cancer", is a highly malignant cancer. If not surgically cured in its earliest stages, it is one of the most dangerous cancers.

### *Are there different types of stomach cancer?*

The overwhelming majority of stomach cancers are in the category of "adenocarcinoma". The discussion in this chapter focuses entirely on the treatment of adenocarcinoma of the stomach. Other malignant tumors of the stomach, such as "gastric lymphoma" or "stromal tumors" are less common, and require very different treatment than the treatment for an adenocarcinoma.

## SYMPTOMS

### What are the symptoms of stomach cancer?

The early symptoms of stomach cancer are often mild. A person may complain of an upset stomach or an uncomfortable feeling in the abdomen.

As the cancer grows larger, it can cause severe and unrelenting pain and significant loss of weight. The cancer may bleed, resulting in blackish stool, or vomiting of material that looks like coffee grounds, or sometimes, bright red blood (see chapter entitled "Upper GI Bleeding"). A large tumor may block the passage of food into, or out of, the stomach and cause difficulty with swallowing or nausea and vomiting. The tumor may bore a hole through the wall of the stomach and cause a sudden, painful peritonitis.

## MAKING THE DIAGNOSIS

### How is the diagnosis of stomach cancer made?

At some point, the mild, or not so mild, symptoms will bring a person to the attention of a physician. The symptoms described to the physician will point to a problem with the stomach. Unless the cancer is far advanced, the physical examination and routine blood tests will not show clear signs of the cancer.

Symptoms of persistent abdominal pain and weight loss are suggestive of a potentially serious problem with the stomach, such as cancer, and will often lead a physician to recommend an "endoscopy". To do this, the physician, who is usually a gastroenterologist, will put an "endoscope" down from the mouth, down the esophagus and into the stomach. Examining the stomach through the endoscope, the gastroenterologist will closely examine the wall of the stomach for abnormalities. The lesion of stomach cancer is usually easy to identify. The gastroenterologist will take several biopsies of the lesion, and send them to the laboratory for analysis by a pathologist. By looking at the tissue under the microscope, a pathologist can make the diagnosis of cancer and determine exactly which type of cancer the person has.

A particularly malignant form of stomach cancer that infiltrates beneath the surface of the stomach may not be visible with endoscopy. When symptoms are very suggestive of stomach cancer, physicians may advise a person to have an old-fashioned "barium swallow" x-ray examination in which the person swallows a chalky tasting substance called "barium", and has x-rays of the abdomen taken. The barium will then give a very good view of the shape of the stomach and might find a type of stomach cancer, called "linitis plastica", in which the wall of the stomach has cancer in it from end to end.

## DETERMINING THE EXTENT TO WHICH THE CANCER HAS SPREAD

*What are the first steps after the making the diagnosis of stomach cancer?*

The most important first issue after making the diagnosis of stomach cancer is to determine whether the cancer has spread and, if it has, how far. If the cancer only involves the stomach, it may be curable with surgery. If the cancer has spread beyond the stomach, it is unlikely that the cancer is curable.

## How is the extent of the stomach cancer determined before an operation?

A very careful physical examination, including a rectal examination (stomach cancer can spread to the wall of the rectum) and a pelvic examination in women (stomach cancer can spread to the ovaries) can occasionally uncover evidence of metastatic cancer.

Routine blood tests will look for evidence of spread of the cancer to the liver or bones. A chest x-ray may identify spread of cancer into the lungs, or may show a malignant pleural effusion (see chapter entitled "Pleural Effusion"). A CT scan of the abdomen can determine whether the cancer has spread beyond the stomach and into other organs such as the liver.

## What is endoscopic ultrasound and when is it helpful?

Occasionally, physicians may recommend that part of the assessment of whether a person's stomach cancer is curable by surgery involve an "endoscopic ultrasound". An ultrasound device uses sound waves that bounce off organs inside the body and transmit images to a screen for evaluation. In endoscopic ultrasound, the ultrasound device is on the end of a thin tube with a light on its end that is passed down the mouth, then down the esophagus, then into the stomach. The ultrasound device inside the stomach transmits images of the tissues surrounding the stomach to a screen for the physician to evaluate for evidence of spread of the cancer beyond the stomach. In particular, the endoscopic ultrasound can also evaluate the lymph nodes to which stomach cancer tends to travel, and help surgeons and people with stomach cancer better assess the options for treatment and the likelihood that the cancer is curable by surgery.

## LAPAROSCOPY TO DETERMINE WHETHER THE CANCER HAS SPREAD

### *What is laparoscopy?*

Laparoscopy is a surgical technique that allows a surgeon to examine the inside of the abdomen without performing a major operation. Through incisions less than an inch in length, a "laparoscope", and surgical tools used to perform the procedure, will be directed through the various parts of the inside of the abdomen. This will permit examination of the inside of the abdomen through images that are projected to a video monitor. Tissues that are abnormal can be biopsied through the laparoscope and sent to the laboratory for analysis.

### *How useful is laparoscopy in evaluating people with stomach cancer?*

Stomach cancer commonly spreads to the "peritoneum", which is the tissue that lines the inside of the abdomen, including the surface of the liver. Small cancer deposits in the peritoneum (called "peritoneal seeding") or tiny spots of cancer on the surface of the liver or intestines may be impossible to identify with a CT scan or with an endoscopic ultrasound, but may be obvious to the surgeon examining images projected by the laparoscope from the inside of the abdomen onto a video monitor. Identification of obvious spread of the cancer can lead to the conclusion that the cancer is surgically incurable, and can save the person from having an unnecessary major operation. With laparoscopy, approximately a quarter of people, previously thought to have a potential to be cured by surgery, are found to have evidence of spread of the cancer and are surgically incurable.

### Is laparoscopy always necessary prior to major surgery?

If a person is having symptoms that require removal of the stomach to relieve serious symptoms, or enable the person to eat and digest properly, there is no point to doing a laparoscopy. At the time of surgery, the surgeon can look directly into the abdomen and assess the extent to which the cancer has spread inside the abdomen. When surgery is not clearly necessary to relieve symptoms, there are differences of opinion as to whether, or when, laparoscopy should precede surgery. Many physicians feel that laparoscopy is important since approximately a quarter of the time the laparoscopy will determine that the cancer is incurable by surgery. A major operation with all its difficulties and complications is not necessary if laparoscopy indicates that the cancer is incurable by surgery.

### How often will evaluation with a CT scan, endoscopic ultrasound, laparoscopy, and other tests lead to the conclusion that the cancer is potentially curable?

Approximately, one in four people with stomach cancer who undergo this thorough evaluation will have no evidence of spread of their cancer, and are potentially curable with surgery.

## <u>SURGERY</u>

### *What is the surgical treatment of stomach cancer?*

The goal of the surgery is to remove and cure the cancer. Depending on the location of the cancer in the stomach, this will involve removal of most, or all, of the stomach. During the operation, the surgeon will examine abdominal organs including the liver for evidence of spread of the cancer.

Stomach cancer can travel to lymph nodes near the stomach. Because of this, the surgeons will remove these lymph nodes and send them to the hospital pathologist for microscopic examination. There are some different points of view as to the extent to which the surgeon should go to find and remove lymph nodes, since the greater the extent of surgery, the greater the risk of complications. It appears that the results of a more extended operation to find, and remove, possibly involved lymph nodes can yield a better outcome, but only if the surgeon is very experienced with this form of complicated cancer surgery.

### *How successful is surgery at curing stomach cancer?*

The success of the surgery depends upon how advanced the cancer was at the time of diagnosis. Overall, the surgery cures only about one in five people with stomach cancer. However, the odds can change quite dramatically depending on where the cancer is located in the stomach, how large it was when identified, the depth to which it penetrated the wall of the stomach, and, quite importantly, depending on whether or not the cancer has spread to lymph nodes near the stomach. Cancers found at their very earliest stages are curable by surgery most of the time. On the other hand, if the cancer has penetrated through the entire wall of the stomach, from the inner lining (the "mucosa") to the outside surface (the "serosa"), or if the cancer has spread to lymph nodes, it is likely that at some point, the cancer will recur.

## TREATMENT AFTER SURGERY TO PREVENT RECURRENCE OF THE CANCER

*Is there therapy that can reduce the odds of recurrence after surgery?*

A combination of local radiation and chemotherapy, given over a period of approximately four months, may reduce the chance of cancer recurrence in people who appear to have had all of their cancer removed by surgery. A commonly used treatment regimen combines radiation therapy with the chemotherapy medications "5-FU" and "Leucovorin". Several new combinations of chemotherapy and radiation given before, or after, or both before and after surgery, are under active investigation in an attempt to improve upon the effectiveness of such treatment.

## WHEN STOMACH CANCER CANNOT BE CURED BY SURGERY

*What is the treatment if, during the operation, the surgeon discovers that the cancer is surgically incurable?*

The portion of the stomach that contains the cancer can produce many serious problems such as bleeding, stomach obstruction, or stomach perforation. Removal of the area of the stomach involved by the cancer can prevent these problems.

After the operation is over, the combination of radiation therapy and chemotherapy may reduce the size of the cancer and may be somewhat helpful in temporarily arresting the growth of the cancer.

## TREATMENT WHEN CANCER HAS SPREAD BEYOND THE STOMACH: CHEMOTHERAPY

*What is the treatment of stomach cancer when it has spread far beyond the stomach and lymph nodes?*

Cancer spread beyond the stomach and nearby lymph nodes is "metastatic stomach cancer", also known as "metastatic gastric cancer" and, with currently available treatments, is incurable. Chemotherapy, given as a combination of medications, can often shrink the cancer, delay the time until the cancer progresses, and slightly extend survival. Still, with currently available chemotherapy treatments, the average survival time once metastatic stomach cancer has developed, is less than one year.

"Herceptin" (manufacturer's product website is www.herceptin. com) is a biotechnology medication developed as a treatment for women with breast cancer whose breast cancer cells are positive for "HER-2 expression". HER-2 expression indicates that the cancer has too many copies of a gene called "HER-2" that is responsible for production of a protein that stimulates growth of breast cancer cells. By interfering with HER-2, Herceptin slows the growth of breast cancer cells and extends the life of women whose breast cancer is positive for HER-2 expression.

Approximately 25% of people with advanced stomach cancer have HER-2 expression on their stomach cancer cells. If a person's stomach cancer cells express HER-2 on their surface, addition of Herceptin to chemotherapy with cisplatin combined with either capecitabine or 5-FU slows the growth of stomach cancer and can extend survival by an average of 2-3 months.

### Are there experimental treatments worth considering?

There are so many unanswered questions with regard to which of the available treatments work best, and whether newer medicines that are being developed can work far better, that enrolling in a clinical trial evaluating new treatments is an important consideration.

## PALLIATIVE TREATMENT FOR ADVANCED GASTRIC CANCER

### What is "palliative treatment" in the context of advanced stomach cancer?

When stomach cancer is growing and is uncontrolled by chemotherapy or radiation, a number of very painful problems can develop. Prevention or treatment of these painful problems is "palliative treatment".

### What is the treatment for severe pain related to advanced inoperable stomach cancer?

Proper pain control with medications such as morphine can greatly relieve the suffering associated with advanced inoperable stomach cancer.

As stomach cancer grows, it can cause a great deal of pain in the center of the abdomen. In an attempt to shrink the cancer, physicians may suggest radiation therapy directed at the area of the cancer.

Pain, as well as nausea and vomiting, may result from a large cancer that is obstructing the flow of food into, or out of, the stomach. There are "stents" which are hollow tubes which can be put down into the stomach and through the obstruction, propping open the obstructed area so that food can flow through. There are also some advanced techniques involving lasers that can open up these obstructions. If these less invasive ways of opening the obstruction are not possible, physicians may recommend an operation to remove or bypass the obstruction. Additional information about this complication is in the chapter entitled "Gastric Outlet Obstruction".

# UTERINE CANCER

## DEFINITION

### What is cancer of the uterus?

Cancer of the uterus is a cancer that begins within the uterus. Most of the time, the cancer begins in the cells which line the inside of the uterus. The inner lining of the uterus is the "endometrium". Cancer that begins in the endometrium is "endometrial scancer".

This chapter will only discuss endometrial cancer.

## SYMPTOMS

### What are the symptoms of endometrial cancer?

The major symptom of endometrial cancer is abnormal vaginal bleeding. Because endometrial cancer is most common in women beyond menopause and no longer having vaginal bleeding from menstrual periods, bleeding will be the major early symptom that brings a woman to her physician for evaluation.

## MAKING THE DIAGNOSIS

### *How is the diagnosis of endometrial cancer made?*

Abnormal vaginal bleeding requires evaluation. When a post-menopausal woman develops vaginal bleeding, a priority of the gynecologist will be to determine whether the cause of the bleeding is endometrial cancer. The simplest method of doing this is with an "endometrial biopsy", a simple procedure done in the gynecologist's office

### *What is a dilatation and curettage and when is it done?*

Sometimes, based upon review of the appearance of the uterus with an ultrasound examination, and based upon experience and intuition, the gynecologist may not be confident that the endometrial biopsy took a sufficient sample of tissue to rule out endometrial cancer. Persistent bleeding after a negative endometrial biopsy can raise the suspicion that the endometrial biopsy, by chance, took a piece of normal tissue and missed a piece of an endometrial cancer causing bleeding. A dilatation and curettage (a "D & C") is a procedure in which an instrument called a "curette", inserted into the vagina, through the cervix and into the uterus, scrapes tissue off the inner wall of the uterus. A pathologist evaluates the tissue removed under the microscope.

An alternative way to examine the uterus is with "hysteroscopy" in which a thin tube with a camera on its end is put into the vagina, through the cervix, and into the uterus. The hysteroscope will then transmit images to a video screen, allowing the physician to carefully examine the inside wall of the uterus and take a biopsy of visibly abnormal areas.

### *What will the pathologist see?*

The pathologist will use the tissue removed to determine whether the diagnosis is endometrial cancer. The appearance of the cancer under the microscope (the "degree of differentiation") can provide critical information about the likelihood that the cancer will spread beyond the uterus.

The pathologist will often report the degree of differentiation by assigning a "grade" to the cancer. Grade 1 cancer is the most likely to be slow growing and to remain confined to the uterus. Grade 2 is intermediate in likelihood. Grade 3 is most likely to grow quickly and spread beyond the uterus.

## DETERMINING WHETHER THE CANCER HAS SPREAD BEYOND THE UTERUS

### *What is done after the diagnosis of endometrial cancer has been made?*

Most of the time, endometrial cancer is only in the inner lining of the uterus at the time the diagnosis is made, and therefore curable with surgery. The priority after the diagnosis of a localized endometrial cancer is to cure the cancer with surgery.

Physical examination, especially in a woman who has had vaginal bleeding for an extended period before seeking medical attention, can occasionally raise the suspicion of uterine cancer that has spread locally or at a distance beyond the uterus. In some circumstances, based upon the results of physical examination suggesting spread beyond the uterus, or the appearance of the cancer cells under the microscope, physicians may prefer to have more information before an attempt at surgical cure. A MRI of the abdomen and pelvis can evaluate the extent of the cancer in the uterus and provide evidence of the presence or absence of spread of the cancer to nearby lymph nodes or to other areas beyond the uterus.

## TREATMENT OF ENDOMETRIAL CANCER CONFINED TO THE UTERUS

*What is the treatment of endometrial cancer confined to the uterus?*

Cancer of the endometrium confined to the uterus is "stage I endometrial cancer".

The treatment of stage I endometrial cancer is total removal of the uterus, the fallopian tubes, and the ovaries (this operation is called a "total abdominal hysterectomy and bilateral salpingo-oopherectomy" or, in short, a "TAH-BSO"). During the operation in which the gynecologist performs the TAH-BSO, the gynecologist will examine lymph nodes inside the pelvis and around the aorta to see whether the cancer has spread. Any suspicious areas will be biopsied.

After the operation, the hospital pathologist evaluates tissues removed.

## What is laparoscopic hysterectomy?

Laparoscopic hysterectomy is removal of the uterus through a laparoscope, which is a narrow tube inserted through a small incision into the abdomen. The laparoscope can then transmit images of the inside of the abdomen via a camera on the laparoscope to a video monitor. Using these images to guide the surgery, the surgeon will insert special small instruments through small incisions in the abdomen and perform the operation. Removal of the uterus and surrounding lymph nodes through the laparoscope can encounter technical difficulties and requires that the surgeon performing this operation have very significant skill and experience in doing this. Since the surgeon, while performing the laparoscopic surgery, occasionally may run into difficulties or complications, it may become necessary to convert the laparoscopic surgery to the standard surgery involving a larger abdominal incision.

The results of performing the operation required to treat, and possibly cure, endometrial cancer either through a standard operation or through a laparoscope appears to be equal, provided the physician performing the operation through the laparoscope has sufficient training and experience to perform both operations properly. With the laparoscope, there is a shorter recovery time, less blood loss from the operation, and a lower risk of surgical complications.

## What will the pathologist look for?

The pathologist will determine the depth to which the cancer has invaded into the wall of the uterus and whether the cancer has spread to lymph nodes, or to any other organs or tissues which have been removed or biopsied by the gynecologist.

## How will the pathologist's report guide treatment?

The pathologist's report enables classification of the endometrial cancer as "low risk", "intermediate risk", or "high risk". The risk category into which a woman's cancer fits helps to guide treatment.

"Low risk" is when the cancer was superficial in the uterus, and the degree of differentiation (see above) of the cancer was either grade 1 or grade 2.

"Intermediate risk" is when the pathologist determines that the cancer has extended sideways into the muscular wall of the uterus or downward into the cervix. "Intermediate risk" is further divided into "low intermediate risk" or "high intermediate risk", based upon several factors including age, the appearance of the cells under the microscope, and the depth to which it has invaded the muscular wall of the uterus (the "myometrium"). Blood drains from tumors through blood vessels and fluid and proteins drain from tumors through lymphatic vessels. Invasion of these blood or lymphatic vessels by endometrial cancer, as discovered by the pathologist under the microscope, is "lymphovascular invasion". This finding moves a woman's disease toward the designation "high intermediate risk".

"High risk" is when the endometrial cancer has spread all the way through the muscular wall of the uterus into the outside surface of the uterus (called the "serosal surface"), or has spread into tissues in the pelvis beyond the uterus, or has spread to the top part of the vagina.

### What treatment is given after surgery to women with low risk or low intermediate risk endometrial cancer?

Approximately 95% of women with low risk or low intermediate risk endometrial cancer are cured by surgery and additional therapy is generally not considered beneficial or required.

### What treatment is given after surgery to women with high intermediate risk endometrial cancer?

Without treatment after surgery, approximately 10-15% of women with high intermediate risk endometrial cancer will develop a recurrence, which usually involves the upper portion of the vagina. Radiation therapy, applied to the upper vagina reduces the risk of recurrence in the upper vagina to less than 2%.

The most effective and safe way of giving this radiation is with "vaginal brachytherapy". Brachytherapy is radiation treatment focused directly on the targeted tissue by putting the radiation source on, or in, the cancer, or in or on the area at risk for spread of the cancer. To give brachytherapy to the area of the vagina at risk for recurrence, a smooth plastic cylinder containing a radioactive source is inserted into the vagina. Through this cylinder, radiation can specifically target the areas at risk for recurrence of the cancer, while sparing nearby normal tissues from exposure to the radiation. Three treatments are usually given, with each treatment session lasting less than two hours.

There could be some diarrhea and local irritation after vaginal brachytherapy. Sexual function after vaginal brachytherapy has been reported as returning to normal after treatment.

### *What is the outlook after vaginal brachytherapy for high intermediate grade endometrial cancer?*

Less than 2% of women who receive vaginal brachytherapy develop a recurrence in the vagina. A risk remains, however, that cancer can recur outside of the area that was irradiated. At the five-year time point commonly used to assess the lasting success of cancer treatment, approximately 85% of women who have received vaginal brachytherapy for high intermediate grade endometrial cancer remain free of cancer.

## TREATMENT WHEN CANCER HAS SPREAD BEYOND THE UTERUS

### *What is done if the endometrial cancer is high risk, that is, it has spread into other organs or tissues in the pelvis?*

Endometrial cancer that has spread beyond the uterus and into other organs or tissues in the pelvis is "stage III endometrial cancer". In the classification of endometrial cancer, involvement of the outermost layer of the uterus ("the serosa") will also put a woman's endometrial cancer into stage III.

Stage III endometrial cancer is very difficult to cure with surgery. Recurrence can occur both in the local tissues in the upper vagina and pelvis, as well as in distant areas of the body.

The best treatment of high-risk endometrial cancer has been the subject of several very large clinical trials, which have yielded some conflicting results. It appears, however, that the most effective way of preventing recurrence of the cancer is with chemotherapy followed by radiation.

The chemotherapy that is given consists of combinations of two or three medications. The common combinations consist of paclitaxel (brand name is "Taxol"), doxorubicin (brand name is "Adriamycin"), and the generic chemotherapy "cisplatin". Other regimens combine carboplatin (brand name is "Paraplatin") with paclitaxel, or cisplatin with doxorubicin. The goal of this chemotherapy is to prevent recurrence anywhere in the body.

After completion of chemotherapy treatment, physicians may suggest additional treatment with radiation to the pelvis, to prevent recurrence of the cancer in the area that surrounded the uterus. The best regimen for administering radiation is currently under investigation in clinical trials.

## TREATMENT OF ADVANCED ENDOMETRIAL CANCER

*What is done if the cancer recurs in the pelvis after treatment with radiation or chemotherapy?*

"Local recurrence", meaning recurrence in the area that surrounded the uterus, can occasionally be truly local and curable by surgery. This is especially true if the recurrence only involves the upper portion of the vagina.

If a woman has a more extensive local recurrence and her underlying health is good, a more extensive operation called a "pelvic exenteration" may be considered. Pelvic exenteration is a very radical operation in which the major contents of the pelvis including the vagina, the rectum, the bladder and other tissues are removed. It is a life-changing operation, associated with many potential complications, but has some chance of curing the recurrent endometrial cancer.

"Surgical debulking", that is, removing as much of the visible cancer as possible, can improve survival time if sufficient cancer is removed such that no visible cancer remains. Radiation therapy, after the surgery, can provide further local control of the cancer.

The more commonly used treatment option for locally recurrent endometrial cancer is radiation therapy delivered to the pelvis. With this treatment, control of the local growth of the cancer often is achieved, and delay or prevention of spread of the cancer is common. There is a wide range in the reported outlook for long-term survival, but it appears that approximately half of women treated with radiation for locally recurrent endometrial cancer are living five years after treatment, with many of these women free of the disease.

### What is the treatment if endometrial cancer has spread beyond the pelvis into distant organs of the body?

Cancer that has recurred despite an attempt at curative treatment is "recurrent disease". Cancer that has spread beyond the pelvis into distant organs of the body is called "stage IV" or "metastatic" disease.

Metastatic disease will require a treatment that can suppress the growth of endometrial cancer cells wherever they may be in the body. At this time, the only treatments that can do this are hormonal therapy or chemotherapy.

## When is hormonal therapy given?

Examination of the woman's cancer cells by the pathology laboratory will indicate whether "progestin receptors" are present on their surface. If progestin receptors are present, response to hormonal therapy is possible and this will be the first "systemic" therapy administered that can affect the cancer wherever it may have spread in the body.

## What type of hormonal therapy can be given?

The hormonal therapy given involves a medicine in the "progesterone" family. The most commonly used medicine is "Megace".

## How effective is the hormonal therapy?

Hormonal therapy can shrink the endometrial cancer approximately 20% of the time. The response to hormonal therapy lasts, on average, for four months, although some responses are quite a bit longer and reflect the appearance of the cells under the microscope.

If hormonal therapy is not effective, the remaining treatment option is chemotherapy.

### What type of chemotherapy is available?

The optimum chemotherapy regimen is under investigation. Chemotherapy that is given consists of combinations of two or three medications. The common combinations consist of paclitaxel (brand name is "Taxol"), doxorubicin (brand name is "Adriamycin"), and the generic chemotherapy "cisplatin" or the combination of carboplatin (brand name is "Paraplatin") with paclitaxel.

### How effective is the current standard chemotherapy in women with metastatic endometrial cancer?

The currently available chemotherapy has minimal effectiveness. Although roughly half of women treated with chemotherapy have shrinkage of their cancer, the toxicity of the chemotherapy is very often severe, and the shrinkage of the cancer is temporary. The majority of favorable responses to chemotherapy last for under a year and the average survival after chemotherapy for metastatic cancer begins is in the range of 12-15 months.

## EXPERIMENTAL TREATMENT

### Where are experimental treatments of endometrial cancer under development?

Several new chemotherapy medicines are under evaluation as potential treatments of endometrial cancer. Pharmaceutical and biotechnology companies in conjunction with the National Cancer Institute or academic medical centers are developing most of these medicines.

The effectiveness of the currently available standard chemotherapy of metastatic endometrial cancer is clearly inadequate. An option for the woman with metastatic endometrial cancer is to enroll in an experimental treatment program at the time of diagnosis of metastatic endometrial cancer.

# COMPLICATIONS
# OF CANCER

# ABDOMINAL
# EMERGENCIES

# ACUTE PANCREATITIS

## DEFINITION

### *What is the pancreas?*

The pancreas is an important abdominal organ that has two major functions. Its "endocrine function" is to deliver critical hormones into the bloodstream, such as "insulin" and "glucagon", which regulate the level of sugar in the bloodstream. Its "exocrine function" is to produce digestive juices and deliver them to the small intestine, where they break down the protein, carbohydrates, and fat in our food.

### *How does the pancreas deliver the digestive juices into the small intestine?*

Digestive juices produced by the cells of the pancreas drain into the "pancreatic duct" which runs through the center of the pancreas. The pancreatic duct joins up with the "common bile duct" which drains bile from the liver and gall bladder. Together, these ducts deliver their contents through the "Ampulla of Vater" into the "duodenum", which is the first part of the small intestine.

### What is pancreatitis and what is acute pancreatitis?

Pancreatitis is an inflammation of the pancreas. When this inflammation appears suddenly, it is "acute pancreatitis". If the inflammation develops slowly and is persistent over a long period, it is "chronic pancreatitis".

The most life-threatening form of pancreatitis is acute pancreatitis.

This chapter will only discuss acute pancreatitis.

## SYMPTOMS

### What are the symptoms of acute pancreatitis?

A person with acute pancreatitis usually has a constant, severe pain in the middle of the abdomen that radiates into the back. Nausea and vomiting are common. Lightheadedness or fainting, when associated with pancreatitis, may indicate a severe form of the disease.

## THE CAUSES OF ACUTE PANCREATITIS

### What usually causes acute pancreatitis?
### Why is this important to treatment?

The most common causes of acute pancreatitis are gallstones and alcohol overuse.

People with cancer certainly can develop pancreatitis from gallstones or from overuse of alcohol. In addition, pancreatitis can uncommonly develop as a side effect of chemotherapy, and is an occasional complication of "hypercalcemia", which is discussed in its own chapter later in this book. Pancreatic cancer or any other cancer that obstructs the pancreatic duct can cause pancreatitis. The medical procedure called an "ERCP", described later in this chapter, is a common component in the evaluation of pancreatic cancer, and can sometimes induce pancreatitis. Roughly 25% of the time, acute pancreatitis develops for no apparent reason.

For all people with acute pancreatitis, it is important to attempt to identify the cause of the acute pancreatitis and, if possible, remove the cause. Identification and removal of the cause of pancreatitis can be critical to survival, recovery, and prevention of recurrence.

## Why can gallstones cause acute pancreatitis?

To understand how gallstones can cause acute pancreatitis it is important to understand the anatomy of what is causing the problem. Bile produced by the left and right side of the liver travels down ducts that join to form the "common hepatic duct". This duct continues downward, joins the duct from the gall bladder, and forms the "common bile duct". The common bile duct travels through the pancreas and empties its bile into the first part of the small intestine (the "duodenum") through the tiny hole called "the Ampulla of Vater". In the duodenum, the bile helps us digest our food.

Gallstones travelling downward from the gall bladder can become stuck in either the common bile duct or the Ampulla of Vater. When this happens, bile from the liver and gall bladder, instead of flowing downward into the intestine, can flow into the open channel which runs sideways, that is, into the pancreatic duct and into the pancreas. This can cause enormous inflammation of the pancreas and pancreatitis.

## <u>MAKING THE DIAGNOSIS</u>

### *How is the diagnosis of acute pancreatitis made?*

Simple laboratory tests that measure levels of "amylase" and "lipase" in the bloodstream, in conjunction with a clear understanding of the person's symptoms and with the results of a physical examination, are usually all that are necessary to make the diagnosis. Amylase and lipase are enzymes normally made by the pancreas that leak into the bloodstream in high concentrations when a person has acute pancreatitis.

### *Can the level of amylase or lipase in the bloodstream indicate the severity of the pancreatitis?*

Elevation of the amylase and lipase (usually to levels more than three times normal) makes the diagnosis. The ultimate height to which serum amylase or lipase will go does not always give an accurate indication of the severity of the attack of acute pancreatitis.

### *Are "imaging tests" such as ultrasound or a CT scan or MRI useful?*

An ultrasound machine bounces sound waves off the body and, with the help of a computer, produces a picture of the liver, the gall bladder, and the pancreas. The ultrasound can often identify gallstones that may be the cause of the episode of acute pancreatitis and can identify the expansion of the bile ducts that occurs when a stone is blocking the flow of bile from the liver into the duodenum, as described earlier in this chapter.

A CT or MRI can give important information about the degree to which the pancreas is inflamed and can assess whether there has been irreversible destruction ("necrosis") of areas of the pancreas.

The MRI provides similar information to that from the CT scan, but can also give important information about the duct which runs through the pancreas and into which a gallstone can get stuck. Some medical centers consider the MRI to be a more accurate and safer imaging tool for pancreatitis than the CT, provided the medical center has the appropriately modern MRI scanner and the trained staff to interpret the images.

## ASSESSING SEVERITY

*What is the "APACHE II" score and how is it useful in evaluating a person with acute pancreatitis?*

"APACHE II" is an abbreviation for "Acute Physiology and Chronic Health Evaluation II". This score assesses the severity of disease of critically ill people, and especially those who are in an intensive care unit. The score derives from evaluating approximately a dozen different factors, such as body temperature, heart rate, blood pressure, kidney function, and the person's age, and assigning points to each factor that add or subtract from the score. The higher the point value, the higher the risk to life.

Many medical centers will assign a person an APACHE II score upon making a diagnosis of acute pancreatitis and revise this score as time proceeds during the hospitalization. Other similar scoring systems are available, such as the "Ranson's score", and are used in many medical centers. These scores are not perfect predictors of outcome, but can give medical professionals a general idea as to the degree to which a person's life is in jeopardy and the likelihood that serious complications may develop.

## TREATMENT OF PANCREATITIS CAUSED BY GALLSTONES

### What is an ERCP?

An ERCP ("endoscopic retrograde cholangiopancreatography") is a type of x-ray test that evaluates the ducts that drain fluid from the pancreas and bile from the liver and gall bladder. This test can be very useful in finding the stone that is blocking the bile ducts and causing bile to run into the pancreas.

In order to do an ERCP, a physician, who is usually a gastroenterologist, will give a person a mild sedative and advance a tube from the mouth to the stomach to the duodenum. In the duodenum, the duct of the pancreas (the pancreatic duct") as well as the bile duct empties their digestive juices into the intestine through the tiny opening called "the Ampulla of Vater". The physician finds the Ampulla of Vater, and, through it, injects a dye that will travel into the bile ducts and the pancreatic duct, making them visible with an x-ray.

### What is "endoscopic sphincterectomy"?

When the ERCP shows that a stone is blocking the pancreatic duct, special instruments can remove the stone, and relieve the obstruction. To do this, during the ERCP, physicians will first pass a wire through the Ampulla of Vater and make a small cut in the sphincter muscle (the "sphincter of Oddi") which surrounds the Ampulla of Vater. This will allow the physician to use special instruments that can reach into the bile ducts and remove the obstruction.

## TREATMENT OF MILD ACUTE PANCREATITIS

### What is the treatment of mild acute pancreatitis?

Attacks that are not severe usually clear up by themselves with the passage of time. Treatment will include medicines to control pain (usually the narcotic "Demerol") and administration of fluid by vein to keep the blood pressure from dropping. In order to rest the pancreas, the person with acute pancreatitis does not take any form of food by mouth.

## SEVERE PANCREATITIS AND NECROTIZING PANCREATITIS

### Why is severe pancreatitis dangerous and what can diminish some of the danger?

People with severe pancreatitis can develop several life threatening medical problems. The severe inflammation in the pancreas creates a situation whereby a very large amount of fluid leaks out of the bloodstream and into the tissues that surround the pancreas. This can result in a dangerous drop of blood pressure, a drop of blood flow to the kidneys, and acute kidney injury. In addition, the severe body stress caused by pancreatitis can trigger "acute respiratory distress syndrome". Information about these life-threatening complications is in this book in the chapters entitled "Acute Respiratory Distress Syndrome" and "Acute Kidney Injury".

Because severe pancreatitis can impair lung function, it is critical for physicians to monitor this carefully, provide supplemental oxygen as needed, and address any lung problems that may develop.

To maintain adequate nutrition, insertion of a tube through the nose, past the stomach and duodenum, and into the part of the small intestine called the "jejunum" enables feeding with a solution containing vital nutrients. This procedure, which is called "enteral nutrition", can reduce the risk of developing serious complications such as "acute kidney injury" (see chapter), "acute respiratory distress syndrome (see chapter), "sepsis" (see chapter entitled "Sepsis and Septic Shock"), and improves the odds of surviving the episode of acute pancreatitis.

Pain control is very important and commonly managed with narcotic pain medications such as "Demerol".

### What is acute necrotizing pancreatitis and how is the diagnosis of acute necrotizing pancreatitis made?

Acute necrotizing pancreatitis means there has been permanent destruction of a significant portion of the pancreas. This tissue, which is now dead or "necrotic", is very susceptible to becoming infected. The diagnosis of acute necrotizing pancreatitis is evident with a CT or MRI scan that can begin to show evidence of the necrotic areas of the pancreas two or three days after the episode began.

## What is the treatment of acute necrotizing pancreatitis?

The major risk to life of a person with acute necrotizing pancreatitis is the risk of infection of the necrotic tissue. When a significant amount of the pancreas has become necrotic, and if the person develops a fever or other signs of infection, powerful antibiotics may prevent development of a very extensive and life-threatening infection in the necrotic tissue.

After several days, despite the best supportive care with fluids and pain medications, a person may still be critically ill with severe pain, unstable blood pressure or other problems. Based upon CT scans or other tests, it may become apparent that, despite antibiotic and other treatment, an infection has developed in the necrosis in the pancreas. It may be necessary for a surgeon or other skilled physician, using a variety of newer techniques that may or may not involve major surgery, to remove necrotic tissue with a procedure called a "necrosectomy". Tissue removed is sent to the laboratory to determine if it is infected. If infection is present, treatment begins with antibiotics that laboratory results will suggest are most likely to be effective.

## OUTLOOK

## What is the outlook for a person who recovers from an episode of acute pancreatitis?

People who recover from an episode of acute pancreatitis can go back to their previous state of health.

If the cause of the acute pancreatitis was gallstones, physicians will generally recommend that the gall bladder be removed to prevent a recurrent episode.

If the episode of acute pancreatitis was due to alcohol, a person is advised to stop, or heavily curtail, drinking of alcohol.

# GASTRIC OUTLET OBSTRUCTION

## DEFINITION

### *What is the gastric outlet?*

The gastric outlet is the area through which food must pass as it travels from the stomach into the small intestine.

### *What is gastric outlet obstruction?*

Normally, partially digested food moves from the stomach to the duodenum (the duodenum is the first part of the small intestine), through an area of the stomach called the "pylorus". Gastric outlet obstruction is means that an obstruction is blocking the movement of digested food either in the pylorus, which connects the stomach to the duodenum, or in the duodenum itself.

### *In people with cancer, what is it that is causing the obstruction?*

Cancer growing on the inside of the stomach or duodenum (an "intrinsic" obstruction) can obstruct the gastric outlet. The most common cancers producing an intrinsic obstruction are stomach cancer and pancreatic cancer that has grown into and obstructed the duodenum.

Widespread cancer inside the abdomen, such as can occur with advanced breast, lung, ovarian, or other cancers, can wrap around or compress the stomach or duodenum. This "extrinsic" compression can narrow the gastric outlet, producing gastric outlet obstruction.

## What are the symptoms of gastric outlet obstruction?

Because, with gastric outlet obstruction, the stomach is not emptying properly, it fills up with fluid and air. This distension causes severe nausea and vomiting along with pain in the upper abdomen just below the breastbone. If not promptly recognized and treated, gastric outlet obstruction will cause significant weight loss, malnutrition, and dehydration.

## How do physicians make the diagnosis of gastric outlet obstruction?

Based upon a person's medical history and an understanding of a person's symptoms, a physician may have a high level of suspicion of the presence of gastric outlet obstruction. A plain x-ray of the abdomen can show a distended stomach with a large air bubble in it. CT scan of the abdomen will give far more detail, including information about the size and location of the cancer causing the obstruction. Examination of the inside of the stomach and duodenum with a flexible instrument called an endoscope will allow a physician to confirm the diagnosis, take biopsies if needed to confirm the presence of cancer, and make an assessment of treatment that is most likely to relieve the obstruction.

# RELIEVING THE OBSTRUCTION

## What is the treatment of gastric outlet obstruction?

The two options available to treat gastric outlet obstruction are enteral stents and surgery.

## What are enteral stents?

Enteral stents are metallic or plastic tube-shaped devices that can prop open the gastric outlet obstruction and relieve the obstruction. A physician inserts an enteral stent during endoscopy.

## What surgery relieves the obstruction?

The surgery to relieve gastric outlet obstruction bypasses the area of obstruction by attaching the stomach to the second part of the small intestine, that is, to the "jejunum". This operation is a "gastrojejunostomy".

## When are enteral stents the preferred treatment?

Although an operation to eliminate the gastric outlet obstruction may be the most effective treatment with the lowest risk of recurrent obstruction, it can be impractical if someone has advanced cancer and a short life expectancy or a high risk for a slow and painful recovery. A stent across the obstruction can be a very effective alternative to surgery to open up the obstructed area, relieve symptoms, and relieve the severe pain and other problems associated with gastric outlet obstruction.

# ILEUS

## DEFINITION

### What is an ileus?

An ileus is a severe weakening or absence of coordinated contractions (called "peristalsis") of the muscles in the intestine. When a person has an ileus, intestinal contents will stop moving forward and the intestine will become distended with fluid and air.

## CAUSES OF ILEUS

### What causes an ileus in people with cancer?

After an abdominal operation, it is very common for a person to develop an ileus. This ileus usually lasts for a few days.

Any disease that suddenly and severely inflames the inside of the abdomen will cause an ileus. Acute pancreatitis and acute appendicitis are just two of the many such diseases that can cause an ileus.

Extensive cancer inside the abdomen can damage the muscles and nerves that are essential for normal peristalsis and produce an ileus

Many other medical problems can cause an ileus. Pneumonia, electrolyte abnormalities in the bloodstream, and a number of medications, including and especially pain medications, all have the potential to produce an ileus.

## SYMPTOMS OF ILEUS

### What are the symptoms of an ileus?

Sometimes, at the time the person develops an ileus, the symptoms of the disease that caused the ileus (such as the symptoms of peritonitis or of a spinal fracture) may be so severe that the symptoms of an ileus are trivial and difficult to identify.

The typical pain of an ileus is in the center of the abdomen and is constant. The person may have nausea and vomiting and have no appetite for food. The abdomen of a person with an ileus will appear distended because of the accumulation of fluid and gas in the intestine.

## MAKING THE DIAGNOSIS OF ILEUS

### How is the diagnosis of an ileus made?

In contrast to mechanical intestinal obstruction (see chapter entitled "Intestinal Obstruction") with its very active gurgling bowel sounds, a physician putting a stethoscope to the abdomen of a person with an ileus will generally hear little or nothing in the way of bowel sounds.

In the context of a person who has just had surgery, the diagnosis of ileus is extremely common and further evaluation is generally not required. If the symptoms are not clearing after a few days, physicians may perform a CT scan of the abdomen to see whether a mechanical obstruction has developed, or to look for signs of an infection inside the abdomen that is perpetuating the ileus.

## TREATMENT OF ILEUS

### What is the treatment of an ileus?

Most of the time, the ileus resolves when the underlying cause of the ileus is successfully treated, or is relieved with the passage of time. If the abdomen is very distended and the person is frequently vomiting, suction through a nasogastric tube or through a long tube put down from the nose to the stomach to the small intestine, can reduce the pressure of fluid and gas in the intestine and encourage the intestine to start contracting normally again. A low level of potassium in the bloodstream ("hypokalemia") can worsen ileus. If the potassium level in the blood is low, adding potassium to the intravenous fluid normalizes the level of potassium in the bloodstream.

### Are there medicines that encourage the ileus to resolve more quickly?

The medicine "Entereg" given before and after an operation can, to some extent, lessen the risk that ileus will cause major symptoms which keep the person in the hospital for a longer period.

# <u>OUTLOOK</u>

*What is the outlook for recovery after an ileus?*

The outlook for recovery will depend largely upon recovery from the illness that caused the ileus. In general, odds of recovery from an ileus are very good. People will usually recover from their ileus without lasting problems with their intestinal system.

# INTESTINAL OBSTRUCTION

## DEFINITIONS

### What is intestinal obstruction?

Food normally passes from the mouth to the stomach, then to the duodenum to the small intestine to the large intestine to the rectum to the anus to the outside world. When a person has "intestinal obstruction", it means that the normal passage of material through the bowels has been blocked somewhere between the duodenum and the anus. Most of the time, this obstruction is in the small intestine, in either the "jejunum" which is the part of the small intestine that immediately follows the "duodenum", or in the "ileum" which follows the jejunum.

## THE CAUSES OF INTESTINAL OBSTRUCTION

### When a person has intestinal obstruction, what is it that is obstructing the intestine?

Two major categories of problems cause intestinal obstruction.

"Mechanical obstruction" means that the inside of the intestine (called the "lumen") is physically blocked. This can occur either because something that is on the outside of the intestine is compressing it (this is more common), or because something growing inside the intestine itself is obstructing it.

"Non-mechanical obstruction" means that the intestine is not propelling its contents forward in a normal manner and that this lack of forward movement creates what amounts to an obstruction of the intestine. The technical word for a non-mechanical obstruction is an "ileus".

This chapter only discusses mechanical intestinal obstruction. The next chapter discusses non-mechanical intestinal obstruction, that is, ileus.

## SYMPTOMS

### What are the symptoms of mechanical intestinal obstruction?

The most common first symptom of mechanical intestinal obstruction is severe pain in the middle of the abdomen. This pain comes and goes, with the person having intense pain, followed by relative comfort, followed by more intense pain, then comfort, and so on. During the painful periods, the person may hear loud gurgles coming from the abdomen. Nausea and vomiting, with the vomit sometimes smelling quite foul, are other major symptoms in most people with mechanical intestinal obstruction.

As time goes by, the pain of mechanical intestinal obstruction may actually diminish or may change in character so that whereas, at first, the pain came and went, the pain becomes steady. This change in the character of the pain may be a sign of severe damage to the intestine and of severe danger to life, unless appropriate and prompt medical treatment is given.

## CAUSES OF MECHANICAL INTESTINAL OBSTRUCTION IN PEOPLE WITH CANCER

*What are the most common causes of mechanical intestinal obstruction in people with cancer?*

The most common causes of mechanical intestinal obstruction in people with cancer are the cancer itself or "adhesions". A less common cause in people with cancer, but more common in people without cancer, is obstruction causes by a "hernia".

Cancer can obstruct the intestine either by growing inside the intestine, which can occur in colon cancer or, more commonly, because of the growth of cancer outside of the intestine. Advanced cancers, such as cancer of the stomach, colon, ovary, or breast can produce large masses of cancer in the abdomen that can compress and obstruct the intestine.

"Adhesions" are bands of fibrous tissue that form inside the abdomen. In some instances, these adhesions have been nicknamed "fiddle-string adhesions" because of their resemblance to the strings of a fiddle. Adhesions occur in people who, at some time in the past, have had an episode of severe inflammation, such as through surgery or peritonitis, inside the abdominal cavity. These adhesions can wrap themselves around the intestine and tie off the intestine obstructing the flow of material through it.

A "hernia" which causes mechanical intestinal obstruction is an abnormal opening in the abdominal wall into which intestine can wedge itself, obstructing the flow of intestinal contents. The most common area for hernia is in the groin. People who have had surgery in the past may also have an opening in their abdominal wall in the line of the scar of an old incision (this is an "incisional hernia") into which intestine can be stuck.

## MAKING THE DIAGNOSIS OF MECHANICAL INTESTINAL OBSTRUCTION

*How is the diagnosis of mechanical intestinal obstruction made?*

The symptoms which a person reports will raise the first suspicion of mechanical intestinal obstruction. Physical examination usually shows a distended abdomen. With a stethoscope, loud, high-pitched gurgling sounds are often heard when the person is feeling the severe pain.

Plain x-rays of the abdomen may show distension of the intestines with fluid and air. This will create an appearance on x-ray of "air-fluid levels" which is characteristic of intestinal obstruction. Most of the time, a person's symptoms, as well as the appearance of the x-rays of the abdomen will be sufficient to make the diagnosis of intestinal obstruction.

A CT scan, especially in people with cancer, can give more precise information about the location and cause of the intestinal obstruction, and can better identify obstruction that requires emergency surgery.

# COMPLICATIONS OF MECHANICAL INTESTINAL OBSTRUCTION

*Why is mechanical intestinal obstruction dangerous?*

There are two major dangers with mechanical intestinal obstruction: loss of fluid and electrolytes, and damage to the intestinal wall.

When the intestine obstructs, fluid and gas will collect in the area of the intestine in front of the obstruction. Because of an unfortunate physiologic reflex, a tremendous amount of fluid leaks out of the body's circulatory system and into the already distended intestine. Additional bodily fluid is lost through vomiting. This loss of fluid can drop the blood pressure. A form of kidney failure called "pre-renal azotemia" (see chapter entitled "Acute Kidney Injury") can develop because of the low blood pressure.

As fluid and gas accumulates in the intestine, the intestine blows up like an elongated balloon. Pressure inside the intestine grows and grows until a point at which blood supply to the wall of the intestine is impaired. This lack of blood supply can cause irreversible damage to the wall of the intestine.

An important and common cause of damage to the intestine in people with mechanical intestinal obstruction is "strangulation", which occurs when the intestine is stuck in a hernia or in an adhesion and the blood supply to that portion of the intestine is completely shut off. This "strangulated obstruction" will cause irreversible damage to the area of the intestine deprived of blood supply. Irreversibly damaged intestine can leak bacteria or intestinal contents into the abdominal cavity and cause a severe inflammation in the abdomen (called "peritonitis") and sepsis (see chapter entitled "Sepsis and Septic Shock").

## TREATMENT OF MECHANICAL INTESTINAL OBSTRUCTION

### *What is the immediate treatment of mechanical intestinal obstruction?*

If there is evidence of significant loss of fluid or potassium from the bloodstream, intravenous replacement will be necessary. If the blood pressure is very low, large amounts of fluid injected rapidly can bring the blood pressure back up. In extreme circumstances, medicines to restore adequate blood pressure such as "dopamine" may be necessary.

High pressure and distension in the intestine is somewhat relieved by putting a tube down the nose and into the stomach, (this tube is a "nasogastric" or "NG" tube) and sucking out the excess fluid and air.

The medication "octreotide" (brand name is "Sandostatin", manufacturer's product website is www.sandostatin.com), given by injection, reduces fluid secretion into the intestine, while, at the same time, helping to slow movement of material through the intestine. This can reduce the nausea and pain associated with intestinal obstruction.

In the context of advanced cancer, treatment decisions take into account the risks and discomforts of surgery to relieve the obstruction, as well as the risks of attempting to treat the obstruction with fluid replacement, NG tube suctioning, and medications.

*If surgery appears to be necessary, how long will physicians generally wait before performing an operation to relieve the obstruction?*

In general, if there is a strangulated obstruction of the intestine, the more quickly the person gets to the operating room, the better the outlook. When possible, surgical intervention to clear the obstruction within 12-24 hours of admission to the hospital is associated with an improved outlook. Prior to getting to the operating room, physicians will do their best, over a period of a few hours, to restore some of the body fluid and potassium that is so commonly lost because of vomiting.

If the obstruction does not appear to be strangulated, it may be possible to hold off on the operation for a while, support the person with intravenous fluids and NG tube suction, and see if the obstruction clears on its own.

Intestinal obstruction in people with cancer is a very serious and life-threatening complication. Both the decision to operate and the decision to attempt to treat the intestinal obstruction without an operation carry significant risks.

*What kind of operation relieves a mechanical intestinal obstruction?*

Just prior to taking a person to the operating room, physicians will commonly give an intravenous dose of an antibiotic to suppress or kill dangerous bacteria that may be growing in the intestine.

The type of operation done to relieve a mechanical intestinal obstruction will depend on the nature of the obstruction.

When adhesions obstruct the intestine, cutting the adhesions and freeing the intestine can relieve the obstruction. When possible, the surgeon can perform this operation using "laparoscopy". Laparoscopy allows a surgeon to examine the inside of the abdomen and cut adhesions that are obstructing the intestine without performing a major operation. Surgeons insert the instrument used, a "laparoscope", into the abdomen through incisions of less than an inch in length. The surgeon directs the instrument through the various parts of the inside of the abdomen and examines it through images projected to a video monitor. Using instruments inserted through the laparoscope, a surgeon will cut or otherwise eliminate adhesions obstructing the intestine.

If solid masses of cancer are the cause of the obstruction, the surgeon will attempt to remove the areas of cancer that are causing the obstruction or release the intestine from its grip.

The surgeon will examine the intestine, and remove irreversibly damaged areas.

## What treatment continues after the operation is over?

After the operation, the person will continue to receive intravenous fluids and will commonly receive antibiotics to prevent bacteria released from the intestine during the operation from growing in the bloodstream. For several days after the operation, the intestines will not have their usual peristalsis (see discussion in the chapter entitled "Ileus") and there may be some continued distension of the intestine. For this reason, suction with a nasogastric tube often continues for several days after the operation.

## ENTERAL STENTS

### What are enteral stents?

Enteral stents are metallic or plastic tube-shaped devices that can prop open an obstructed segment in the stomach, small intestine, or large intestine. Enteral stents are inserted in the radiology department with guidance of "fluoroscopy", which allows the physician to see moving images of the catheters, guide wires and balloons used to find the obstruction, get across the obstruction, and insert the stent.

### When are enteral stents most useful?

Although an operation to eliminate the cause of the obstruction may be the most effective treatment, it can be impractical if someone has advanced cancer or another serious disease that causes a major operation to have a high risk for life-threatening complications, or for a slow and painful recovery. A stent across the obstruction can be a very effective alternative to open up the obstructed area, relieve symptoms, and prevent fatal complications of the intestinal obstruction.

# BLOOD CLOTS IN DANGEROUS PLACES

# ACUTE DISSEMINATED INTRAVASCULAR COAGULATION

## DEFINITIONS

### *What is coagulation?*

Coagulation is the process by which blood clots form to stop bleeding from injured blood vessels.

### *How does coagulation occur?*

In good health, when a blood vessel is cut or otherwise injured and is leaking blood, a component of the blood called "platelets" stick together at the site of the injury and form a temporary plug which stops the bleeding. This initial plug is a very loose one, and requires additional strengthening.

The strengthening of the plug that permanently stops the bleeding requires production of "fibrin", which is a tough protein that is the major component of a good, firm blood clot. Production of fibrin is dependent upon a series of events called a "coagulation cascade", in which the damage to the blood vessel triggers a sequence of chemical reactions involving sequential activation of "coagulation factors" that, at the end, produce fibrin and a good healthy blood clot.

### What is acute disseminated intravascular coagulation?

When a person is critically ill or injured, incorrect signals, sent throughout the body, tell blood to coagulate. This causes small blood clots to develop throughout the circulatory system, abnormally plugging small blood vessels and consuming the platelets and coagulation factors blood needs to form clots. This depletion of platelets and coagulation factors makes a person extremely susceptible to sudden and life-threatening internal bleeding. At the same time, blood clots can form in the small arteries feeding the kidney, leading to kidney failure.

## SYMPTOMS

### What symptoms or other observations lead to the suspicion that a person has acute disseminated intravascular coagulation?

People with cancer who develop acute disseminated intravascular coagulation are usually in the hospital because of a serious illness such as sepsis (see chapter "Sepsis and Septic Shock"), or have recently undergone major surgery.

A first sign of acute disseminated intravascular coagulation may be bleeding around intravenous catheters or from surgical or other traumatic wounds. Bleeding may occur under the skin and appear as large purple-colored blotches. Sudden, life-threatening bleeding can also occur in the gastrointestinal tract and manifest as vomiting of bright red blood or the passage of blood in the stool. Bleeding in or around the brain can occur (see chapter "Brain Hemorrhage: Intracerebral Hemorrhage"). Bleeding in the lung can cause a person to spit up blood.

Small blood clots and deposits of fibrin can develop in the bloodstream and travel to the arteries of the kidney, lung, liver and brain. This can block the normal blood flow to these vital organs causing serious injury.

Fibrin, the tough protein that forms because of the coagulation cascade, can form sharp bands in the circulatory system that can slice up red blood cells that are passing by. This destruction of red blood cells will cause a type of anemia called "hemolytic anemia". The release of a substance called "bilirubin" from the damaged red blood cells into the bloodstream can cause a person's skin to appear yellow, indicating that the person has jaundice.

## MAKING THE DIAGNOSIS

*How is the diagnosis of acute disseminated intravascular coagulation made?*

Physical examination as well as blood tests reflecting abnormalities of the blood's coagulation ability makes the diagnosis of acute disseminated intravascular coagulation. A particularly important blood test looks for "fibrin degradation products", whose level is usually elevated in the presence of acute disseminated intravascular coagulation.

## TREATMENT

### *What is the treatment of acute disseminated intravascular coagulation?*

The treatment of acute disseminated intravascular coagulation is to treat the underlying cause and to provide supportive care for the life-threatening complications that may develop. If the underlying disease driving acute disseminated intravascular coagulation is treated, the abnormal consumption of coagulation factors can stop, with resolution of the condition.

When there is severe bleeding and evidence of major consumption of coagulation factors and platelets, emergency replacement of these essential clotting factors with infusions of platelets, "fresh frozen plasma", and "cryoprecipitate" can help control or prevent further bleeding.

Current available medications do not appear to accelerate recovery from acute disseminated intravascular coagulation.

## OUTLOOK

### *What is the outlook for a person with acute disseminated intravascular coagulation?*

The outlook for survival from acute disseminated intravascular coagulation depends upon the severity of the underlying disease or injury and the person's age. If the cause of the disseminated intravascular coagulation is sepsis or septic shock, the outlook for survival depends upon how rapidly the underlying illness is controlled. Depending on these factors, the likelihood for survival can cover a broad range, from a high likelihood of survival to a high likelihood that the episode of disseminated intravascular coagulation proves fatal.

# ACUTE MESENTERIC ISCHEMIA

## DEFINITION

### What is acute mesenteric ischemia?

The mesenteric arteries are responsible for delivery of blood to the intestines. Acute mesenteric ischemia means that an inadequate flow of blood through one or more of the major mesenteric arteries is causing injury to the intestines.

Lack of blood supply to any organ produces a type of early organ injury called "ischemia". If tissue remains without adequate blood supply, "infarction", that is, death of the tissue will result.

### Why is acute mesenteric ischemia dangerous?

Acute mesenteric ischemia can damage the wall of the intestine and allow dangerous bacteria and toxins to get into the bloodstream. In addition, damage to the wall of the intestine can perforate it, causing intestinal contents, including bacteria, to leak out of the intestine and into the abdomen. Bowel perforation produces a highly dangerous inflammation and infection inside the abdomen called "peritonitis".

# THE CAUSE OF MESENTERIC ISCHEMIA

## What causes acute mesenteric ischemia?

The most common cause of acute mesenteric ischemia is a blood clot that is blocking the flow of blood through the "superior mesenteric artery". The superior mesenteric artery has major responsibility for the blood supply of the entire small intestine and for over half of the large intestine.

Low blood pressure, usually in the context of another critical illness, can diminish the flow of blood through the mesenteric arteries, and, by doing so, cause mesenteric ischemia. In elderly people with already compromised blood flow because of narrowed atherosclerotic arteries, this reduction of blood flow can be sufficient to trigger acute mesenteric ischemia.

## What types of blood clots can block the mesenteric arteries?

The two types of blood clots that block mesenteric arteries are an "embolus" and a "thrombosis". An "embolus" is a blood clot that travels through the bloodstream and lodges in an artery elsewhere in the body. The superior mesenteric artery, because of its size and location, is prone to catching blood clots that arise in the heart and travel downstream. The most common cause of acute mesenteric ischemia is an embolus into the superior mesenteric artery.

A "thrombus" is a clot that develops in a blood vessel that can block the flow of blood through that blood vessel. A thrombus can develop in a mesenteric artery, block its blood flow, and cause mesenteric ischemia.

### *In people with cancer, what is a common source of the blockage of an artery delivering blood to the intestine?*

Most commonly, an embolism causes the blockage. This embolism often arises in the heart because of a condition called "nonbacterial thrombotic endocarditis".

### *What is nonbacterial thrombotic endocarditis?*

Nonbacterial thrombotic endocarditis means that small, fragile growths called "vegetations" have developed on the heart valves. Most commonly, this occurs in the setting of advanced cancer. These vegetations can easily break off the valve and float into blood vessels feeding the brain, heart, kidneys or intestines.

## SYMPTOMS

### *What are the symptoms of acute mesenteric ischemia?*

The symptoms depend upon the cause of the acute mesenteric ischemia.

An embolus to the mesenteric arteries will usually cause sudden severe pain throughout the abdomen. A thrombus in the mesenteric arteries produces the same type of pain, although the onset is a bit slower. The pain is usually associated with nausea and vomiting.

When acute mesenteric ischemia is a complication of low blood pressure (and not of a blocked artery), the symptoms can be milder and can be obscured by the other major medical problems which are causing the low blood pressure.

## MAKING THE DIAGNOSIS

*How is the diagnosis of acute mesenteric ischemia made?*

Acute mesenteric ischemia caused by an embolus or thrombus that is blocking an artery can be diagnosed with an "angiogram". To do this, a radiologist will advance a catheter through an artery in the groin, or the arm, and into the area of the aorta from which the mesenteric arteries originate. The radiologist will then give an injection of a special dye that can very clearly identify any obstruction that exists in the mesenteric arteries. Newer forms of the angiogram that are easier and safer to perform using CT and MRI scans have become available which may eventually replace the older, more conventional forms of angiography.

Acute mesenteric ischemia caused by low blood pressure can be very difficult to diagnose, although the angiogram can give some information about areas of the intestine to which blood flow seems to be inadequate. Abdominal pain and the rigidity of the abdominal wall seen with peritonitis that may develop, raises the suspicion of mesenteric ischemia in a person with a very low blood pressure.

## TREATMENT

*What treatment can begin when it appears that a person has acute mesenteric ischemia?*

Acute mesenteric ischemia can cause the blood pressure to drop to dangerously low levels. The physician will monitor blood pressure very closely and give fluid or medications as needed to keep the blood pressure in the normal range. Monitoring a person's output of urine will give the physician information regarding the adequacy of blood flow to the kidneys.

A tube passed from the nose into the stomach (a "nasogastric tube") can pull air and liquid out of the stomach and relieve some of the bloating and pressure in the abdomen.

Because damaged, ischemic intestine can leak bacteria into the bloodstream, or into the inside of the abdomen, physicians will commonly prescribe intravenous antibiotics to kill bacteria that may be leaking out of the intestine.

### How is an embolus in the mesenteric arteries treated?

An operation called an "embolectomy" can remove the embolus from the blocked mesenteric arteries. The surgeon will also remove any area of intestine that appears irreversibly damaged and sew the remaining normal healthy ends back together. This will restore the continuity of the intestine.

A medicine called "papaverine", which relieves spasm of arteries, may be used to help improve blood flow to the intestines.

In some medical centers, when an angiography identifies an embolus, and severe damage to the intestine requiring surgical repair is not present, injection of a "thrombolytic agent", which is a medicine that could break up the clot, is given. This treatment can be effective in breaking up the clot and restoring blood flow to the intestines.

## What is the treatment of a thrombus causing acute mesenteric ischemia?

The treatment of a thrombus in the mesenteric arteries is very similar to the treatment of an embolus in the mesenteric arteries. Because the thrombus may develop on a bed of severe atherosclerosis and narrowing in the artery, it may be possible to insert a "stent" into the artery that props it open, allowing blood to resume its flow.

## What is the treatment of acute mesenteric ischemia caused by low blood pressure?

The treatment of acute mesenteric ischemia caused by low blood pressure is to bring the blood pressure back up with fluid and medication. If there is evidence that the intestine has sustained significant damage, an operation to repair the damaged intestine will be necessary.

## OUTLOOK

## What is the outlook for a person who has acute mesenteric ischemia?

The outlook depends upon the speed with which the diagnosis was made and treatment begun. Other major factors that effect odds of recovery are the person's age (the younger, the better) and the person's underlying health at the time the acute mesenteric ischemia developed. Even under the best of circumstances, acute mesenteric ischemia is extremely dangerous and life-threatening.

# DEEP VEIN THROMBOSIS AND PULMONARY EMBOLISM

## DEFINITIONS

### What is a deep vein thrombosis?

Deep vein thrombosis is a blood clot that develops in veins that are deep within the body, often in the legs or pelvis, and, less commonly, in other areas of the body. The development of deep vein thrombosis is particularly common in people with cancer.

### What is a pulmonary embolism?

A pulmonary embolism is a blood clot that has traveled through the bloodstream from the vein in which it originated, and that has wedged into, and blocked an artery in the lung.

### Where does the pulmonary embolism usually come from?

Most of the time, the embolus arises from a large blood clot (the blood clot is a "thrombus") in the leg between the knee and the hip. A piece of the thrombus breaks loose, travels up the inferior vena cava (the "inferior vena cava" is the major vein in the abdomen), into the right side of the heart, and is pumped into the pulmonary arteries delivering blood to the lung.

## DEEP VEIN THROMBOSIS AND PULMONARY EMBOLISM AND CANCER

*Why is deep vein thrombosis and pulmonary embolism so common in people with cancer?*

Three factors, commonly known as "Virchow's triad", are the major causes of deep vein thrombosis and pulmonary embolism. These three factors are changes in the consistency of the blood such that it clots more easily, abnormalities or impediments to the normal flow of blood through the veins, and injury to the inner lining (called the "endothelium") of the veins. Cancer affects each of these components of the triad, leading to a much higher risk of developing deep vein thrombosis and pulmonary embolism.

Cancer cells release substances into the bloodstream, and induce normal cells to release substances into the bloodstream, that can cause the blood to clot more easily. These substances are "pro-coagulant" or "pro-thrombotic" factors, and induce "cancer-associated hypercoagulability".

Bed rest or limited mobility, can slow the flow of blood through the veins of the legs and cause "venous stasis", which is, slowing of blood flow through the veins. The growth of cancer in the abdomen or pelvis can compress veins draining the legs, slowing the movement of blood upstream from the legs to the major veins returning blood to the heart. This "venous stasis" greatly increases the risk of deep vein thrombosis and pulmonary embolism.

The various forms of cancer treatment can injure the lining of blood vessels, increasing the risk of clots developing within them.

## DETECTION OF DEEP VEIN THROMBOSIS

### *What are the symptoms of deep vein thrombosis?*

Often, the deep vein thrombosis produces no symptoms. If the deep vein thrombosis produces symptoms, it reflects the blockage of the vein in which it is located along with some local inflammation. Since most of the time the deep vein thrombosis involves the deep veins of the leg, it is often associated with pain and swelling of the leg. If a pulmonary embolism develops because of the deep vein thrombosis, chest pain and shortness of breath, as described later in this chapter, can develop.

### *How do physicians and medical professional make the diagnosis of a deep vein thrombosis?*

The most common test used to detect a deep vein thrombosis is a test called "duplex ultrasound imaging" in which, sound waves bounced off the legs generates images of the leg veins which can be evaluated by physicians and ultrasound technicians. These images can show clear evidence of deep vein thrombosis in leg veins. In circumstances in which duplex ultrasound imaging yields uncertain results, physicians may recommend an MRI scan of the area suspected of having a deep vein thrombosis. The MRI scan can be especially useful in identifying blood clots involving the deep veins of the pelvis or the large vein in the abdomen called the "inferior vena cava".

## SYMPTOMS OF PULMONARY EMBOLISM

*What are the symptoms of pulmonary embolism?*

When a person develops a pulmonary embolism there usually is sudden, severe shortness of breath associated with pain in the chest area. Blood pressure can fall and the person may feel dizzy and faint. Because many medical problems other than a pulmonary embolism can produce identical symptoms, a number of tests will be necessary to establish the diagnosis.

## MAKING THE DIAGNOSIS OF A PULMONARY EMBOLISM

*When pulmonary embolism is a possibility, what can physicians do to assess whether the likelihood is high or low that a pulmonary embolism has occurred?*

There is a numerical measure, called the "Modified Wells Criteria" which assigns a person a "score" indicating a high, low, or moderate probability that a pulmonary embolism has occurred. This scale takes into consideration symptoms suggestive of a blood clot in the veins of the leg or pelvis such as a painful or swollen leg, the lack of other likely reasons for a person's symptoms, a history of predisposing factors, the heart rate, and the presence or absence of a history of spitting up blood. If the score is high, the likelihood is high. If the score is low, the likelihood is low.

## What is the blood test called the "d-dimer" test?

D-dimer is a substance derived from blood clots that is generally elevated in the bloodstream if a person has a pulmonary embolism. Because many other conditions can cause d-dimer elevation in the bloodstream when a person is seriously ill, an elevated d-dimer level does not alone make the diagnosis of a pulmonary embolism. Because of this, if the person appears to have a moderate or high likelihood of having a pulmonary embolism, physicians will generally proceed rapidly to the more definitive testing described below without waiting for the results of a d-dimer test.

When the person appears to have a low likelihood of having a pulmonary embolism and the d-dimer concentration in the bloodstream is not elevated, it is very unlikely that a pulmonary embolism has occurred.

## How is the certain diagnosis of pulmonary embolism made?

The most helpful test for a pulmonary embolism is a specialized type of CT scan called a "multidetector CT" along with the injection of a "contrast material" which enables physicians to examine the arteries feeding into the lungs for abnormalities consistent with blockage of blood flow. An "ultrasound examination", using harmless sound waves, scans the legs for evidence of a source of blood clots that may have travelled to the lung.

In some medical centers, and especially in smaller community hospitals, the sophisticated multidetector CT scanner is not available. In addition, some people are allergic to the "contrast material" required by the CT scan to detect evidence of a pulmonary embolus, or have serious kidney disease that can limit the use of contrast material. In this case, a type of lung scan, called a "ventilation-perfusion scan" can be done in which radioactive material is inhaled and radioactive material is intravenously injected. Normally, radioactive material that is inhaled or injected will distribute relatively evenly through the lungs from top to bottom. When an artery, or when several arteries of one or both lungs are blocked, portions of one or both lungs will not pick up the radioactive material and will appear to the radiologist as "defects" suggestive of a pulmonary embolism.

There are times, now relatively uncommon, when symptoms, laboratory tests, multidetector CT and ventilation-perfusion scans are all suggestive of a pulmonary embolism, but the diagnosis remains in doubt. The most precise method available to diagnose a pulmonary embolism is a pulmonary angiogram. To perform this test, a radiologist will advance a catheter from an arm or groin vein, to the major vein leading to the right side of the heart and into the pulmonary arteries. The catheter goes with the flow, so it is usually easy for the radiologist to get the catheter into the pulmonary arteries. When the catheter arrives at the pulmonary arteries, the radiologist's dye, injected into the pulmonary arteries, will not be able to get into blocked branches, confirming the diagnosis of pulmonary embolism.

## COMPLICATIONS OF PULMONARY EMBOLISM

### *Why is a pulmonary embolism dangerous?*

In our circulatory system, blood from the veins throughout our body flows into the "superior vena cava" and "inferior vena cava" and, from there, to the heart, into the right atrium, that then pumps the blood to the right ventricle. The right ventricle then pumps the blood into the "pulmonary arteries" which deliver our blood to the lungs to receive oxygen. The bright red blood, full of oxygen, is then returned to the heart from the lungs, into the left atrium from which it is pumped into the left ventricle and then to the entire body. Separating the right and left ventricle is an area of tissue called the "interventricular septum" which normally remains in its fixed location with each heartbeat.

The most important function of the lungs is to provide a continuous supply of oxygen to the blood. In order for blood to pick up oxygen, it must flow into the lung, pick up oxygen and flow out again. When a pulmonary embolism blocks blood flow into a large portion of one or both lungs, the amount of oxygen in the bloodstream will drop.

A shower of emboli (blood clots can break into pieces) to both lungs, or a huge embolus that sits in an anatomic saddle astride the large arteries leading to both lungs, can block blood flow into the lungs and put a great deal of strain on the right ventricle. As the right ventricle tries to pump blood past the obstruction, the pressure inside of its chamber can rise dangerously and cause the "interventricular septum" to bulge into the left ventricle. This can compromise the ability of the left ventricle to fill properly with blood, dramatically reducing the amount of blood pumped with each heartbeat to the rest of the body. The combined effect of this can be sudden severe heart failure and sudden death.

# TREATMENT

*What immediate steps will physicians or emergency medical professionals take when a person appears to have had a pulmonary embolism?*

"ABC" is the abbreviation for airway, breathing, and circulation. In every medical emergency, and a major pulmonary embolism is definitely a medical emergency, proper movement of air in and out of the lungs and proper blood circulation must be maintained.

The "A" is the airway and the "B" is for breathing. In the context of pulmonary embolism, the airway is clear and the person is rapidly breathing, but an insufficient amount of oxygen is getting into the bloodstream. Supplemental oxygen is given.

The "C" stands for circulation that must be maintained for life to continue. If the blood pressure is far too low as a consequence of the severe heart failure that can follow a pulmonary embolism, medication and fluids can be administered which can help to bring the blood pressure up to a much safer level.

## *What is anticoagulation?*

Anticoagulation is treatment to prevent the formation of new clots that have the capability of traveling to the lung. Although anticoagulation can also prevent expansion of a clot that has already traveled to the lung, it does not have the ability to break apart that clot.

*What medicines provide anticoagulation when a person has deep vein thrombosis or pulmonary embolism?*

The medicine used to provide immediate anticoagulation to a person who has deep vein thrombosis or pulmonary embolism is a form of heparin. Most commonly, this heparin will be in the category of a "low molecular weight heparin" which, given intravenously, provides anticoagulation within minutes after intravenous injection.

After the first couple of days of heparin treatment, physicians may prescribe different anticoagulants depending on whether or not the cancer is in complete remission at the time the deep vein thrombosis or pulmonary embolism developed.

If the deep vein thrombosis or pulmonary embolism do not appear to be related to the presence of an active cancer, after a couple of days or so of heparin treatment, an oral medicine from the family of medicines that are known as "vitamin K antagonists" such as "Coumadin" may be initiated. It takes several days for the Coumadin to provide effective anticoagulation. The adequacy of the anticoagulation achieved by Coumadin is determined by a blood test that measures the "international normalized ratio", abbreviated as "INR", which, once it is in the range of 2.0 to 3.0, indicates that a person is properly anticoagulated. Once a person has reached the proper INR range, treatment with Coumadin alone will continue.

In the presence of an active cancer, coumadin is not as effective as heparin in preventing recurrence of a deep vein thrombosis or pulmonary embolism. If cancer is still evident, or if a person who has had a deep vein thrombosis or pulmonary embolism is receiving chemotherapy, physicians will often prescribe a form of heparin, usually "low molecular weight heparin", as a daily injection for six months or longer.

### Is there anything that can break apart or remove the clot that is blocking the flow of blood into the pulmonary arteries feeding the lung?

When a person's blood pressure is very low, or if a person has severe heart failure, physicians may attempt to use thrombolytic medicines (see the description of thrombolytic therapy in the chapter entitled "Heart Attack: Acute Myocardial Infarction") which may help dissolve a large, life-threatening pulmonary embolism. There is a small but significant risk of developing dangerous internal bleeding with thrombolytic medicines. Thrombolytic medicines can, however, be dramatically life saving when a person has had a huge pulmonary embolism which is causing a major blockage of circulation of blood to the lungs, and dangerously low blood pressure or heart failure.

### Can surgery remove a major pulmonary embolism?

Surgical removal of a pulmonary embolism is an "embolectomy". This is a very difficult operation with a high potential for complications and is performed in large medical centers with sophisticated cardiac surgery capabilities. Because of the risks associated with embolectomy, it is reserved for people who have failed to respond to thrombolytic therapy, or who cannot safely be given thrombolytic therapy, and whose lives are in immediate jeopardy because of the pulmonary embolism.

## RISKS OF ANTICOAGULANT TREATMENT

### *What are the risks of anticoagulant treatment?*

A person receiving anticoagulant medicines is at risk for developing serious internal bleeding. Bleeding into the stomach or intestines is usually controllable. Bleeding into the brain can cause serious and occasionally lethal brain damage. For this reason, blood tests may be done at regular intervals to monitor the degree to which the blood is anticoagulated, and to make sure that excessive anticoagulation has not inadvertently occurred.

### *Are there contraindications to anticoagulant treatment?*

A recent episode of serious internal bleeding may be a contraindication to anticoagulant treatment.

## WHEN ANTICOAGULANT TREATMENT IS CONTRAINDICATED

### *What is the treatment when anticoagulant treatment is not safe, or not adequately effective?*

There are tiny filtering devices (sometimes called an "umbrella"), inserted by a surgeon or a radiologist into the inferior vena cava, that can catch an embolism that is travelling from the leg through the vena cava before it reaches the lung. Insertion of one of these devices is a useful treatment when anticoagulant therapy is contraindicated, or when a person appears to be having additional pulmonary emboli despite anticoagulant treatment.

## OUTLOOK

### What is the outlook for someone who has had a pulmonary embolism?

Most deaths from pulmonary embolism are a result of a massive pulmonary embolism that is lethal within 24 hours of the onset of symptoms.

With prompt diagnosis and treatment, odds in favor of surviving a pulmonary embolism and returning to the prior state of health are very high. The concern that remains is that of recurrence of deep vein thrombosis and having another pulmonary embolism.

## DVT PROPHYLAXIS

### What puts a person at risk of recurrence of a pulmonary embolism or deep vein thrombosis?

Any hospitalization or surgical procedure or illness that requires a person to remain in bed or have limiting mobility for an extended period is associated with a higher risk of deep vein thrombosis and pulmonary embolism. Because of this, hospitalized people with cancer are often given a form of heparin. The administration of an anticoagulant to prevent development of blood clots in the deep veins of the legs or pelvis is called "deep vein thrombosis prophylaxis" or "DVT prophylaxis". DVT prophylaxis, when required, will strongly reduce the risk of a dangerous blood clot developing in the legs or elsewhere.

*Should everyone with cancer receive DVT prophylaxis,
even without ever having had a deep vein
thrombosis or pulmonary embolus?*

At this time, the major groups of experts who have reviewed this question have recommended against routine anticoagulation, unless a person has previously had a deep vein thrombosis or pulmonary embolism or is considered to be "non-ambulatory", that is, unable to walk around sufficiently to prevent venous stasis in the legs.

# ISCHEMIC STROKE

## <u>DEFINITIONS</u>

### *What is an ischemic stroke?*

An ischemic stroke is a sudden loss of neurologic function caused by lack of normal blood flow to the brain. The severity of an ischemic stroke can vary from minor, hardly detectable symptoms to massive loss of neurologic function leading up to irreversible coma, or death.

## <u>HOW AN ISCHEMIC STROKE DEVELOPS</u>

### *What causes an ischemic stroke?*

The entire brain needs an uninterrupted flow of oxygen-rich arterial blood in order to remain healthy and alive. When there is interruption of the blood supply to an area of the brain, the deprived area of the brain will almost immediately stop functioning. If the area of the brain lacks blood supply for more than a few minutes, there can be irreversible damage. This irreversible brain damage is an ischemic stroke.

## Where does the blood supply of the brain come from?

Four major arteries carry oxygen-rich arterial blood from the heart to the brain. These large arteries–the left and right internal carotid arteries in the front of the neck and the left and right vertebral arteries in the back of the neck–travel up the neck, through the bottom of the skull and into the brain. The carotid and vertebral arteries and the arteries that branch off from them are responsible for feeding blood to the brain.

## If a brain artery is blocked, does the area of the brain it feeds always die?

Each artery in the brain has the job of supplying blood to a specific area of the brain. There is, however, some overlap such that more than one artery may be able to supply blood to a particular area of the brain. This overlap in blood supply to areas of the brain is "collateral circulation". Collateral circulation can be life saving if there is a block to blood flow through an artery in the brain.

## What is it that blocks the arteries of the brain and causes strokes?

When an artery of the brain is blocked, it is usually by a blood clot. These clots come in two different forms: "a therothrombosis" and a "thromboembolus". There are important differences between an atherothrombosis and a thromboembolus in both treatment and outlook.

Atherothrombosis is a blood clot that forms on top of an area of narrowing in an artery. As a person ages, and particularly if a person has high blood pressure or diabetes, a fatty material is driven into the walls of arteries. As the wall of the artery bulks up with this material, the channel in the center of the artery through which blood flows becomes narrow. In a healthy person, blood flows smoothly through the artery. When hardening of the artery narrows the arterial channel, blood flows turbulently through the artery. When blood is agitated like this, clots can form in the area of turbulent blood flow and plug the arterial channel shut. This is an "atherothrombosis".

A "thromboembolus", often abbreviated as an "embolus" or "embolism", is a blood clot that travels through the bloodstream from one area of the body to another and lands in an artery and plugs it shut. The embolus that travels to an artery in the brain, causing an ischemic stroke, usually began in the heart, broke loose, and traveled up into the head. People with some forms of heart disease are at risk for developing clots within the heart that can break loose and travel up into the circulation of the brain. These travelling clots are dangerous wherever they may travel and when they travel to the brain, they cause strokes.

### In people with cancer, what is the most common cause of blockage of an artery delivering blood to the brain?

Most commonly, an embolism causes the blockage. This embolism often arises in the heart because of a condition called "nonbacterial thrombotic endocarditis".

### What is nonbacterial thrombotic endocarditis?

Nonbacterial thrombotic endocarditis means that small, fragile growths called "vegetations" have developed on the heart valves.

Most commonly, this occurs in the setting of advanced cancer. These vegetations can easily break off the valve and float up into the brain or into blood vessels feeding the heart, kidneys or intestines.

## SYMPTOMS

*What are the symptoms of an ischemic stroke?*

The symptoms of an ischemic stroke depend upon the size and location of the area of the brain deprived of blood supply. Commonly, but by no means always, the area of the brain which is damaged by an ischemic stroke controls the ability to move one side of the body. The stroke may simultaneously affect the area of the brain that controls the ability to speak, or to understand spoken words. Other symptoms that may indicate an ischemic stroke include diminished sensation on one side of the body, inability to understand, or accurately process information, sudden problems with vision, and loss of balance.

## MAKING THE DIAGNOSIS

*How is the diagnosis of stroke made? How can a physician tell the difference between symptoms of an embolic stroke and symptoms caused by spread of cancer to the brain?*

The signature of embolic strokes is the speed with which the neurologic symptoms appear. Embolic strokes generally cause symptoms that appear all of a sudden and reach their peak of severity in seconds. Spread of cancer to the brain ("brain metastasis") causes neurologic symptoms that worsen gradually over a period of days or weeks. An important exception to this is sudden bleeding into an area of brain metastasis, which can cause the abrupt appearance of life-threatening symptoms.

The most important information the physician will assess are the symptoms, physical examination, the electrocardiogram, chest x-ray, a CT scan of the brain, and, in some circumstances, an echocardiogram. With this information, the experienced physician can generally make a diagnosis of an embolic stroke, and can rule out the possibility that the symptoms reflect spread of cancer to the brain.

## TRANSIENT ISCHEMIC ATTACK

### What is a transient ischemic attack?

A transient ischemic attack is a brief episode in which transient lack of blood flow to an area of the brain causes sudden, reversible, neurologic symptoms. The most common symptoms of a transient ischemic attack are numbness and weakness on one side of the body and, often, garbled speech. These symptoms usually last for less than an hour. A transient ischemic attack is a very important signal that blood circulation in the brain is in jeopardy. If appropriate treatment is not given, the person is at risk for developing a stroke.

### What is the difference between a transient ischemic attack and an ischemic stroke?

The symptoms of a transient ischemic attack completely disappear within 24 hours, and usually within one hour after they begin. The symptoms of an ischemic stroke remain for days or are permanent.

## TRANSIENT ISCHEMIC ATTACK CAUSED BY AN EMBOLISM

*If a blood clot travelled into the brain and caused a stroke, where did the clot come from?*

The embolus that floats up into the brain usually developed in a blood clot within the chambers of the heart. Many forms of heart disease, including prior heart attacks, can damage the smooth inner lining of the heart and allow blood clots to build up on the inner surface of the heart (the "endocardium"). These clots can break free, float upward into the brain, and cause devastating strokes.

Nonbacterial thrombotic endocarditis, as discussed earlier in this chapter, is associated with "vegetations" on the heart valves that can be seen with a test called "transesophageal echocardiogram".

When a person has an embolic stroke, it is critical to determine the reason that clots are forming inside the heart. A cardiologist may help determine the source of the blood clots and manage their treatment.

### What is a transesophageal echocardiogram?

A transesophageal echocardiogram is a test in which, through the mouth, a device that gives off sound waves is advanced through the mouth into the esophagus (the tube between the mouth and the stomach). Since the esophagus is located inside the chest next to the heart, these sound waves will bounce off the heart and back to the device, which transmits an image onto a screen. This test permits the physician to evaluate heart valves and can make the diagnosis of nonbacterial thrombotic endocarditis.

## What is atrial fibrillation?

Atrial fibrillation is a common cause of embolic strokes. With atrial fibrillation, the chambers of the heart called the "left atrium" and the "right atrium", continually quivers instead of pumping, and do not perform their fundamental job of pumping blood into the ventricles. The lack of normal rhythmic contraction of the left atrium produces abnormal currents in the left atrium's chamber that can cause blood in the left atrium to clot. This clot can very easily travel from left atrium to left ventricle, to the aorta, up the carotid artery and into the brain.

## How is a transient ischemic attack or an ischemic stroke caused by an embolus treated?

Unless the clot in the heart stops growing, chunks of the growing clot will break off and float up into the brain or into the arteries feeding other major body organs such as the kidney and the intestines. Emboli that lodge in these major arteries can have catastrophic effects. Anticoagulant medicines prevent new emboli from travelling to the brain and causing devastating problems.

When nonbacterial thrombotic endocarditis is responsible for emboli to the brain or elsewhere, physicians will often prescribe a form of heparin, given as an injection one or more times daily.

In people with atrial fibrillation, dabigatran (brand name is "Pradaxa", manufacturer's product website is www.pradaxa.com)

is a new and very effective anticoagulant that many experts believe will replace the anticoagulant "warfarin" that physicians have been prescribing for over 50 years. Dabigatran prevents strokes caused by an embolism more effectively than warfarin, while exposing a person to a lower risk of serious internal bleeding. An additional major advantage of dabigatran is that, unlike warfarin, dabigatran does not require frequent blood tests to monitor for excessive or insufficient anticoagulation.

## STROKE: IMMEDIATE TREATMENT

*What immediate treatment will a physician administer when a person has an ischemic stroke?*

The goal of treatment is to re-establish blood flow to the entire brain and to prevent any area of the brain from suffering irreversible damage.

Immediately after a severe stroke, a person may be very confused or may fall into a coma. Normal reflexes, such as cough reflexes, or normal breathing patterns, may be lost. In these circumstances, initial treatment assures that breathing is not impaired and that there is adequate oxygen in the bloodstream. It may be necessary to put a tube into the trachea (called "intubation") and support breathing with a mechanical ventilator. Control of blood pressure and the blood glucose level, and any infections that may be causing a person to have a fever, will also be critical.

After this rapid assessment, the immediate consideration will be whether to attempt to open the artery with an injected medicine that can possibly dissolve or break up the blood clot (called "thrombolytic therapy").

### Who can benefit from thrombolytic therapy?

The major benefit from thrombolytic therapy is if the treatment begins within three hours of development of the symptoms of an ischemic stroke. There still is some benefit, although smaller, if the thrombolytic therapy is begun after 3 hours but before 4 ½ hours. After 4 ½ hours, there is no apparent benefit from the thrombolytic therapy, while risks from the thrombolytic therapy itself remain.

### What is the risk of thrombolytic therapy?

The major risk of thrombolytic therapy is an increased risk of serious bleeding, and most dangerously, bleeding into the brain (see chapter entitled "Brain Hemorrhage"). The risk of brain hemorrhage is small, and is considered by experts to be worth taking in order reduce the high risk that a blocked cerebral artery will produce extensive permanent brain damage after an ischemic stroke.

### How do physicians reduce the risk of bleeding in the brain after thrombolytic therapy?

Occasionally, a person who appears to have an "ischemic stroke" may actually have had a "brain hemorrhage" (see chapter entitled "Brain Hemorrhage"). If a person with a brain hemorrhage receives thrombolytic therapy, the results are likely to be catastrophic. A CT scan will clearly show whether the person has sustained a brain hemorrhage or another form of bleeding in or around the brain. For this reason, an emergency CT scan is essential before administering thrombolytic therapy.

### How do physicians administer thrombolytic therapy?

The most common thrombolytic therapy is a medicine called "Activase", administered intravenously over a period of one hour.

### How effective is thrombolytic therapy?

Thrombolytic therapy approximately doubles the chance of having a complete, or almost complete, recovery of brain function if given within three hours of first developing symptoms. The earlier the thrombolytic therapy, the more likely it is that full, or almost full, recovery will happen.

### Is thrombolytic therapy effective in people who are elderly?

Clinical trials have evaluated the effectiveness of thrombolytic therapy in people up to the age of 90. In all age groups, thrombolytic therapy improves the likelihood of a favorable outcome, that is, it reduces the risk of serious disabilities after the stroke.

### OUTLOOK

### What is the outlook for a person with cancer who has had an embolic stroke?

Most commonly, when embolic stroke occurs in a person with cancer, the cancer is advanced and not responding well to treatment. For this reason, survival after an embolic stroke is often only a few months. This relatively short survival in people who have had an embolic stroke in the setting of advanced cancer is an important consideration for the person and their family in deciding whether to accept the intensive treatments given for this condition.

# BRAIN AND SPINAL CORD COMPLICATIONS

# DELIRIUM, STUPOR AND COMA

## DEFINITIONS

### What is delirium?

Delirium is the sudden development of severe confusion. Delirium can take two forms:"hypoactive delirium" in which a person appears quiet, apathetic, drowsy, and depressed and "hyperactive delirium" in which a person appears agitated, sometimes with combative, euphoric, or other inappropriate behavior.

### What is stupor and coma?

Coma is a state of complete unconsciousness from which a person cannot be aroused. Closely related to coma is "stupor" in which a person's state of consciousness is altered, but in which arousal by voice, touch, or some other stimulus is still possible. The appearance of either coma or stupor is a medical emergency that can rapidly lead to death or permanent brain damage unless the cause of stupor or coma is promptly treated.

# DELIRIUM, STUPOR, OR COMA IN PEOPLE WITH CANCER

## What causes delirium, stupor, or coma in people with cancer?

The most common causes of delirium, stupor, or coma in people with cancer are problems with blood chemistry, spread of cancer to several areas in the brain (see chapter entitled "Brain Metastases"), side effects of medications, and infections (see chapters in the section of this book called "Infections"). Often, however, evaluation will uncover more than one possible cause of the delirium, stupor, or coma. Even so, identification of each of the conditions contributing to the delirium, stupor or coma is important, since correction of any one contributing factor can greatly improve or possibly reverse the delirium, stupor or coma.

# IDENTIFYING THE CAUSE OF DELIRIUM, STUPOR OR COMA

## How is the cause of delirium, stupor or coma identified?

The events that led up to the confusion or alteration of the state of consciousness are of critical importance. Any piece of the story that might shed light on the cause of the alterations in consciousness is important. This includes the speed with symptoms developed, any immediately preceding symptoms, history of recent or ongoing illness, use of any kind of medications that can alter consciousness such as pain medication or antidepressants, and a history of any symptoms consistent with those described in the chapter entitled "Brain Metastasis".

## *How does the physical examination help in making the diagnosis when a person has fallen into a coma?*

Measurement of the blood pressure, pulse, breathing rate, and body temperature can rapidly narrow the range of possible or probable causes of coma. High fever and coma implies meningitis. Brain swelling associated with a brain hemorrhage, can cause the pressure inside the skull to rise quickly and the pulse rate to drop way down. Very low blood pressure suggests that circulatory shock may have caused the coma.

Examination of the back of the eye with an ophthalmoscope (this is a "fundoscopic examination") can show evidence of brain hemorrhage, brain swelling, or longstanding problems with diabetes or high blood pressure. Evaluation of eye movements and the reaction of the pupils to light give information about the integrity of the brainstem and, at times, can pinpoint the exact location of an area of brain damage that is causing coma.

A detailed neurological examination can provide extremely useful information that could suggest the cause of the coma.

A rapid, complete physical examination, may uncover problems with the heart, liver, lungs or other organs that explain the reason for the coma.

## *How are blood and urine tests helpful in determining the cause of coma?*

If the cause of the coma is not obvious from the history and physical examination, blood tests may very quickly spot the problem.

High or low blood sugar, liver failure, and kidney failure are easy to identify with blood tests. Measurement of the level of oxygen in the blood in the arteries (the "arterial blood gas") determines whether the lungs are delivering an adequate amount of oxygen to the bloodstream.

Urinary tract infections, especially in people who are in frail health, are a common cause of changes of mental status. Analysis of the urine makes the diagnosis.

### How is an overdose with pain medication identified and treated?

Medicine used to treat cancer-related pain is usually in the family of medications, such as morphine and codeine, called "opiod" medication. If there is a question about an overdose, whether accidental or intentional, of opiod pain medication, injection of the antidote medication "naloxone" can rapidly reverse the symptoms and identify the cause of the coma.

### How can x-rays be helpful?

If the person has a fever, a chest x-ray can show evidence of pneumonia.

A CT scan of the brain is a rapid and very important test that gives physicians a remarkably precise image of a person's brain. A CT scan can identify structural lesions or bleeding inside or around the brain, that is causing the coma.

### When is a spinal tap useful?

A spinal tap (see description of a spinal tap in the chapter entitled "Bacterial Meningitis") is a critical test when a person has fever and is in a coma, and meningitis is a significant possibility.

When the cause of coma appears to be something other than infection, the spinal tap may provide useful information as to the likely cause of coma when the history, physical examination, and CT or MRI scan fail to make the diagnosis.

### When is an electroencephalogram (EEG) useful?

Occasionally, even in the absence of jerking movements, a person with brain metastases may be having recurring seizures that are causing or contributing to delirium. In addition, a condition called "non-convulsive status epilepticus" can be a cause of coma in a person with brain metastases. The EEG identifies the presence of these seizures. If present, treatment of these seizures with medications can stop the seizures and reverse the symptoms or delirium, stupor, or coma. For additional information, please see the chapter entitled "Seizures".

## IMMEDIATE TREATMENT OF COMA: ABC AND MORE

### What steps will physicians or emergency medical professionals take when a person falls into a coma?

"ABC" is the abbreviation for airway, breathing, and circulation. Without the proper movement of air in and out of the lungs, or without proper blood circulation, life could end in minutes.

The "A" is the airway. In the context of emergency treatment of a person in coma, the "airway" at greatest risk is the path air takes from the mouth to the throat to the windpipe (the "trachea") and down to the bronchial tubes. Removal of anything that could obstruct movement of air into the airway, such as vomit, secretions, or dentures, clears the airway. To assure that the airway remains clear, it may be necessary to insert a breathing tube into the trachea (an "endotracheal tube) and then attach the endotracheal tube to a mechanical ventilator.

The "B" stands for breathing which can stop when injury occurs to vital areas of the brain. If breathing is at risk, an endotracheal tube (see above) and attachment to a mechanical ventilator will be necessary.

The "C" stands for circulation. If the heart is beating too fast or too slow or the blood pressure is far too low, circulation of blood through the body can be dangerously inadequate. If the blood pressure is far too high, a person can have a condition called "hypertensive encephalopathy" which can present itself as stupor or coma. Any significant circulatory compromise will require medications or other appropriate treatment.

Glucose can reverse the coma quickly if the cause of coma is a severely low blood sugar. The antidote for a narcotic overdose, as described earlier in this chapter, is naloxone. For this reason, it is common for physicians to administer intravenous injections of glucose and naloxone when a person with cancer unexpectedly falls into in coma.

# TREATMENT

## *What is the treatment of delirium, stupor or coma?*

The most effective treatment is to identify the causes of the new symptoms and, to the extent possible, correct them. This can involve correction of blood chemistry problems, correction of dehydration, discontinuation of medicines that affect brain functioning ("psychoactive medicines") such as sedatives, removal of large masses of blood or tumor in the brain, cure of meningitis (see chapter entitled "Bacterial Meningitis"), or reversal of any of the other many medical problems that can induce coma.

## *What can treat delirium if no effective treatment is available?*

Evaluation to determine the cause of delirium may reveal an irreversible problem such as liver or kidney failure. When delirium has an irreversible cause, treatment to relieve symptoms can be helpful.

If a person has "hyperactive delirium" and is very agitated, the medication "haloperidol" (common brand name is "Haldol") can calm a person down, reducing their risk of injury to themselves or others.

If a person has "hypoactive delirium", the medication "methylphenidate", better known as "Ritalin", can improve a person's thinking ability and ability to communicate.

# HYPOXIC ENCEPHALOPATHY

## What is hypoxic encephalopathy?

Hypoxic encephalopathy is brain damage caused by lack of delivery of adequate oxygen to the brain. With interruption of the supply of oxygen to the brain for more than three minutes, irreversible brain damage can occur.

## What can interrupt oxygen delivery to the brain?

When the heart temporarily stops beating, that is, if a person has a cardiac arrest, or when for any other reason there is an interruption of blood supply to the brain, oxygen delivery to the brain temporarily stops.

Even if the heart is beating and circulation through the brain is normal, the blood must have enough oxygen in it to keep brain cells alive. When breathing stops, or if there is obstruction of the airway, the amount of oxygen in the blood will drop very steeply. A few minutes of inadequate supply of oxygen to the brain will cause hypoxic encephalopathy.

## Can anything prevent irreversible brain damage after an episode of cardiac arrest?

If the person does not immediately awaken after cardiac arrest, "induced hypothermia" can reduce the risk of permanent brain damage from hypoxic encephalopathy. Induced hypothermia means that a person's body temperature is lowered to approximately 90 degrees Fahrenheit by artificial means, such as a cooling blanket.

*Are there treatments other than induced hypothermia that might improve the outlook of hypoxic encephalopathy?*

The only known treatment of hypoxic encephalopathy is to reverse the medical problem that led to the inadequate supply of oxygen to the brain. This type of treatment can prevent further damage but cannot repair damage that has already occurred.

No medicines are available that improve the outlook for survival and recovery of people with hypoxic encephalopathy.

*What happens to people who wake up after hypoxic encephalopathy?*

People who make a full recovery from hypoxic encephalopathy usually begin waking up within hours of the beginning of the episode. The longer a person is in coma, the greater the amount of neurological damage that is likely to be evident if the person ever regains consciousness.

There are areas of the brain that are extremely sensitive to lack of oxygen. Some of these areas control the ability to organize thought. Others control the ability to coordinate movements of the body. Damage to these areas of the brain can result in major permanent neurological disabilities.

## PERSISTENT VEGETATIVE STATE

*What is a persistent vegetative state?*

A "persistent vegetative state" is when a person appears to be awake but has no awareness of anything that is around them and no ability to respond in any meaningful way to the environment around them. The longer someone remains in a persistent vegetative state, the worse the outcome. Although some people who have sustained a head injury can make a remarkable recovery after an extended period in a persistent vegetative state, significant recovery from a prolonged period in a persistent vegetative state after hypoxic encephalopathy is very uncommon.

## BRAIN DEATH

### *What is brain death?*

Brain death indicates the total destruction of the brain from top to bottom, along with lack of blood flow or electrical activity in the brain. To make the diagnosis of brain death, two evaluations 24 hours apart confirm the conclusion that brain death, and, therefore, death has occurred.

## OUTLOOK

### *What is the outlook for survival and recovery for a person in coma?*

It can be very difficult, in the first days after the onset of a coma, to predict with certainty the outlook for survival and recovery from coma. Largely, the outlook for recovery depends upon the medical problem that caused the coma and the degree to which treatment of the underlying medical problem prevented permanent brain damage.

There are "coma scales", the most common of which is the "Glasgow coma scale", which give a grade to certain symptoms that are indicative of the depth of coma. The Glasgow coma scale has three key components related to the ability to understand and respond to the spoken word, the ability to move in an appropriate way to verbal or physical stimuli and the ability to open the eyes upon verbal or physical stimuli. The Glasgow coma scale runs from 3 to 15, with 3 being the worst possible score and 15 being the best. A score of 8 or less indicates severe brain damage. The person's Glasgow coma scale score and the length of time that the person stays deeply in coma, can give important information about the probability that the person will regain consciousness and regain normal brain function.

## What does it mean when a person moves their arms and legs while in a coma?

Two major types of arm and leg movements are indicative of major brain damage. In "decorticate posturing", a person's wrists and elbows flex and turn inward. In "decerebrate posturing", the arms and legs rigidly extend and turn outward. When a person spontaneously makes these movements while in a coma, it is indicative of a very serious brain injury.

The muscles of the body may twitch ("myoclonus") and arms, legs or hands may move. This reflex is neither a positive nor a negative prognostic sign.

The most significant body movement is when a person makes a willful movement in response to a command such as "blink your eyes" or "squeeze my hand". When a person can do this, they have a possibility of making a very significant, or, perhaps, total recovery.

# INCREASED INTRACRANIAL PRESSURE

## DEFINITION

### What is increased intracranial pressure?

Intracranial pressure is the pressure inside the skull transmitted to the brain. When elevated, the intracranial pressure can rapidly cause severe and potentially lethal brain injury.

## SYMPTOMS

### What are the symptoms of increased intracranial pressure?

The major symptom of increased intracranial pressure is a severe headache, which is sometimes associated with vomiting. As the increased intracranial pressure worsens, a person can become confused or sleepy, and ultimately fall into a coma.

## MAKING THE DIAGNOSIS

### When a person has cancer, what causes an increased intracranial pressure?

The most common cause of increased intracranial pressure in a person with cancer is the presence of one or more areas of brain metastasis, or growth of a glioblastoma and the swelling around it (see chapters discussing "Brain Metastasis" and "Brain Cancer: Glioblastoma").

### How do physicians identify the presence of increased intracranial pressure?

The presence of increased intracranial pressure is often obvious, based upon a person's symptoms, and neurologic examination. A CT scan showing a glioblastoma or areas of metastasis and surrounding brain swelling ("cerebral edema") makes the diagnosis.

## TREATMENT OF INCREASED INTRACRANIAL PRESSURE AND HERNIATION

### Why is a rise in intracranial pressure dangerous?

The increased pressure exerted on the brain by increased intracranial pressure can cause damage to compressed regions of the brain.

The inside of the skull is not like the smooth inside of a rubber ball. There are compartments inside the skull surrounded by sharp ridges and grooves that neatly cradle and protect the normal brain. When the brain swells, areas of the brain may push into areas in the skull where they do not belong and cannot fit. When this happens, (this is "herniation") compression of the brain against sharp ridges in the skull or against other areas of the brain can develop. Herniation can rapidly damage vital areas of the brain and is a medical emergency.

## What is the initial treatment of increased intracranial pressure?

The initial treatment is a medication in the family of steroids called "dexamethasone", or, more commonly known by its old brand name "Decadron". Decadron relieves brain swelling, and by doing so, reduces intracranial pressure. Radiation therapy directed at areas of a brain tumor, whether a glioblastoma or brain metastasis, and occasionally surgery to remove a large area of tumor and surrounding brain swelling, may be useful.

## What is the treatment of a severely increased intracranial pressure or of herniation?

The goal of treatment of severely increased intracranial pressure or herniation is to reduce brain swelling and reduce the size of any structural lesion in the brain that has caused the herniation. The hope is that by reducing the swelling and the size of any structural lesion, the brain can shift within the skull so that the herniation is relieved.

A medicine called "mannitol" can be given by vein, takes about an hour to begin to work, and can take down some of the brain swelling. Putting the person on a mechanical ventilator and increasing the breathing rate ("mechanical hyperventilation") can also bring down some of the brain swelling. If surgery can relieve the herniation by removing a large brain tumor, emergency surgery may be necessary. Herniation is very dangerous and, although sometimes reversible, carries a very high risk of causing death.

# SEIZURES

## DEFINITION

### What is a seizure?

A seizure is a sudden change in brain function caused by electrical malfunction of the brain. When people with cancer begin, for the first time, to have seizures, the most serious and life threatening seizures are "grand mal" seizures.

## SYMPTOMS

### What happens with a grand mal seizure?

When a person has a grand mal seizure, abruptly and usually without warning, consciousness is lost and, if standing, the person will go crashing down to the floor. Muscles throughout the body stiffen, the head draws back, the hands clench, and for a brief period, breathing may stop and the person may turn blue. Within moments, the arms and legs start jerking rhythmically and in unison. After another short period, the jerking stops and the muscles relax. Unconsciousness persists for a period of several minutes or hours. Slowly and by degrees, the successive veils of unconsciousness and confusion lift until the person becomes alert and oriented.

## IMMEDIATE TREATMENT

### What is the treatment of a grand mal seizure?

While a person is having a seizure, practical steps such as moving furniture or clearing broken glass can prevent the person from being injured while the seizure is causing the body to thrash about. Trying to hold the arms and legs still can be dangerous. If the person has vomited, rolling the person onto their side may prevent a person from "aspirating" that is, breathing their vomit into their lungs. Although it is not possible for a person to "swallow their tongue" during a seizure, the tongue can block the movement of air into the lungs. By rolling the person on their side, the tongue usually drops to the side of the mouth, clearing the airway.

Seizures will most often stop on their own. Once the seizure has stopped, it will be necessary to figure out the cause of the seizure and try to prevent seizures from happening again.

## THE CAUSE OF GRAND MAL SEIZURES

### What causes grand mal seizures in people with cancer?

The most common reason for a person with cancer to have seizures is the presence of cancer in the brain.

In the absence of evidence of cancer in the brain, a seizure in a person with cancer can be a sign of other serious medical problems. "Bacterial meningitis", "ischemic stroke", "intracerebral hemorrhage", "acute kidney injury", and metabolic complications are other possible causes when a person with cancer develops a seizure for the first time. These complications are discussed in their own chapters elsewhere in this book. Occasionally, seizures can develop as a side effect of medications, or as a side effect of radiation therapy.

After identification of the problem causing the seizure, specific appropriate treatment of the underlying disease, if possible, can begin. Successful treatment of the underlying disease can permanently prevent the seizures from recurring.

### How is the cause of the seizures identified?

A CT or MRI scan can usually identify "brain metastases", that is, areas of the brain containing cancer. The CT or MRI scan can also identify areas of hemorrhage within the brain that might have triggered the new onset of seizures.

When brain metastases or hemorrhage are not evident with the CT or MRI scan, blood tests and physical examination may reveal infections, or serious kidney, liver, metabolic, or other problems causing or contributing to the seizures.

## TREATMENT WHEN THE CAUSE OF SEIZURES IS CURABLE

### What happens if the problem causing the seizures is treatable?

When the problem is easily treatable, such as problems with the chemistry of the blood, correction of the underlying problem will remove the cause of the seizures. When the cause is an infection that can be cured with appropriate treatment, there is some risk of a lingering effect of the infection that can trigger another seizure, and physicians may recommend that a person take medication for a period of time to prevent further seizures.

## TREATMENT WHEN THERE IS NO EFFECTIVE TREATMENT FOR THE CAUSE OF SEIZURES

*What happens if there is no effective treatment for the cause of the seizures? For example, what happens if there is an incurable brain tumor and the risk of seizures remains?*

Medications are available that are quite effective in controlling seizures. An antiepileptic called "levetiracetam", (brand name is "Keppra XR", and manufacturer's product website is www.keppraxr.com) is a common choice for a person with a primary or metastatic brain tumor who requires antiepileptic medication. Other commonly used medicines are lamotrigine (brand name is "Lamictal", manufacturer's product website is www.lamictal.com) and valproic acid (which has several brand names including "Depakote", manufacturer's product website is www.depakote.com). Other medicines that are sometimes used include Dilantin, Phenobarbital, and Tegretol. Each drug has advantages and each has side effects. The choice of which medication or combination of medications to use can be complex, requiring consultation with a neurologist with special expertise in treating seizures.

## STATUS EPILEPTICUS

*What is status epilepticus?*

Status epilepticus is when seizures occur one directly after another without any intervening period of consciousness.

In the absence of jerking movements characteristic of grand mal seizures, a person with brain metastases may be have a condition called "non-convulsive status epilepticus" which can cause coma and greatly endanger life. The EEG identifies the presence of non-convulsive status epilepticus.

## How is status epilepticus treated?

The treatment of status epilepticus is to administer medications that will stop the seizure. As treatment begins, physicians will pay close attention to the all-important abbreviation remembered in emergency medical situations: ABC. "ABC" is the abbreviation for airway, breathing, and circulation. Without the proper movement of air in and out of the lungs, or without proper blood circulation, life could end in minutes.

The "A" is the airway. In the context of emergency treatment of a person in status epilepticus, the "airway" at greatest risk is the path air takes from the mouth to the throat to the windpipe (the "trachea") and down to the bronchial tubes. Blood, vomit, food, or anything else which is blocking the airway will be removed, if necessary manually, and, if possible and readily available, with suction. To be sure that the airway remains clear, it may be necessary to insert a breathing tube into the trachea (an "endotracheal tube"),

The "B" stands for breathing which can stop when vital areas of the brain are affected. If breathing is at risk, an endotracheal tube (see above) and attachment to a mechanical ventilator will be necessary.

The "C" stands for circulation that must be maintained for life to continue. If the heart is beating too fast or too slow, or the blood pressure is far too low, circulation of blood through the body can be dangerously inadequate. Medicines can correct circulation problems that can immediately jeopardize life.

## *What medicines stop the status epilepticus?*

Lorazepam, a drug commonly used for anxiety under the brand name is "Ativan", has the powerful ability to break status epilepticus when given intravenously. This medication often stops the immediate problem, provided there is correction of the underlying problem, such as a problem with some aspect of the person's blood chemistry, which caused the status epilepticus.

If the intravenous Lorazepam does not stop the status epilepticus, other medications such as Dilantin, valproic acid, and phenobarbital given one at a time and sequentially, will usually break the seizure.

Occasionally the seizures are terribly resistant to these medicines and large doses of barbiturates or other anesthetic medicines will stop the seizures. These powerful medicines can stop breathing, and will generally require insertion of a breathing tube in the lungs ("intubation") and mechanical ventilation.

## OUTCOME OF STATUS EPILEPTICUS

### *What is the outcome of status epilepticus?*

The outcome depends upon how quickly status epilepticus responds to treatment. Serious permanent brain damage can occur after a prolonged episode of status epilepticus. Most people make a full recovery from the episode if treatment begins promptly and if the status epilepticus is quickly controlled. Depending upon the cause of the status epilepticus, there could be a significant risk of recurrence; therefore, medication to prevent this may be necessary.

# MALIGNANT SPINAL CORD COMPRESSION

## DEFINITION

### What is malignant spinal cord compression?

Malignant spinal cord compression means compression of the spinal cord by a malignant tumor. Compression of the spinal cord by a malignant tumor is a medical emergency that, unless treated promptly, can lead to paralysis and premature death.

## THE SOURCE OF THE COMPRESSION AND ITS CONSEQUENCES

### What causes malignant spinal cord compression?

A tough fibrous membrane called the "dura" and the thick bony wall of the vertebral column surround the spinal cord, protecting it from harm. Cancer in, or adjacent to, the vertebral bones can grow and bulge into the space (called the "epidural space") between the dura and unyielding bony wall of the interior of the spinal column and compress the spinal cord. In addition, when a vertebral bone is extensively involved with cancer, the bone can fracture, sending bone fragments into the epidural space, where they can compress the spinal cord.

## Why does this compression cause spinal cord damage?

Cancer that is growing in the epidural space can obstruct the flow of blood through the veins in the epidural space that are responsible for carrying blood away from the spinal cord. Just as an arm or a leg with a tight band around it will swell, the obstruction of blood flowing away from the spinal cord will cause swelling ("edema") of the spinal cord. This swelling can compress and obstruct blood vessels supplying the spinal cord. Without adequate blood supply, the spinal cord will "infarct", that is, the area of spinal cord inadequately supplied with blood will die. Infarction of the spinal cord has the same effect as trauma that cuts the spinal cord in two: all function below the area infarcted is lost.

## Which cancers are most likely to cause malignant spinal cord compressions?

Cancers of the lung, breast, and prostate, commonly spread to the bones of the vertebral column and are the most likely cancers to produce malignant spinal cord compression. Most cancers, however, can spread to bone and can produce spinal cord compression if they have spread to the vertebral column.

## SYMPTOMS

## What are the symptoms of spinal cord compression?

The first symptom of spinal cord compression is usually pain in the area of the neck or back that is directly over the area of spinal cord compression. If the area of spinal cord compression is in the neck, pain may radiate into the shoulders or down the arms. If the area of spinal cord compression is in the upper back, pain may radiate around the chest. If the area of spinal cord compression is in the lower back, pain may radiate down the legs or into the groin. The pain usually worsens while lying down and lessens a bit when sitting or standing.

When compression begins to injure the spinal cord, a person will feel weakness, difficulty walking, and a loss of sensation in those areas of the body that are supplied with nerve fibers originating from the endangered portion of the spinal cord. As the spinal cord damage becomes more severe, paralysis, loss of sensation, and loss of all function of the spinal cord below the level that is compressed, can occur.

### How are the symptoms of spinal cord compression different from the symptoms of arthritis of the spine?

Arthritis of the spine (called "degenerative joint disease") usually has been going on for quite a while and usually produces the same symptoms that have already been troubling someone for several years. In addition, whereas the pain of spinal cord compression usually worsens when lying down, the pain of degenerative joint disease usually lessens when lying down.

Evaluation of symptoms alone is usually inadequate to make a firm diagnosis of spinal cord compression. Establishment of an unequivocal diagnosis of spinal cord compression requires additional testing.

*How urgent is it to be evaluated if new back
pain develops in a person with cancer?*

Malignant spinal cord compression is a medical emergency and new back pain or weaknesses in the legs are its major symptoms. Prompt evaluation is critically important.

## MAKING THE DIAGNOSIS

*How is the diagnosis of malignant spinal
cord compression made?*

The most useful test in making the diagnosis is the MRI scan. The MRI can show the size and location of the tumor that is pressing on the spinal cord as well as give important information about destructive effects that the cancer may be having on the vertebral bone. Occasionally, cancer can grow in the "epidural space" at more than one level along the spinal column. For this reason, physicians will commonly suggest that an MRI scan evaluating the entire extent of the spinal cord from the upper neck at the top of the "cervical spine to the area where the spinal cord ends, in the lower back in the "lumbar spine".

## TREATMENT

*What is the treatment of spinal cord compression?*

The immediate treatment of spinal cord compression is to give high doses of steroids. The most commonly used steroid medication is "dexamethasone" (commonly called by its older brand name

"Decadron"). Decadron can relieve a good deal of the swelling in the spinal cord and reduce the risk that compromised blood flow to the spinal cord will cause irreversible damage.

After starting treatment with steroids, surgery may be necessary to relieve the compression of the spinal cord. This surgical approach can be challenging, requiring a highly skilled and experienced surgeon to carry it out effectively. The tumor compressing the spinal cord is usually located in front of the spinal cord in an area that is technically challenging for a surgeon to reach. When an appropriately skilled surgeon and medical care facility is available, surgery to relieve the compression caused by the cancer from around the spinal cord can improve outcome, that is, it reduces the risk of paralysis or inability to walk properly. After the surgery, radiation therapy, given to the involved area, will further reduce the risk of permanent spinal cord damage.

When spinal cord compression develops in a person with a very advanced cancer and very little time left to live, a major operation may not be the best treatment.

When surgical treatment is not technically possible or appropriate, high doses of steroids in combination with radiation therapy can sometimes be quite effective in shrinking the tumor and relieving the spinal cord compression.

## **OUTLOOK**

*What is the outlook for recovery for a person with spinal cord compression?*

Radiation treatment can often relieve back pain.

The outlook with regard to paralysis and ability to walk depends upon the severity of the spinal cord damage at the time of the diagnosis of spinal cord compression. Most people who are able to walk at the time of the diagnosis are still able to walk after treatment. The greater the degree of weakness or paralysis at the time treatment begins, the lower the chances of recovery. In general, approximately one in three people, who are unable to walk because of weakness at the time of diagnosis of malignant spinal cord compression, will regain the ability to walk normally. Approximately, one in twenty people paralyzed at the time of diagnosis, regain the ability to walk. The odds are somewhat better if the cancer is of a type, such as prostate cancer or breast cancer, which is sensitive to the cancer-killing effects of radiation.

The outcome in people who begin treatment after they have major symptoms of weakness or paralysis is not favorable. This emphasizes the critical importance of immediate evaluation by a skilled physician if, in the setting of a previous diagnosis of cancer, severe back pain develops. Back pain and new leg weakness in a person with cancer is a medical emergency which needs prompt and thorough evaluation and, if necessary, treatment.

# CANCER THERAPY COMPLICATIONS

# BONE MARROW SUPPRESSION

## DEFINITIONS

### What is the bone marrow?

The bone marrow is the tissue on the inside of the bones that produces blood cells. The bone marrow produces white blood cells, red blood cells and platelets and then releases them into the bloodstream.

### What does it mean when someone has bone marrow suppression from chemotherapy?

Bone marrow suppression from chemotherapy means that the chemotherapy is preventing the normal production of white and red blood cells and platelets.

## THE REASON CHEMOTHERAPY SUPPRESSES THE BONE MARROW

### Why does chemotherapy suppress the bone marrow?

The formation of blood cells in the bone marrow begins with an immature cell called a "stem cell" that divides and undergoes a transformation into cells that are committed to give rise to red blood cells, white blood cells, or platelets. As committed cells undergo further division, they go through a maturation process, resulting in the release of mature white and red blood cells and platelets into the bloodstream.

Chemotherapy damages rapidly dividing cells anywhere in the body. Because of this, the most powerful chemotherapy medications or combinations of these medicines, can suppress cell division anywhere in the body, whether it is in cancer cells, bone marrow cells, or dividing cells in the gastrointestinal tract. The suppression of cell division in the bone marrow is the cause of the bone marrow suppression caused by chemotherapy.

## RISKS OF BONE MARROW SUPPRESSION

*Why is bone marrow suppression potentially dangerous?*

Inadequate white blood cells in the bloodstream ("leukopenia") will put a person at a higher risk of developing serious infections. A lower amount of red blood cells produces anemia, is associated with fatigue, and can cause serious problems related to inadequate delivery of oxygen to the major organs. A reduced number of circulating platelets in the bloodstream reduces the effectiveness with which blood can clot, and exposes a person to the risk of major bleeding.

*When does bone marrow suppression from chemotherapy appear and how long does it last?*

Signs of bone marrow suppression usually appear within a few days of receiving chemotherapy, with the maximal suppression of the number of white blood cells in the bloodstream (the "nadir") appearing roughly ten days (plus or minus two or three days) after treatment. The duration of the bone marrow suppression is variable, and depends upon the intensity of the chemotherapy, whether it is given with radiation therapy at the same time, and many factors related to the underlying health of the person receiving the chemotherapy. Bone marrow suppression, along with its potential for causing serious problems, usually lasts for only a few days.

## INADEQUATE WHITE BLOOD CELLS: "LEUKOPENIA"

### *What is leukopenia?*

Leukopenia means that the total amount of white blood cells in the bloodstream is lower than it should be. In the context of leukopenia caused by chemotherapy, the types of white blood cells most dangerously reduced in number are the "neutrophils" and the "lymphocytes".

## NEUTROPENIA

### *What is the function of the neutrophils and what is "neutropenia"?*

Neutrophils are the major defense system our body has to destroy bacteria or fungal organisms that have gained access to the inside of the body. Neutropenia is a reduction of the number of neutrophils in the blood.

Thresholds have been set, below which a person is at a low, moderate, or high risk of developing serious infections. Specifically, if the neutrophil count is "less than 500 cells per microliter", the person is at a high risk of developing very serious bacterial or fungal infections. If the laboratory determines the neutrophil count is "less than 100 cells per microliter", the person is at a very high risk of developing very serious bacterial or fungal infections.

## What are the symptoms of neutropenia?

In the absence of symptoms, routine blood tests identify neutropenia that follows chemotherapy treatment.

Symptoms of neutropenia result from the infectious problems caused by the neutropenia, rather than the neutropenia itself. These symptoms may include fevers, chills, difficulty breathing, confusion, and dizziness and often reflect the serious infections discussed in the section of this book discussing infectious complications of cancer. Other symptoms can include local pain, redness, and swelling associated with infection of intravenous or "central venous catheters" used for administering chemotherapy.

Fever that develops in a person with neutropenia is "febrile neutropenia". Serious infection in a person with neutropenia is "neutropenic sepsis".

*Febrile neutropenia is a very important and dangerous complication of chemotherapy, and for this reason, is discussed separately in the chapter entitled "Febrile Neutropenia and Neutropenic Sepsis".*

## What can a person do to reduce the risk of infection after chemotherapy?

Depending upon the type of chemotherapy given, the level of white blood cells in the bloodstream is likely to diminish at some point in time. When there is maximal suppression of the number of white blood cells in the bloodstream (the "nadir"), the susceptibility to infection is the greatest. It is therefore important for a person to ask their physician when their expected white blood cell nadir will be, so that when the nadir occurs, there is extra attention to prevention of infection and to signs of infection.

Perhaps the most important way of preventing infection is to keep the hands clean through frequent hand washing, especially after touching anything that is unclean. If there is an intravenous access line in place, it is critical to give strict attention to keeping the area clean and to not touching the area unless the hands are very clean or have a sterile glove on them.

The most common sign of infection to look for is a fever of over 100.4 degrees Fahrenheit that lasts for over an hour, or any fever over 101. If this degree of fever occurs during a nadir, it could be a sign of a serious infection: this requires immediate evaluation by a physician. Other common signs of infection are chills, redness around catheters, difficulty breathing, a new persistent cough, a sore throat, or a change in mental clarity.

### Which medicines prevent development of neutropenia after chemotherapy?

A family of biotechnology medicines called "colony stimulating factors" stimulates the bone marrow to produce neutrophils and can prevent complications related to neutropenia. The most convenient of these medications to administer has the brand name is "Neulasta" (manufacturer's product website is www.neulasta.com) and requires only one injection of the medication 24 hours after beginning a cycle of chemotherapy.

### What factors encourage physicians to give Neulasta along with chemotherapy?

Neulasta is very expensive, and, as with all potent medications, has its own risk of side effects. Neulasta is particularly useful for people who are receiving chemotherapy that is likely to cause serious neutropenia, and for people receiving potentially curative chemotherapy, where interruption of treatment because of neutropenia would reduce the chance of achieving a cure.

### Are antibiotics always necessary to prevent infection if a person has neutropenia but no fever or other evidence of infection?

If, based upon an understanding of the chemotherapy given and a person's underlying condition, it appears that the neutropenia will only last for a few days, antibiotics are not routinely given. If, however, there is an expectation that the neutropenia will persist for an extended period, an antibiotic in the family of medications called "fluoroquinolones" may prevent development of a serious infection.

## LYMPHOCYTOPENIA

### What are lymphocytes? What is lymphocytopenia?

Lymphocytes are white blood cells that, among other functions, help to protect the body against infections with viruses and other microscopic organisms. Lymphocytopenia means that there is a reduced number of "lymphocytes" in the bloodstream. The consequence of this is that there is a reduced ability to fight infections.

### What is the treatment of chemotherapy-induced lymphocytopenia?

No specific treatment accelerates the production of lymphocytes in people who have lymphocytopenia caused by chemotherapy. "Opportunistic" viral infections (see chapter entitled "Opportunistic Infections") that emerge because of the lymphocytopenia are treated, as necessary, with antiviral medications.

## ANEMIA CAUSED BY CHEMOTHERAPY

### What are the symptoms of anemia caused by chemotherapy?

Anemia is a low number of red blood cells in the bloodstream. The major symptoms of anemia associated with chemotherapy are severe fatigue and shortness of breath.

## Why can chemotherapy cause anemia?

Chemotherapy can directly suppress the production of all blood cells by the bone marrow, including red blood cells. Powerful chemotherapy medications, such as "docetaxel" (brand name is "Taxotere") which is commonly used for breast and lung cancer, can cause significant anemia.

In addition, some forms of chemotherapy, such as the commonly used chemotherapy medication "cisplatin", can cause toxicity to the kidney. Because the kidney produces a hormone called "erythropoietin" that helps to regulate production of red blood cells, kidney damage from chemotherapy, by reducing production of erythropoietin, can impair the ability of the bone marrow to make red blood cells.

## What is the treatment of anemia caused by chemotherapy?

In evaluating a person who has developed anemia while receiving chemotherapy, a physician may first perform blood tests that will determine whether there is evidence of vitamin B12 or folic acid deficiency that may be causing the anemia. If blood tests find vitamin B12 or folic acid deficiencies, appropriate supplements can restore red blood cell production and correct the anemia.

When anemia is causing severe symptoms, a blood transfusion with "packed red blood cells" can correct much of the anemia and relieve its symptoms.

There are biotechnology medicines that stimulate production of red blood cells. Production of red blood cells is "erythropoiesis" and medicines that stimulate red blood cell production are "erythropoiesis stimulating agents".When anemia is causing severe weakness or other difficult symptoms, "erythropoiesis-stimulating agents" with the brand names of "Epogen" (manufacturer's product website is www.epogen.com) and "Procrit" (manufacturer's product website is www.procrit.com) and "Aranesp" (manufacturer's product website is www.aranesp.com), can accelerate recovery from symptoms by increasing production of red blood cells.

### What are the advantages and disadvantages of treating severe anemia with a blood transfusion or an erythropoiesis-stimulating agent?

Blood transfusions rapidly correct the anemia and cause a relatively rapid reduction in the fatigue associated with anemia. Disadvantages of blood transfusion include the risk of viral infection from contaminated blood, and the risk of an "infusion reaction" to the blood transfusion (see chapter entitled "Infusion Reactions").

The advantage of the erythropoiesis-stimulating agents is the avoidance of the potential complications of a blood transfusion. The disadvantages of erythropoiesis-stimulating agents are a slower recovery from fatigue, a higher risk of developing serious blood clots, and the possibility that the medication may accelerate the growth of the cancer and shorten survival.

## LOW PLATELET COUNT ("THROMBOCYTOPENIA") CAUSED BY CHEMOTHERAPY

### What is the danger of low platelet counts?

Low platelet counts impair the clotting ability of the blood and expose a person to a risk of serious internal bleeding.

## Can medicines stimulate production of platelets?

No available medicine stimulates the production of platelets. Platelet counts depressed by chemotherapy generally recover within a few days.

## What is done if platelet counts are sufficiently depressed to expose a person to a high risk of bleeding?

If platelet counts are very low and the person is at high risk of bleeding, a blood transfusion with platelets can rapidly elevate the platelet count and reduce the risk of bleeding. Because platelets are very expensive and in short supply, and because platelet transfusions can cause serious side effects such as allergic reactions, transfusion of platelets is reserved for situations in which the risk of serious bleeding is very high. When the platelet count in the bloodstream drops to the level of "5000 per cubic millimeter", a platelet transfusion is generally required.

# INFUSION REACTIONS

## DEFINITION

### What is an infusion reaction?

An infusion reaction is a side effect that can develop within two hours of the intravenous injection of a medication. The severity of this reaction can range from mild and slightly annoying to very serious and life threatening.

## SYMPTOMS

### What are the symptoms of an infusion reaction?

Mild infusion reaction symptoms might include reddening and itchiness of the skin, along with a bit of shortness of breath, nausea, and light-headedness. If the reaction is severe, a person may develop the severe skin rash commonly known as "hives", along with swelling of the face, extreme shortness of breath, severe dizziness, chest pain, palpitations and loss of consciousness.

## CANCER MEDICATIONS THAT CAUSE INFUSION REACTIONS

*Which cancer medications can cause infusion reactions?*

The most common cancer medications that can cause infusion reactions are the biotechnology medications called "monoclonal antibodies". The most frequently used monoclonal antibodies, "Rituximab" (brand name is "Rituxan", manufacturer's product website is www.rituxan.com), and "trastuzumab" (brand name is "Herceptin", manufacturer's product website is www.herceptin.com), frequently cause infusion reactions, which though usually mild, can sometimes be very serious and life threatening.

Among the chemotherapy medications, the most likely to induce infusion reactions include paclitaxel (brand name is "Taxol"), docetaxel (brand name is "Taxotere", manufacturer's product website is www.taxotere.com), cisplatin (which is generic), carboplatin (brand name is "Paraplatin"), and oxaliplatin (brand name is "Eloxatin", manufacturer's product website is www.eloxatin.com).

## PREVENTION OF INFUSION REACTIONS

*Is there a way to reduce the risk of having a severe infusion reaction?*

The monoclonal antibodies used in cancer treatment carry different risks of infusion reactions. For monoclonal antibodies such as Rituxan, or for people who have had prior infusion reactions, premedication with "acetaminophen" (brand name is "Tylenol") and "diphenhydramine" (brand name is "Benadryl") can reduce the severity of an infusion reaction that might occur. Some physicians may also prefer to administer a steroid medication such as "dexamethasone" (brand name is "Decadron") before the infusion.

The risk of having an infusion reaction is very different between the different chemotherapy medications. With medications such as Taxol and Taxotere, physicians will generally administer "diphenhydramine" (brand name is "Benadryl") and "dexamethasone" (brand name is "Decadron") before the infusion. Although infusion reactions can occur after cisplatin, carboplatin and oxaliplatin (as described above), premedication does not clearly prevent them and is therefore not routinely given.

## TREATMENT OF INFUSION REACTIONS

### What is the treatment of mild infusion reactions?

When a person is having a mild infusion reaction, the medical professionals administering the infusion will often interrupt the infusion and make a careful assessment of the severity of the infusion reaction, specifically looking for any sign that the infusion reaction may become very severe. When symptoms resolve, the infusion resumes at a slower rate and with very close observation. Intravenous administration of "diphenhydramine" (brand name is "Benadryl") is helpful to relieve some of the symptoms associated with the mild infusion reaction.

### What is the treatment of severe infusion reactions?

The onset of symptoms of severe infusion reactions may be an indication of "anaphylaxis", which is a rapidly progressive allergic reaction that could cause swelling of the airways and seriously drop the blood pressure and prove fatal within minutes unless properly treated.

When symptoms of severe infusion reactions or anaphylaxis appear, medical professionals will stop the infusion of monoclonal antibody or chemotherapy. An injection of "epinephrine", also known as "adrenaline", will immediately be given into a large muscle, such as the muscle of the thigh. To keep oxygen-rich blood flowing to the head, supplemental oxygen is given and the person will lie on their back, with the bed in a flat position. The antihistamine "diphenhydramine", given intravenously, helps relieve symptoms and accelerate recovery. If blood pressure has dropped, it may be necessary to give intravenous fluids and, occasionally, blood pressure raising medications.

**What is done after a severe infusion reaction if the medication causing it, such as Rituxan, is vitally important for improving the odds of a cure of the person's malignant disease?**

There are "desensitization protocols" that can induce tolerance to the medications. By first giving diphenhydramine and other medications, with emergency medicines and other measures at the bedside, and with slowly escalating doses of the monoclonal antibody, a person can be "desensitized" such that they tolerate the treatment.

Carrying out "desensitization protocols" does have some risk of producing a very serious infusion reaction, although this risk is lower in a center with extensive experience in carrying out these protocols. In considering treatment options when a person has had a previous serious infusion reaction, the risk of desensitization is balanced against the risk of stopping treatment with a medication that may be able to control the growth of a person's malignant tumor.

# NAUSEA AND VOMITING

## DEFINITION

### What is chemotherapy-induced nausea and vomiting?

Chemotherapy-induced nausea and vomiting, is a common side effect of cancer chemotherapy that can occur anytime, starting from when a person anticipates getting the chemotherapy to days after administration of chemotherapy. This nausea and vomiting poses a danger not only because of the severity of the symptoms and discomfort, but because it can interfere with the ability to give chemotherapy that is critical to obtaining control of a life-threatening cancer. About 80% of people who receive chemotherapy develop some nausea or vomiting.

## ASSESSING THE RISK OF SEVERE NAUSEA AND VOMITING

### Is it possible to predict who will develop nausea or vomiting after chemotherapy?

Each chemotherapy medication fits into a category in which it is classified as having a "high", "moderate", "low" or "minimal" risk of inducing nausea and vomiting. "High risk" chemotherapy nearly always causes nausea and vomiting, "moderate risk" usually causes nausea and vomiting, "low risk" sometimes causes nausea and vomiting, and "minimal risk" rarely causes nausea and vomiting.

Other factors that make vomiting with chemotherapy more likely include a younger age, being female, a history of motion sickness, and never or rarely drinking alcohol. People who have had nausea and vomiting with previous chemotherapy treatments are more likely to have the same symptoms with new chemotherapy regimens.

Based upon the category into which the prescribed chemotherapy medicines fit and other risk factors, an assessment is made regarding the likelihood of nausea and vomiting after chemotherapy. This information will prompt physicians and other caregivers to give appropriate treatment before and after chemotherapy that can prevent or diminish this side effect.

### *Why does some chemotherapy cause nausea and vomiting?*

The lining of the digestive tract contains "enterochromaffin cells" whose normal function is to produce hormones that regulate the functioning of the intestines. One of the most important hormones produced by these cells is "serotonin", which can help remove irritants from the digestive system by either triggering vomiting or diarrhea.

When certain types of chemotherapy are given, they can damage the enterochromaffin cells, causing them to release serotonin. This serotonin binds to "serotonin receptors" that send a signal to the lowermost part of the brain called the "brainstem". Within the brainstem, there is an area called "the vomiting center" which, when triggered, stimulates vomiting.

Other biological mechanisms also contribute to chemotherapy-induced nausea and vomiting. Chemotherapy can directly stimulate the vomiting center in the brain by stimulating the "NK-1 receptors" in the vomiting center of the brain.

## PREVENTION AND TREATMENT OF CHEMOTHERAPY-INDUCED NAUSEA AND VOMITING

*What types of medications prevent or control nausea and vomiting with chemotherapy?*

Four building blocks create the foundation upon which treatment regimens to control nausea and vomiting with chemotherapy are constructed. The goal of the treatment regimen will be to prevent the nausea and vomiting that can occur both immediately after chemotherapy and in the hours and days after receiving chemotherapy.

The first building block is medication that interferes with activation of the vomiting center by the "serotonin receptor". These medicines, the "5-HT3 receptor antagonists", are "ondansetron" (brand name is "Zofran", manufacturer's product website is www.gsk.com/products/prescription-medicines/zofran), "granisetron" (brand name is "Kytril", manufacturer's product website is www.kytril.com), and the most potent and newest medication in this category, "palonosetron" (brand name is "Aloxi", manufacturer's product website is www.aloxi.com). The FDA has issued a warning that a related medication called "dolasetron" (brand name is "Anzemet", manufacturer's product website is www.anzemet.com), when given by injection, can cause dangerous heart rhythm disturbances, and should not be used to prevent chemotherapy-associated nausea and vomiting.

The second building block is medication that prevents stimulation of the "NK-1 receptors" and, is therefore an "NK-1 antagonist". There is one NK-1 antagonist medication, "aprepitant", that is available in pill and injectable forms. The oral form of "aprepitant" has the brand name is "Emend" and the injected medicine has the brand name is "Emend for injection". Additional information about both forms of Emend is at the manufacturer's product website www.emend.com.

The third building block is the steroid medication "dexamethasone", better known by its brand name is "Decadron".

The fourth building block consists of the older, milder, and inexpensive anti-nausea medicines "metoclopramide" (brand name is "Reglan") and prochlorperazine (brand name is "Compazine").

*Which medicines are given if the chemotherapy is considered "highly likely" to produce nausea and vomiting?*

Giving a single dose of one of the medicines that block the serotonin receptor ("5-HT3 receptor antagonists") as well as three days of treatment with the oral or injected medicine that blocks the NK-1 receptor ("Emend" or "Emend for injection") and the steroid medication "dexamethasone" ("Decadron") effectively prevents or greatly diminishes nausea or vomiting most of the time. When given as a component of this three-drug combination, it is not clear whether any one of the 5-HT3 receptor antagonists is superior to the others.

### Which medicines are given if the chemotherapy is considered "moderately likely" to produce nausea and vomiting?

Giving a single dose of one of the medicines that block the serotonin receptor ("5-HT3 receptor antagonists") along with up to three days of treatment with the steroid medication "dexamethasone" ("Decadron") effectively prevents, or greatly diminishes, nausea or vomiting most of the time.

When a 5-HT3 receptor antagonist is given along with Decadron but without Emend, it appears that "palonosetron" (brand name is "Aloxi", manufacturer's product website is www.aloxi.com) is effective in preventing the vomiting that can occur one or more days after the chemotherapy is given.

### Which medicines are given if the chemotherapy is considered "low risk" to produce nausea and vomiting?

If there is a low risk of developing nausea and vomiting with chemotherapy, dexamethasone or one of the older anti-nausea medicine such as "metoclopramide" (brand name is "Reglan") or prochlorperazine (brand name is "Compazine") is usually effective in preventing nausea and vomiting.

### Is preventive medicine helpful if the chemotherapy has "minimal risk" to produce nausea and vomiting?

Medications to prevent nausea and vomiting are often unnecessary if the chemotherapy is of minimal risk to produce nausea and vomiting. If mild nausea or vomiting was a problem with previous minimal risk regimen, dexamethasone or one of the older anti-nausea medicines such as Reglan or Compazine often prevents the nausea or vomiting.

### What is "anticipatory nausea and vomiting" and how is it treated?

"Anticipatory nausea and vomiting" means that even before chemotherapy is given, the thought of chemotherapy provokes nausea and vomiting. This can occur in the hours, minutes, or seconds before the chemotherapy is given.

Anticipatory nausea and vomiting is often reduced by giving a medicine that can relieve the very significant anxiety that a person may feel about being injected with chemotherapy. The medication "lorazepam" (brand name is "Ativan") can be very helpful in preventing or reducing anticipatory nausea and vomiting.

## RADIATION-INDUCED NAUSEA AND VOMITING

### What types of radiation are most likely to cause nausea and vomiting?

Radiation to the upper part of the abdomen, as well as radiation to large areas of the body, is most likely to cause nausea and vomiting. Nausea and vomiting, however, can be a troublesome symptom with almost any form of radiation administered as cancer treatment.

### How is radiation-induced nausea and vomiting prevented and treated?

If the radiation oncologist administering the radiation believes that nausea and vomiting is likely, a treatment commonly used will be a 5-HT3 antagonist, as described earlier in this chapter, sometimes along with the medication "Decadron". If the form of radiation administered is unlikely to cause nausea and vomiting, physicians will often defer preventive medication and only administer the preventive medications if nausea and vomiting develop.

*What preventive treatment is helpful if a person receives treatment with a combination of chemotherapy and radiation that is very likely to produce nausea and vomiting?*

Treatment given to prevent nausea and vomiting will reflect the more intensive treatments used to prevent nausea and vomiting from chemotherapy as described earlier in this chapter.

# SEVERE DIARRHEA

## DEFINITIONS

### What is chemotherapy-induced diarrhea?

Chemotherapy-induced diarrhea is loose, watery stool passed several times in a day that develops because of receiving chemotherapy. The diarrhea is often associated with cramping abdominal pain, a sense of bloating of the abdomen, and a frequent urgent sensation of a need to run to the bathroom. The severity of the diarrhea can range from very mild to extremely severe, to the point where it is life threatening.

### What does it mean to have "severe chemotherapy-induced diarrhea"?

Physicians grade the toxicity associated with chemotherapy on a scale from "0" which means no symptoms to "4" which means life-threatening symptoms. Severe diarrhea refers to "grade 3" or "grade 4" diarrhea. "Grade 3" diarrhea is when a person is moving their bowels 7 or more times a day, cannot control their bowels before they reach the bathroom, and has severe cramping abdominal pain. "Grade 4" diarrhea is when the person is moving their bowels more than 10 times a day, and needs intravenous fluid to keep up with the fluid lost in stool that may also be bloody.

# THE RISKS OF SEVERE CHEMOTHERAPY-INDUCED DIARRHEA

## *Why can diarrhea be dangerous?*

The loss of large volumes of fluid in the stool can cause severe dehydration and deplete the bloodstream of essential salts and minerals such as sodium and potassium. Severe dehydration can contract the amount of fluid in the bloodstream, causing a dangerous drop of blood pressure and inadequate circulation of blood to the kidneys and other vital organs. Inadequate blood flow to the kidneys can produce "pre-renal azotemia" (see chapter entitled "Acute Kidney Injury") and is a serious complication of severe diarrhea.

Reductions of chemotherapy dose or delays of chemotherapy treatment can diminish the effectiveness of the treatment and reduce the chance of having the desired response to treatment.

## *What is the cause of severe chemotherapy-induced diarrhea?*

In good health, the cells lining the intestine both secrete fluid into the intestine and absorb fluid from the intestine. The proper balance between secretion and absorption allows us to absorb nutrients from our food and excrete unneeded waste products.

Chemotherapy can damage the cells lining the intestine and disrupt the normal balance between secretion and absorption, such that secretion dominates. When this happens, diarrhea develops. This can be a problem with the medications "5-FU", "capecitabine" (brand name is "Xeloda", manufacturer's product website is www.xeloda.com), "irinotecan" (brand name is "Camptosar"), and "oxaliplatin" (brand name is "Eloxatin", manufacturer's product website is www.eloxatin.com).

## TREATMENT OF SEVERE CHEMOTHERAPY-INDUCED DIARRHEA

### What first steps will be taken in treating chemotherapy-induced diarrhea?

Severe chemotherapy-induced diarrhea usually requires immediate hospitalization.

As a first step, a person's fluid and electrolyte status are evaluated to determine if there is significant dehydration or loss of sodium and potassium. If these problems are present, medical professionals will administer fluid and electrolytes by mouth or by vein. Because glucose encourages absorption of sodium from the intestine, drinking a glucose-containing solution such as "Gatorade", is very useful.

### Which medication reduces the severe diarrhea?

Although the medicine "loperamide" (brand name is "Imodium") is useful and effective for mild or moderate chemotherapy-induced diarrhea, it may not work well enough or quickly enough when a person has severe chemotherapy-induced diarrhea.

The medication "octreotide" (brand name is "Sandostatin", manufacturer's product website is www.sandostatin.com), given by injection, reduces fluid secretion and enhances fluid absorption in the intestine, while, at the same time, helping to slow movement of material through the intestine. Octreotide is a very potent medication in the treatment of severe chemotherapy-induced diarrhea. When necessary, octreotide is administered in increasing doses until the diarrhea stops and remains under control for at least 24 hours.

Chemotherapy may cause damage to the lining of the intestine. Because damaged intestine may permit entry of bacteria into the bloodstream, intravenous antibiotics may be necessary. Antibiotics may be particularly important if, along with the diarrhea, a person is susceptible to bacterial infections because of "chemotherapy-induced neutropenia" (see chapter entitled "Bone Marrow Suppression"). Antibiotics commonly given belong to the family of powerful "broad spectrum" antibiotics called "fluoroquinolones".

# SEVERE ORAL MUCOSITIS

## DEFINITION

### *What is severe oral mucositis?*

Severe oral mucositis is a very painful inflammation of the tissues lining the inside of the mouth and the throat. The severity of oral mucositis can range from mild to severe and is a common side effect of chemotherapy. When oral mucositis occurs, it begins causing symptoms within a few days of receiving chemotherapy, gets to its worst point about a week after getting chemotherapy, and is usually much better or resolved a week after it reaches its peak severity. Severe oral mucositis commonly occurs with intensive chemotherapy, such as the chemotherapy given for colorectal cancer, or with the chemotherapy used for people undergoing bone marrow transplantation.

## THE CAUSE OF SEVERE ORAL MUCOSITIS

### *Why can intensive chemotherapy cause severe oral mucositis?*

Intensive chemotherapy suppresses rapidly dividing cells anywhere in the body. Because of this, the most powerful chemotherapy medications or combinations of these medicines, can suppress cell division anywhere in the body, whether it is in cancer cells, bone marrow cells, or dividing cells in the mouth and throat. The damage to the cells lining the mouth and throat is the cause of the severe oral mucositis caused by chemotherapy. When the effects of the chemotherapy wear off, the cells in the mouth will begin to function normally again, and the oral mucositis will heal.

## RISKS OF SEVERE ORAL MUCOSITIS

### Why is severe oral mucositis dangerous?

Severe oral mucositis is very painful and could lead to reductions in the doses of chemotherapy given, which could lead to reduced effectiveness of chemotherapy.

When severe oral mucositis breaches the protective barrier formed by the lining of the inside of the mouth and throat, dangerous bacteria or fungus infections can get into the bloodstream and cause sepsis (see chapter "Sepsis and Septic Shock").

## TREATMENT OF SEVERE ORAL MUCOSITIS

### What is the treatment of severe oral mucositis?

No treatment clearly accelerates recovery from severe oral mucositis. The treatments of severe oral mucositis are palliative, that is, they relieve the pain associated with it and include vigilant observation for signs of infection that could spread from the damaged tissues in the mouth into the bloodstream.

Many different forms of specially prepared "mouthwashes" contain medications including anesthetic solutions, baking soda, calcium phosphate (this solution has the brand name "Caphosol", manufacturer's product website is www.caphosol.com), as well as chalky material that can coat the ulcers in the mouth and relieve their associated pain. These forms of mouthwash can significantly relieve symptoms.

The severe pain in the mouth often requires the use of powerful or injected narcotic painkillers, such as "Demerol" or "morphine". These medications can be enormously helpful in getting a person through the difficult week when the oral mucositis is severe.

If swallowing is difficult, a liquid diet with nutritional supplements may be required. Intravenous nutrition or fluids may be necessary if the pain associated with swallowing is too severe to permit eating or drinking.

# COMORBIDITIES: COMMON INDEPENDENT COEXISTING CONDITIONS

# COPD: CHRONIC OBSTRUCTIVE PULMONARY DISEASE

## DEFINITIONS

### What is chronic obstructive pulmonary disease?

Chronic obstructive pulmonary disease, abbreviated as "COPD", is a disease in which narrowed airways in the lungs obstruct the flow of air into and out of the lungs. In contrast to asthma, in COPD the obstruction of airflow into the lungs is only partially reversible with medications or with the passage of time.

### What is the association of COPD with cancer?

Although cancer does not cause COPD, people who were smokers and who have developed cancer, and especially lung cancer, very commonly have COPD. Depending upon its severity, COPD can have an important effect on a person's ability to withstand rigorous cancer treatments.

### How does air normally flow into the lungs?

Air enters the mouth or nose and travels down the trachea that divides into the large bronchial tubes that deliver air to each lung. The bronchial tubes send off smaller and smaller branches that eventually stop branching at the "terminal bronchioles" and "respiratory bronchioles". These bronchioles deliver air to microscopic airspaces called "alveoli" that transfer oxygen to the bloodstream.

## What is chronic bronchitis?

Chronic bronchitis is a chronic inflammation of the bronchial tubes that lasts for several months or longer. This inflammation can cause a serious problem with excess production of thick mucus that interferes with the ability to move air into and out of the lungs.

## What is emphysema?

With emphysema, there is damage to the walls of the bronchioles, alveoli and surrounding lung tissue. Destruction of lung tissue around the bronchioles can cause the bronchioles to collapse or become compressed, interfering with their ability to move air out of the lungs, and making it difficult for a person to exhale normally.

## THE CAUSE OF COPD

## Who gets COPD?

COPD is almost entirely a disease of smokers. Rarely, a genetic disease called "alpha one antitrypsin deficiency" causes COPD.

# SYMPTOMS

## *What are the most common symptoms of COPD?*

The most common early symptom of COPD is shortness of breath with exertion. This shortness of breath, which at first may be very slight, can progress over many years to the point where mild exertion leaves the person feeling short of breath. People with COPD have a chronic cough that produces thick sputum. As time passes, the cough gets worse and there is an increasing amount of sputum coughed out of the lungs. The cough and increasing sputum are signs of chronic bronchitis, and as this worsens, the inflamed bronchial tubes get swollen and narrowed and severe airway obstruction can develop.

# MAKING THE DIAGNOSIS

## *What tests confirm the diagnosis of COPD?*

A physician can often make a tentative diagnosis of COPD based on a history of smoking, the symptoms a person is experiencing, and the history a person provides regarding the evolution of their symptoms over the previous months or years. A test called "spirometry" will make the definitive diagnosis.

# DETERMINING THE SEVERITY OF DAMAGE TO THE LUNGS

## *What is spirometry?*

Spirometry is a test that measures the amount of air that a person can inhale and exhale, and the speed with which a person can exhale air over time.

One of the most important tests during spirometry will measure the maximum volume of air a person can forcefully exhale in one second. This test is a "FEV1", which stands for "forced expiratory volume, one second". The FEV1 is measured before and after the person inhales a medicine that widens or "dilates" the bronchial tubes (a "bronchodilator"). If the FEV1 is less than half what would be expected for a person of the same age, and if there is a lack of significant improvement of the FEV1 after a bronchodilator (discussed later in this chapter), and if the person's smoking history, symptoms and history of symptoms are consistent with COPD, the diagnosis of COPD is made. The FEV1 gives very important information about the severity of the disease and determines, over time, whether the disease is getting better or worse, and whether the disease is responding to treatment.

Another important measurement done with spirometry is the "FVC" or "forced vital capacity". FVC is a measurement of the amount of air that a person can expel from their lungs after taking a full deep breath. The relationship between the FEV1 and the FVC in a ratio called the "FEV1/FVC ratio" provides important information about the severity of the person's disease and helps to provide guidance with regard to appropriate treatment.

## How is the severity of the disease characterized?

Based upon the FEV1 and the FVC as well as an experienced physician's judgment a person can be characterized as having either mild ("stage I"), moderate ("stage II"), severe ("stage III"), or very severe (stage IV") COPD. This categorization of people with COPD into four stages provides a framework for decisions made about treatment.

# TREATMENT OF COPD
# BRONCHODILATORS

## What are inhaled bronchodilators?

Bronchodilators used to treat COPD are inhaled medicines that relax the muscles in the walls of the bronchial tubes and allow their air channels to "dilate" or become wider. This will help air to flow more easily through abnormally narrow airways. Although bronchodilators cannot entirely relieve the obstruction caused by the damage to the airways, they clearly provide some relief of symptoms and can be particularly helpful when shortness of breath suddenly worsens.

There are two major types of bronchodilators: short-acting bronchodilators and long acting bronchodilators.

## What are short-acting bronchodilators and when are they useful?

Short-acting bronchodilators are "rescue inhalers" used to immediately dilate the bronchial tubes and treat rapidly worsening shortness of breath. These rescue inhalers can be carried in a pocket or a purse and allow a person to deliver the medicine directly into their lungs by putting the mouthpiece of the device in the mouth, pressing on the canister, and taking a deep breath as a puff of medicine comes out of the mouthpiece. The device used to do this is a "metered dose inhaler" or "MDI". In order to achieve maximal benefit from the metered dose inhaler, it is essential that the person master the technique of inhaling deeply the moment there is release of a puff of medicine from the mouthpiece of the canister. The most commonly used medicine inside the metered dose inhaler is "albuterol", which is a "short-acting beta agonist".

The short-acting bronchodilators are commonly prescribed to be used on an "as needed basis" for people with mild (stage I) COPD who may be intermittently troubled by symptoms of shortness of breath.

## What are long-acting beta agonist bronchodilators and when are they useful?

Unlike the short-acting bronchodilators, long-acting bronchodilators do not rapidly relieve symptoms of shortness of breath. Long-acting beta agonists gradually relax the muscle around the bronchiole tubes and keep them relaxed for several hours during which there will be relief of symptoms. The two most commonly used long-acting beta agonist bronchodilators (sometimes abbreviated as "LABA"), are "formoterol" (brand name is "Foradil", manufacturer's product website is www.foradil.com) and "salmeterol" (brand name is "Serevent", manufacturer's product website is www.serevent.com). These medications are usually prescribed when a person arrives at the stage of having moderate (stage II) COPD.

A once-daily long-acting beta agonist called "indacaterol" was recently approved by the FDA and is expected to become available in the United States in early 2012 under the brand name "Arcapta Neohaler" (manufacturer's product website is www.arcapta.com). Indacaterol modestly improves lung function, and reduces the risk of developing an "acute exacerbation" of COPD, as described later in this chapter.

### What are anticholinergic agents?

Anticholinergic agents are also bronchodilators administered with an inhaler, and relax the muscle around the bronchioles, improving the flow of air back and forth. They also can reduce, to some extent, the mucus in the lungs that can make it more difficult to breathe.

### What is the difference between short-acting and long-acting anticholinergic medications?

The most common short-acting anticholinergic, "ipratropium" (brand name is "Atrovent") clearly relieves shortness of breath and enhances a person's ability to tolerate physical exertion. Ipratropium has an effect that is relatively rapid in onset but not sustained, and requires administration several times a day to have its best effect on breathing.

The most commonly used long-acting anticholinergic medication, "tiotropium" (brand name is "Spiriva", manufacturer's product website is www.spiriva.com), has a slower onset in improving symptoms, but the effect is sufficiently sustained such that it can be given only once per day. Like the long-acting beta agonists, long-acting anticholinergic medications are usually prescribed when a person arrives at the stage of having moderate (stage II) COPD.

### Is tiotropium useful when given indefinitely to people with COPD?

A clinical trial involving approximately 6000 people with COPD followed over a period of 4 years compared the effectiveness of tiotropium with that of a placebo. The people who took the tiotropium clearly did better than people receiving placebo, with better lung function, better quality of life, and fewer hospitalizations and episodes of acute respiratory failure (described later in this chapter). Largely because of this study, tiotropium is an every day treatment for many people with COPD.

## Is it useful to give beta agonist and anticholinergic medications together?

Beta agonists given with anticholinergic medications may further reduce symptoms and the risk of developing acute exacerbations of COPD (described later in this chapter). The inhaled medicine with a brand name of "Combivent" (manufacturer's product website is www.combivent.com) combines ipratropium with albuterol. As separate medications, the long-acting beta agonist formoterol (brand name is "Foradil") may be taken twice daily along with the once daily long-acting anticholinergic tiotropium (brand name is "Spiriva").

## Can these medications slow progression of COPD or do they only treat the symptoms?

Beta agonist and anticholinergic medications relieve symptoms of COPD, but do not slow or stop progressive lung damage associated with COPD. The only intervention that can slow the progression of COPD is smoking cessation. In people with advanced COPD, there commonly is progressive deterioration of lung function even after a person has stopped smoking, although not as rapid deterioration as in a person who keeps smoking.

## STEROIDS

### When are inhaled steroids useful?

Inhaled steroid medications are useful when beta agonists, anticholinergic medications, and respiratory therapy are not working well and the person is having severe or increasing difficulty breathing. These are often people who have moderate or severe or very severe (stage II, III, or IV) COPD or who are having episodes where their symptoms of shortness of breath suddenly worsens. The inhaled steroids most commonly used are "fluticasone" (brand name is "Flovent", manufacturer's product website is www.flovent.com) or "beclamethasone" (brand name is "Q-Var", manufacturer's product is www.qvar.com) or "budesonide" (brand name is "Pulmicort", manufacturer's product website is www.pulmicort.com).

Inhaled steroids, when combined with an inhaled bronchodilator, can be much more effective in relieving a person's symptoms of shortness of breath. It is more convenient and a lot easier to take two inhaled medications combined in the same canister and inhaled into the lungs with the same puff. There are inhaled medications that combine budesonide with formoterol (brand name is "Symbicort", manufacturer's product website is www.symbicort.com) and fluticasone and salmeterol (brand name is "Advair", manufacturer's product website is www.advair.com).

### Are steroids in a pill as safe as an inhaled steroid?

The benefit of an inhaled steroid is that there is not a great deal of absorption of the steroid from the lungs into the bloodstream. In contrast, orally administered steroid medicine is absorbed into the bloodstream, exposing the entire body to steroids. When given over a period of weeks or months, steroids taken as a pill can have a great deal of side effects.

### What are the side effects of long-term use of steroids when taken orally, that is, as a pill by mouth?

Side effects of oral steroids can include high blood pressure, diabetes, cataracts, and weakening of the bones ("osteoporosis"). People taking oral steroids may complain about not thinking clearly and often feel very restless and moody.

## OXYGEN THERAPY

### What is oxygen therapy?

Oxygen therapy, in the setting of COPD, refers to the use of oxygen for 12 hours or more per day or the routine use of oxygen during any significant physical exertion.

### When is oxygen therapy useful?

When a person has very severe COPD, physicians commonly will measure the amount of oxygen in a person's bloodstream. If this is very low, it can indicate that supplemental oxygen can be helpful.

### How effective is oxygen therapy?

When the level of oxygen in the bloodstream drops significantly, a person with COPD is at a higher risk of death, including sudden death, from COPD. The supplemental oxygen helps relieve some of the symptoms of breathlessness, and reduces the risk of death from COPD.

## ACUTE EXACERBATION OF COPD

### What is an acute exacerbation of COPD?

An acute exacerbation of COPD means a sudden worsening of shortness of breath associated with an increased production of sputum that may have changed its color to a deeper yellow or green. The severity of this exacerbation can range from a mild worsening treated with medicine at home, to worsening requiring treatment in a hospital and sometimes in an intensive care unit. Severe exacerbations are life threatening and are a common cause of death for people with COPD. Rapidly worsening fatigue, or any new symptoms of confusion, are particularly dangerous symptoms and may indicate that the person with COPD is not only having an exacerbation but is in imminent danger of a complete failure of ability to breathe ("acute respiratory failure").

## IMMEDIATE ACTION NEEDED WHEN SYMPTOMS OF ACUTE RESPIRATORY FAILURE DEVELOP

### What can a person with COPD or their family do when symptoms suggestive of impending acute respiratory failure develop?

Acute COPD exacerbation requires prompt treatment. Sudden worsening of shortness of breath can occur with acute COPD exacerbation and can rapidly progress to acute respiratory failure, and an inability to breathe, with life-threatening consequences.

People with COPD and their families should have a well-organized plan that will allow them to get treatment promptly if very severe difficulty breathing, suggesting impending acute respiratory failure, develops. If these symptoms develop, immediate transportation to a nearby well-equipped hospital will be essential.

A systematic emergency plan for dealing with acute respiratory failure should include exactly how to call an ambulance and, in some cities, which ambulance company to call. In working out these plans, it is good to consult with the person's physician and other medical professionals regarding how to arrange to have an ambulance bring the person with a severe exacerbation and impending respiratory failure to the hospital that is best equipped to treat this medical emergency.

### *Why do people with COPD develop exacerbations?*

People with COPD are very prone to developing lung infections. When a person already has limited lung function because of COPD, these infections can trigger an acute exacerbation. In addition, exposure to environmental pollutants including smoke from any source can irritate the lungs and trigger an exacerbation.

## PREVENTION OF COPD EXACERBATIONS

### *How are COPD exacerbations prevented?*

The risk of developing COPD exacerbations is lower with appropriate vaccinations against some types of infection, and immediate treatment with antibiotics at the first sign of a bacterial infection in the lungs. Adherence to the prescribed regimens of inhaled bronchodilators and inhaled steroids can also reduce, although not eliminate, the risk of developing exacerbations.

A medication very recently approved by the FDA called "roflumilast" (brand name is "Daliresp", manufacturer's product website is www.daliresp.com), can reduce the incidence of exacerbations in people with severe COPD who have had previous exacerbations. In the two large studies upon which the FDA's decision to approve the marketing of Daliresp was largely based, Daliresp, given as a once-daily pill for a year, reduced the risk of a person having a COPD exacerbation by 15-18%. The possible side effects of Daliresp include weight loss, nausea, diarrhea, and development of psychiatric problems such as depression and suicidal tendencies.

### What can help deal with all the thick mucus in the lungs?

A respiratory therapist can teach a person or their family techniques of using gravity and hands clapping on the back to loosen mucus in the lungs so that it easier to cough the mucus up and out.

The over-the-counter cough medicines containing "guaifenesin" (one of many brand names of this is "Mucinex", manufacturer's product website is www.mucinex.com) as well as a special liquid formulation of potassium iodide called "SSKI" (SSKI is an abbreviation for "saturated solution of potassium iodide") appear to have some ability to thin the thick mucus. This makes it easier to cough the mucus up from the lungs and spit it out. These medicines, which are "mucolytic agents", appear to have a small, but real, effect in reducing the risk of developing serious exacerbations and, if exacerbations develop, reduce the number of days that symptoms are severe and disabling. Mucolytic agents appear to be most effective in people who have many exacerbations and in people who are not already taking inhaled steroids.

Breathing in vaporized water or salt water does not clearly have benefit and can sometimes irritate the airways. Drinking an excessive amount of fluid to try to loosen the mucus does not have any clear benefit either.

## What vaccinations should a person with COPD regularly receive?

The "influenza vaccine" can reduce the risk of developing the flu ("influenza"), which is a common trigger of exacerbations. The "pneumococcal vaccine" is useful for people with severe COPD or who are over 65 years of age, as it can prevent pneumonia caused by bacteria called "pneumococcus".

## Since people with COPD are so prone to lung infections, should they take antibiotics all the time?

Wide varieties of bacteria are normally present in the airways. These bacteria may not cause disease (they are "non-pathogenic bacteria") and may suppress the growth of bacteria that do cause disease (called "pathogenic bacteria"). Antibiotics given for a very long period can encourage the growth of pathogenic bacteria that are resistant to antibiotics. Prompt treatment with antibiotics is important, however, when new symptoms appear that suggest that a lung infection has developed.

A recent study evaluated over 1000 people with COPD, randomly assigning half to receive the antibiotic "azithromycin" and the other half to receive a placebo. In addition to its antibiotic effect, azithromycin has an anti-inflammatory effect that researchers thought could possibly be helpful. The people receiving azithromycin clearly had a reduced incidence of exacerbations and a longer time between when they began treatment and had their next exacerbation. Azithromycin, however, encouraged the growth of some antibiotic resistant bacteria in the nose and throat. Based upon this study, some physicians suggest every day treatment with azithromycin for people with COPD who are having frequent acute exacerbations.

## TREATMENT OF ACUTE COPD EXACERBATION

*What is the treatment of an acute exacerbation of COPD?*

In order to improve breathing, modifications to the dose and type of bronchodilators the person is receiving may be useful. An oral steroid, in the form of a medicine called prednisone, can shorten, to a mild extent, the length of time it takes for recovery.

Because bacterial infection is a common trigger of an acute exacerbation, antibiotic treatment begins when it becomes evident that a person is having a COPD exacerbation.

Despite all these treatments, a person may be too short of breath and in too much distress to receive treatment at home. Hospitalization for COPD exacerbations is a common event as a person's COPD progresses into its most severe stages.

*In addition to bronchodilators, steroids, and antibiotics, what is the treatment in the hospital during an acute COPD exacerbation?*

We breathe in oxygen, and we breathe out carbon dioxide. When we are not breathing out properly, the carbon dioxide accumulates in the blood stream and leads to a condition called "respiratory acidosis" which can be dangerous.

To support a person's ability to breathe, a tight mask applied to the mouth and nose and attached to a machine, will push air into the lungs and help a person to breathe. This is "non-invasive positive pressure ventilation", abbreviated as "NPPV", and will greatly reduce a person's feeling of breathlessness, help take some of the carbon dioxide out of a person's bloodstream, and alleviate the respiratory acidosis that may have developed.

## ACUTE RESPIRATORY FAILURE

*What happens if despite these treatments, the situation worsens and a person still cannot breathe adequately?*

Despite best efforts with bronchodilators, antibiotics, non-invasive ventilation, and other medications, some people with severe COPD will develop a worsening of their condition to the point where it is impossible for them to breathe on their own. At this stage, a person has developed "acute respiratory failure" and will need "mechanical ventilation".

Mechanical ventilation requires a tube in the trachea (an "endotracheal tube") attached to the machine called a "ventilator" which pushes air into the lungs.

The insertion of the endotracheal tube, as well as maintaining the endotracheal tube in place, commonly causes anxiety and discomfort. To help relieve this, physicians may give sedatives before and after insertion of the endotracheal tube.

## GETTING A PERSON OFF A VENTILATOR

*How does a person get off the mechanical ventilator?*

Getting off the mechanical ventilator, (called "weaning off the ventilator") can be a difficult process. Physicians will try to decrease the person's dependence on the ventilator by gradually decreasing the work the mechanical ventilator does to support breathing. Once the person gets to the point where he or she can breathe independently and maintain their level of oxygen without the mechanical ventilator, the tube in the trachea can be removed (removal of the endotracheal tube is called "extubation") and support with the ventilator discontinued.

## THE RISK OF TOO MUCH OXYGEN

*Why can excessive oxygen trigger acute respiratory failure?*

The reflex to breathe depends upon the body's ability to sense the amounts of oxygen and carbon dioxide in the bloodstream.

People with COPD can develop an increased amount of carbon dioxide in their bloodstream because of their inability to move air in and out of their lungs normally. Over time, this chronic high amount of carbon dioxide in the bloodstream eliminates the reflex that stimulates breathing when the amount of carbon dioxide in the bloodstream gets too high. This leaves the person dependent on a reflex to breathe triggered by the body's sensing the amount of oxygen in the bloodstream. In this circumstance, if too much administered oxygen artificially raises the level of oxygen in the bloodstream, the reflex to breathe disappears, breathing slows down, and the person may develop acute respiratory failure.

## COR PULMONALE: A MAJOR HEART PROBLEM CAUSED BY COPD

### What is cor pulmonale?

In our circulatory system, blood returns to the heart from the top of the body via the superior vena cava and from the bottom of the body via the inferior vena cava. The superior and inferior vena cava delivers blood to the right side of the heart in the "right atrium". The right atrium empties the blood into the right ventricle and the right ventricle pumps blood to the lungs through the pulmonary artery. This large pulmonary artery divides left and right into smaller and smaller branches ("arterioles") until the arterial circulation of blood in the lungs reaches the microscopic capillary stage where the blood picks up its oxygen.

When there is extensive damage to the lungs associated with advanced COPD, structural abnormalities and constriction of the arteries in the lung develops and impedes the flow of blood through the arteries of the lungs. This is "pulmonary hypertension".

In order to overcome the increasing resistance of the arteries in pulmonary hypertension, the right ventricle must pump harder and harder. This causes the wall of the right ventricle to thicken (this is called "right ventricular hypertrophy") and the chamber inside the right ventricle to get larger. Eventually the right ventricle can no longer carry out its pumping function adequately and effectively. This is "cor pulmonale".

## What are the symptoms of cor pulmonale?

People with cor pulmonale are troubled by shortness of breath, fatigue, and occasionally by fainting with mild exertion.

Because in cor pulmonale the heart has difficulty with pumping blood through the lungs, there is an inadequate transfer of oxygen into the bloodstream. Lips, fingertips, and eventually the skin may begin to acquire a bluish tinge. This bluish tinge is "cyanosis".

The inability of the heart to pump blood into the lungs will cause a back up of pressure in the veins throughout the body. This increased pressure can cause the neck veins to bulge, the liver to enlarge, and the legs to swell.

## How is the diagnosis of cor pulmonale made?

A physician will have a strong suspicion of cor pulmonale based upon a person's medical history, symptoms, and physical examination. An echocardiogram, which bounces harmless sound waves across the heart and transmits images to a video screen, can provide details regarding the structure of a person's heart and provide clear evidence of right ventricular hypertrophy and of a failure of the right side of the heart to pump properly.

## What is the treatment of cor pulmonale?

The most effective treatment of cor pulmonale is for the person to receive supplemental oxygen for the majority of their day. Special small oxygen tanks are available that are carried like a knapsack or walked alongside the person with a cart.

Diuretics, given cautiously, can take down some of the swelling in the legs (see chapter entitled "Heart Failure").

A medication called "theophylline" may have modest ability to relieve constriction in the pulmonary arterial circulation and may improve the ability of the weakened right ventricle to forcefully contract.

## <u>OUTLOOK</u>

### *What is the outlook for a person with COPD?*

The outlook depends upon the degree of lung damage already done and on whether the person stops smoking.

As the FEV1 decreases, and if cor pulmonale develops, the outlook for a good quality of life and long survival worsens.

Continued smoking accelerates lung damage and is associated with a shortened survival.

# HEART FAILURE

## DEFINITIONS

### *What is heart failure?*

Heart failure occurs when the heart cannot pump blood with sufficient strength to keep pace with the needs of the body. Heart failure causes significant and possibly disabling symptoms and has the potential to greatly reduce lifespan and cause sudden death.

### *How does the heart pump blood normally?*

The heart consists of four chambers surrounded by muscle and filled with blood. These chambers are the right atrium, right ventricle, left atrium and left ventricle.

Contraction of the heart muscle (the "myocardium") surrounding the blood will abruptly compress blood in the heart's chambers. The heart's contractions push blood from the right atrium to the right ventricle, from the right ventricle to the lungs, then, after the blood returns to the heart from the lungs, from the left atrium to the left ventricle and from the left ventricle to the entire body.

"Valves" protect the forward movement of blood during heart muscle contraction by snapping shut at appropriate split seconds, preventing blood from rushing backward in the wrong direction as the heart muscle contracts and relaxes. These valves are located between the right atrium and right ventricle (the "tricuspid valve"), right ventricle and pulmonary artery ("pulmonary valve"), the left atrium and left ventricle (the "mitral valve") and the left ventricle and aorta (the "aortic valve").

## THE CAUSES OF HEART FAILURE

### *What can cause the heart to fail?*

For heart failure to occur there must be some event which initiates damage to the muscle or the valves of the heart. This initiating event can be a sudden event, such as an acute myocardial infarction (see chapter entitled "Heart Attack: Acute Myocardial Infarction") which suddenly and irreversibly damages a significant amount of heart muscle. The initiating event can also have evolved over an extended period, such as the strain, that high blood pressure puts upon the heart to pump blood throughout the body. Other initiating events include viral infections of heart muscle, chronic exposure to high levels of alcohol, or diseases involving the valves of the heart.

### *What causes heart failure in people with cancer or who have received treatment for cancer?*

Several chemotherapy medications can directly damage heart muscle and cause heart failure. Among chemotherapy medications, the medications with the highest risk of causing heart muscle damage and heart failure are in the "anthracycline family". The most widely used anthracycline is "doxorubicin", also known by its brand name "Adriamycin".

Some of the newer life-saving cancer medications discussed elsewhere in this book that are "monoclonal antibodies" and "targeted therapies" could damage heart muscle and cause heart failure. Among the more important medications with this potential side effect are "trastuzumab" (brand name is "Herceptin") and bevacizumab (brand name is "Avastin").

Radiation therapy, applied to the area of the chest beneath which, or adjacent to which, the heart is located, exposes the heart to radiation and can increase the risk of damage to the coronary arteries, the heart muscle, or to the valves inside the heart. Symptoms from radiation damage to these areas of the heart may appear many years, or even decades, after the radiation treatments.

*Other than cancer treatments, which other diseases of heart muscle may cause heart failure in people with cancer or who have received treatment for cancer?*

The most common cause of heart muscle damage leading to heart failure is a myocardial infarction (see chapter entitled "Heart Attack: Acute Myocardial Infarction"). A myocardial infarction will produce some permanent damage and scarring of heart muscle. If there is damage to a large area or several areas of heart muscle, there can be a weakening of the heart's pumping action.

The damage caused by a myocardial infarction can be sudden and massive, provoking sudden heart failure. On the opposite end of the spectrum, a slow and progressive narrowing of the heart's arteries and chronic lack of blood flow to the heart can gradually damage heart muscle and, over time, produce heart failure. People with diabetes, hypertension, or both, are particularly prone to silently progressive heart muscle damage that can lead to heart failure.

Less common causes of heart muscle problems are viral infections of the heart (called "viral myocarditis") and an assortment of uncommon diseases of heart muscle called "cardiomyopathies".

## WHEN VALVE PROBLEMS CAUSE HEART FAILURE

### Why can valve problems cause heart failure?

The valves in the heart normally flip open, allowing blood to flow forward and then snap shut, preventing blood from flowing backward. When there is damage or scarring of heart valves, serious problems can develop.

Valves that do not shut normally allow blood to flow backward or "regurgitate". When blood regurgitates backward, it strains the heart by forcing it to compensate for the blood pumped in the wrong direction. The regurgitation of blood into a chamber of the heart will also force that chamber to accommodate a volume of blood that is greater than its normal capacity. This will stretch the wall of the heart. Although at first, the strains and stretches caused by regurgitation may actually stimulate the heart to pump with greater strength, at some point the stretch is just too much for the heart to handle and the heart begins to fail.

Blood must flow past the scarred valves. Sometimes the valves are so scarred and immovable that they narrow the opening between the atrium and ventricle or between the ventricle and pulmonary artery or aorta. The narrowing of the valve ("stenosis") can create a partial blockade to normal blood flow. The heart, determined to carry out its essential function of pumping blood forward throughout the body, will pump harder to send blood past this partial blockade. At a point, the heart may no longer have the strength to push blood past this obstacle and heart failure can develop.

**What diseases can damage the valves in people with cancer or who have received treatment for cancer?**

Several diseases can cause scarring or damage to heart valves.

People who have had radiation therapy for cancer many years before can uncommonly develop a scarring of their heart valves that could lead to or contribute to heart failure.

In older people, the valves or the ring of tissue that surrounds the valves may collect calcium, harden ("calcify"), and interfere with the valves' ability to open and shut.

Acute bacterial infection of the heart valves (see chapter entitled "Infective Endocarditis") can cause serious damage to heart valves.

## SYMPTOMS OF HEART FAILURE

**What is the most common early symptom of heart failure?**

The most common symptom of heart failure is shortness of breath, which in medical terms is "dyspnea". Initially, this shortness of breath occurs mainly with mild physical exertion. As heart failure worsens, the shortness of breath develops with less and less physical activity (referred to as "dyspnea on exertion"). Shortness of breath may be particularly noticeable when lying flat, and may require the person to sleep propped up with several pillows or to sleep sitting up in a chair. When a person awakens in the middle of the night with sudden, severe difficulty breathing, medical people refer to it as "paroxysmal nocturnal dyspnea".

As the left ventricle weakens, it fails to deliver blood adequately to meet the needs of the entire body. Because of this, fatigue may become a prominent problem, which generally worsens as the day proceeds.

The development of a new, chronic cough, which usually does not produce sputum, is another common early symptom of heart failure.

## Why does a person with heart failure get shortness of breath?

Blood flows from the right ventricle to the lungs to the left atrium to the left ventricle. When the failing left ventricle is unable to adequately pump blood forward, there will be a pressure back-up which is transmitted backward from the left ventricle to the left atrium and then to the blood vessels in the lungs. This will engorge the blood vessels of the lungs with blood and cause a clear fluid to leak out of the blood vessels into the substance of the lung (called "interstitial pulmonary edema"). The combined effect of engorged lung blood vessels and interstitial pulmonary edema impairs the transfer of oxygen into the bloodstream and, in addition, makes the lungs stiff, increasing the effort it takes to breathe in and out.

## MAKING THE DIAGNOSIS

*How is the diagnosis of heart failure made?*

A skilled and experienced physician will have a very high suspicion that a person has heart failure based upon their medical history and their symptoms. In a physical examination, the physician can notice distension of the external neck veins along with characteristic pulsations in these veins that are indicative of heart failure. By touch, the physician can find that the area on the chest where the heartbeat is best felt shifted significantly to the left, indicating an enlargement of the heart. With a stethoscope, the physician can hear a subtle additional heart sound added to the "lub-dub" normal sounds, such that the heartbeat sounds a bit like a horse's gallop (this sound is an "S3 gallop"). With the stethoscope, the physician can hear heart murmurs indicating valve problems and detect the presence of fluid in the lungs. Leg swelling ("leg edema") is commonly present in people with heart failure.

The chest x-ray of a person with heart failure often shows some enlargement of the heart and engorgement of the blood vessels in the lungs.

A blood test is available measuring the "BNP". BNP is an abbreviation for "brain natriuretic peptide, and is a hormone that was first found in the brain (hence its name) but that is released primarily from the heart. The heart produces an excess of BNP in people with heart failure, elevating the levels of BNP in the bloodstream.

## How are the cause and the degree of heart failure determined?

An echocardiogram, a test using harmless sound waves, can examine the functioning of the heart valves as well as determine how effectively and symmetrically the heart muscle contracts. When the cause of heart failure is in doubt, the echocardiogram can often pinpoint or strongly suggest an underlying cause of the heart failure, such as a new myocardial infarction, and better direct treatment.

A standard electrocardiogram (often abbreviated as either "EKG" or "ECG") can provide vital information about the existence of heart muscle damage related to a new or old myocardial infarction. In addition, with chronic high blood pressure, which is a common cause of heart failure, the wall of the left ventricle thickens (called "left ventricular hypertrophy"). Left ventricular hypertrophy is readily evident with the electrocardiogram.

When the cause is in doubt, and inadequate blood flow to the heart is a significant possibility, the physician may recommend "exercise testing" or "stress testing". With exercise testing, evaluation of the electrocardiogram during physical exertion such as running or walking on a treadmill can identify evidence of inadequate blood flow to the heart muscle. If this test indicates a problem, physicians may suggest a cardiac catheterization (described in the chapter entitled "Heart Attack: Acute Myocardial Infarction") to evaluate the heart's arteries (the "coronary arteries") and determine whether there is a blockage or blockages that need to be relieved by surgery. Surgery to relieve blockage in coronary arteries is a "coronary artery bypass graft" or "CABG" (pronounced like the word "cabbage"). More information about this surgery is in the chapter entitled "Heart Attack: Acute Myocardial Infarction".

### *What is the "ejection fraction"?*

Using the echocardiogram, the physicians can calculate the "ejection fraction" which is a percentage of the blood within the heart ejected with each beat. A percentage of 55% or over is in the normal range. An ejection fraction of 35% or less can indicate significant heart failure.

## IDENTIFYING PROBLEMS WHICH WORSEN HEART FAILURE

### *What initial steps will a physician take after making a diagnosis of heart failure?*

Initially, the physician will consider whether the person is in any acute danger because of heart failure and whether there are any conditions at that moment in time that are suddenly and severely weakening the heart.

A new myocardial infarction can cause a sufficient amount of heart muscle damage so that the heart begins to fail. When heart failure develops suddenly, a myocardial infarction may have occurred recently despite the person not recalling having had the typical symptoms such as chest pain. More information about myocardial infarction is in the chapter entitled "Heart Attack: Acute Myocardial Infarction".

Several forms of irregular heart rhythm can produce heart failure. These rhythms can take the form of very slow heart rates (bradycardia) or very fast heart rates (tachycardia). Pneumonia (see chapters entitled "Community-Acquired Pneumonia" and "Hospital-Acquired Pneumonia") or a pulmonary embolism (see chapter entitled "Deep Vein Thrombosis and Pulmonary Embolism") can also provoke sudden, severe or worsening heart failure. If these conditions are present, their successful treatment can reverse the signs and symptoms of heart failure.

## TREATMENT OF CHRONIC HEART FAILURE

### Is heart failure curable?

There are several curable causes of heart failure. The most striking of these are the problems with heart valves. Cardiac surgeons can replace diseased valves with artificial valves and return heart function to normal. Erratic heart rhythms can greatly diminish the heart's effectiveness. Correction of these rhythms with appropriate treatments can greatly improve heart function.

Most of the time, however, after treatment of acute heart failure, a person will be left with some degree of irreversible heart disease and some degree of chronic heart failure.

### What drives the progression of heart failure?

Continued damage to heart muscle because of lack of adequate blood supply (ischemia), or because of uncontrolled high blood pressure, viral infection, or exposure to toxins, or other insults, can continually weaken the heart muscle and drive progression of heart failure.

In the past few years, it has become apparent that for many people, the factors that are most likely to be driving a person's heart failure, such as high blood pressure, seem to be under reasonable control, but the heart failure worsens anyway and eventually proves fatal. An additional critical factor, called "remodeling", takes place in a failing heart that can steadily worsen heart function.

## What is remodeling?

In the earliest stages of heart failure, the body tries to compensate for the inadequate pumping of the heart by releasing a series of hormones that help the heart pump more strongly and effectively. These hormones also signal the kidneys to take less fluid out of the bloodstream, and make less urine. This helps keep the volume of blood high enough to sustain a good blood pressure. People without heart failure produce these hormones every moment of the day and they are essential for maintaining normal heart function.

When the heart begins to fail, excessive production of these hormones can alter the shape of the chambers of the heart as well as scar the muscle of the heart. As the shape of the heart changes and the chambers of the heart enlarge, and as there is scarring of heart muscle, the heart pumps less efficiently. Less efficient pumping produces more hormones, which further remodels the heart, and causes worsening heart failure. This process is "remodeling". A critical goal of therapy is to prevent remodeling by using medications that interfere with the damaging effects of these hormones.

### *What is the treatment of chronic heart failure?*

The treatment of chronic heart failure depends upon the severity of the heart failure. A number of measures can make a person feel much better, prevent or delay remodeling, and reduce the short and long-term risk of death from heart disease.

The treatment of heart failure is a science that has a mass of literature as its foundation. There is, however, a divergence of opinion on some specific issues in the treatment of heart failure among the top cardiologists in the world, and the guidelines for treatment of heart failure are evolving. Cardiologists and other physicians may initiate medications in very different sequences and in very different doses. These differences could reflect the different causes of heart failure, as well as the different abilities people may have to adhere to their treatment schedules. The following discussion of the treatment of heart failure provides information regarding a treatment plan that is commonly used.

## TREATMENT OF MILD HEART FAILURE

### *What is mild heart failure?*

Mild heart failure, discovered during a routine physical examination, can exist without any significant symptoms. When this occurs, a person has "New York Heart Association class I" or "NYHA class I" heart failure.

When mild heart failure is associated with shortness of breath, fatigue or palpitations with normal exertion, the person has "NYHA class II" heart failure.

A person with mild heart failure can usually continue working full time at a job that does not require significant physical exertion.

## What is the treatment of mild heart failure?

Strenuous physical activity may put harmful strain on the heart, but moderate exercise, such as walking or riding an exercise bike, can help minimize symptoms of heart failure, and can prevent or slow worsening of heart failure.

With heart failure, a person is prone to retaining too much fluid in their body, which can strain the heart and, because of excess fluid in the tissues of the lungs, cause shortness of breath. Salty food or putting extra salt on food will cause the body to retain fluid and worsen the heart failure. It will be very important for the person with heart failure to restrict their intake of salt. Limiting the amount of fluid that a person drinks during the day is generally not necessary.

"Diuretics", "ACE inhibitors" and "beta blockers", are medicines commonly prescribed for the person with mild heart failure.

## THE NEED FOR DIURETICS

### Why do people with heart failure retain fluid?

In the aorta, which is the major artery emerging from the heart, and in the carotid arteries, which are the arteries feeding the brain, are "baroreceptors" which detect the pressure of blood flowing through these vessels. These baroreceptors send signals to the brain indicating whether the pressure in these blood vessels, which reflects the volume of blood flowing through our circulatory system, is too low, too high, or normal. Based upon these signals, the brain releases hormones that control the amount of water and sodium that the kidney absorbs back into the bloodstream. By this means, the healthy body maintains a steady blood pressure and an appropriate volume of blood in our bloodstream, despite day-to-day changes in our intake of water and sodium.

When the heart is failing, the "baroreceptors" detect a lower blood pressure and, incorrectly sense that the blood volume is too low. This triggers the kidneys to prevent the loss of water and sodium from the bloodstream. This excessive fluid retention expands the volume of fluid in the bloodstream too much, and can lead to excess fluid in the lungs and difficulty with breathing. This excessive fluid also leads to swelling of the legs.

### What are diuretics?

Diuretics are medicines which help the body to get rid of excess sodium by preventing the kidney from fully absorbing the sodium back into the bloodstream. The increased amount of sodium eliminated by the kidneys carries water along with it. This increases the volume of urine eliminated from the body by urination, and helps relieve the "fluid overload" which causes difficulty with breathing and leg swelling.

### When does treatment with diuretics begin?

Diuretics are an initial treatment when a person with heart failure appears to have "fluid overload" that is causing leg swelling or shortness of breath with exertion or when lying down.

## Which diuretics relieve the fluid overload associated with heart failure?

The three major types of diuretics prescribed are the "loop diuretics", "thiazides", and "aldosterone antagonists". Each of these diuretics has a unique way that it interferes with the kidney's ability to absorb sodium.

The most commonly used diuretics in heart failure are the "loop diuretics" and the most commonly used has the generic name "furosemide" (brand name is "Lasix"). Depending on the symptoms a person is experiencing, the physician will generally start treatment with a low dosage and gradually increase the dosage to a level that removes the excess fluid from the body and relieves the associated symptoms. If Lasix fails to do the job adequately, other "loop diuretics" may substitute for Lasix, or a thiazide diuretic or aldosterone antagonist diuretic may replace or supplement Lasix treatment.

## DANGERS OF DIURETICS

## What are the dangers of diuretics?

Loop diuretics and thiazide diuretics can cause the level of potassium in the bloodstream to go down. A low level of potassium in the bloodstream can cause very dangerous heart rhythm problems and can increase the risk of developing dangerous side effects from digoxin (see below). For this reason, the person taking these diuretics may be advised to take supplemental potassium in order to keep blood potassium levels in the normal range.

The aldosterone antagonist diuretics have the opposite effect on potassium and can have the side effect of raising the level of potassium in the bloodstream, occasionally to worrisome levels. This can also cause dangerous heart rhythm problems.

Diuretics, by pulling fluid out of the bloodstream, can produce an excessive contraction of the amount of fluid in the bloodstream and can drop the blood pressure and the flow of blood to the kidneys. Too much contraction of the blood volume can result in a type of kidney failure called "pre-renal azotemia" (see chapter entitled "Acute Kidney Injury").

For these reasons, it is very important that a person with heart failure receiving diuretics have regular visits with their health professionals and not increase their own dose of diuretics without medical supervision.

## ACE INHIBITORS

### *What are ACE inhibitors?*

There is a hormone produced by the body called "angiotensin" which constricts the arteries of the body and elevates the blood pressure. This puts a strain on the heart since it has to pump harder to drive the blood through constricted, high-pressure blood vessels. In addition, angiotensin has a direct toxic effect on the heart, thickening the wall of the heart and playing a key role in causing the "remodeling" of the heart that was discussed earlier in this chapter.

The full name of medications called "ACE inhibitors" is "angiotensin converting enzyme inhibitors". ACE inhibitors slow down the production of angiotensin by the body, reduce the amount of angiotensin in the bloodstream, free the arteries from the constricting influence of angiotensin, and prevent or slow the thickening of the heart muscle (called "hypertrophy") and the remodeling that are so damaging in heart failure.

## Are ACE inhibitors always useful in heart failure?

There is a solid body of information, based upon well-designed clinical trials, which show that medicines in the ACE inhibitor family relieve symptoms, prevent remodeling, reduce hospitalizations and reduce the risk of death from heart failure. Once diuretics have relieved excess fluid, which generally is accomplished in days or a few weeks, ACE inhibitors are recommended indefinitely for almost every person with heart failure regardless of its severity.

## Are ACE inhibitors safe?

ACE inhibitors have a low risk of side effects and most people can easily tolerate them indefinitely. Most of the side effects relate to slightly excessive drops in blood pressure at the beginning of treatment, and generally go away on their own. ACE inhibitors can also cause a person to retain more potassium, especially if they are taking a potassium supplement or receiving diuretics called "aldosterone antagonists". Occasionally, these side effects may require a reduction of the dose, and then, if possible, gradual increase to the higher optimal dose levels later on.

Approximately one in eight people who start treatment with ACE inhibitors develops a persistent, annoying cough, and less than one person in one hundred develops a swelling of the tissues in the head and neck area (this swelling is called "angioedema") that can be dangerous.

As with almost all medicines, there is a potential for a broad range of side effects, however, the ACE inhibitors usually have few, if any, side effects, and have played a critical role in improving and extending life in people with heart failure. For this reason, physicians encourage people with heart failure take to ACE inhibitors whenever possible.

### What is the alternative treatment when a person cannot tolerate ACE inhibitors?

An alternative way of blocking the angiotensin that is so damaging to the heart is to give a medicine in the family of "angiotensin receptor blockers", which are also nicknamed "ARB's". When ACE inhibitors cause significant problems with persistent cough or angioedema, substitution of ARB's will have a similar benefit to that of the ACE inhibitors.

### What are the names of the ACE inhibitors that are used?

ACE inhibitors that improve the health of people with heart failure include enalapril (brand name is "Vasotec"), captopril (brand name is "Capoten"), and ramipril (brand name is "Altace", manufacturer's product website is www.altace.com).

### What are the names of ARB's that are useful in heart failure?

ARB's that have proven to be useful in heart failure include valsartan (brand name is "Diovan", manufacturer's product website is www.diovan.com), losartan (brand name is "Cozaar", manufacturer's product website is www.cozaar.com), irbesartan (brand name is "Avapro", manufacturer's product website www.avapro.com), and candesartan (brand name is "Atacand", manufacturer's product website is www.atacand.com).

## BETA BLOCKERS

### What are beta-blockers?

It is the common human experience that when we are frightened or angered or put under great stress, our hearts beat more quickly and with sufficiently greater force such that we feel the pounding of our heart in our chest. In good health, this "fight or flight response" is a good thing, as it prepares our bodies to react to sudden severe emergencies.

The "fight or flight response" happens because, when exposed to stress, our bodies suddenly release the hormones called "epinephrine" and "norepinephrine" in high amounts into our bloodstream. Among other things that they do, the epinephrine and norepinephrine bind to "beta adrenergic receptors" which are present on the heart and blood vessels, and stimulate the acceleration of heart rate and other heart and blood vessel changes that go along with the "fight or flight" response.

In heart failure, there is excessive stimulation of the "beta adrenergic receptors" leading to increases in heart rate and blood pressure. This causes the heart to work harder which, with increasing heart failure, puts further strain on the heart. Beta-blockers block the effects of epinephrine on the beta-adrenergic receptors and can prevent their stimulation and the problems this can cause.

## How effective are beta-blockers?

After diuretics, if they were necessary, have corrected a person's fluid retention, and if the person is taking an appropriate dose of an ACE inhibitor or ARB medication, beta-blockers can be clearly effective in relieving symptoms, improving heart function, and reducing the risk of death from heart failure.

## How do physicians initially prescribe treatment with beta-blockers?

When a person begins treatment with beta-blockers, physicians generally initially prescribe a very low dose and gradually increase the dose, taking each step upward in dose every 2 to 4 weeks. The reason for this is that too rapidly increasing the beta-blocker dose can itself be harmful to blood pressure levels and heart function.

## Which beta-blockers are effective treatments of heart failure?

Beta-blockers proven effective in heart failure include bisoprodol (brand name is "Zebeta, manufacturer's product website is www.zebeta.com), carvedilol (brand name is "Coreg", manufacturer's product website is www.coreg.com) and a long-acting form of metoprolol (brand name is "Lopressor").

## HYDRALAZINE AND NITRATES

### What is hydralazine and what are nitrates?

Hydralazine is a medication that relaxes arteries, which allows the heart to work less hard to push blood through them and around the body

Nitrates also relax blood vessels, but work mainly on the veins and can help keep blood in the veins longer and reduce the volume of blood returning to the heart. This will reduce the volume of blood that the heart must pump with each beat. This reduces strain on the heart and allows the heart to beat more effectively.

Hydralazine is a generic medicine sold under that name. The nitrate that is usually used is "isosorbide dinitrate", sometimes sold under the brand name "Isordil". There is a more expensive tablet called "BiDil" (manufacturer's product website is www.bidil.com) that combines the two medications, in proper doses in one pill. Hydralazine and nitrates given together reduce the effort that the heart has to make to push blood through the body and can be helpful for people with heart failure.

## When are hydralazine and nitrate prescribed?

Hydralazine and nitrates are useful if a person is intolerant of ACE inhibitors or ARBs or if these medications do not seem to be adequately controlling a person's symptoms of heart failure.

African American people with heart failure appear to respond better to combination treatment with hydralazine and nitrates than people of other races, and for this reason, physicians commonly prescribe hydralazine and nitrates in conjunction with other heart failure medications for people with heart failure who are African American.

# ALDOSTERONE ANTAGONISTS

## *What is aldosterone and what are aldosterone antagonists?*

Aldosterone is a hormone made in the adrenal glands that stimulates the absorption of sodium from the kidneys. In heart failure, there is excessive production of aldosterone. Excessive aldosterone in the bloodstream has a direct damaging effect on the heart, promoting remodeling, weakening the heart, and worsening heart failure.

Aldosterone antagonists block the binding of aldosterone to its "receptor" on heart muscle cells, thereby preventing aldosterone from causing further damage. Aldosterone antagonists also inhibit sodium absorption in the kidney, and have a powerful effect in reducing excess fluid in the body by driving sodium and fluid into the urine.

## *When is an aldosterone antagonist useful?*

A recent large and important clinical study indicated that an aldosterone antagonist called "eplerenone" (brand name is "Inspra"), has the potential to reduce the risk of death from heart failure and the risk of sudden worsening of symptoms requiring hospitalization. This important benefit was evident when Inspra was included in the treatment of people with mild symptoms of heart failure and with evidence from the echocardiogram of serious weakening of the left ventricle as indicated by an "ejection fraction", as described earlier in this chapter, of less than 35%. Because of this and other clinical trials evaluating the use of aldosterone antagonists, the use of aldosterone antagonists has become more common in people with mild or moderate heart failure.

## What is the major side effect of aldosterone antagonists?

Aldosterone antagonists cause the body to retain potassium and can lead to dangerous elevations of potassium in the bloodstream. This elevated level of potassium in the bloodstream is called "hyperkalemia" and can lead to a dangerously irregular heartbeat and, if severe, to cardiac arrest. Frequent blood tests assure that this complication does not develop.

## DIGOXIN

## What is digoxin?

Digoxin is a medicine that stimulates the heart to beat with greater strength.

Digoxin has been around for a long time. Over 200 years ago, "digitalis", prescribed in the herbal form called "foxglove", was a treatment of "dropsy", which we now call "heart failure". Today, the most common form of digitalis prescribed is "'digoxin" which can be given by mouth or, in an emergency, by intravenous injection.

## When is digoxin helpful?

Digoxin is often prescribed when, despite treatment with ACE inhibitors, angiotensin receptor blocking medication, a beta blocker and diuretics, a person's heart failure appears to be worsening.

## Is digoxin a safe medicine?

Digoxin can be a useful medicine that reduces the risk of hospitalization for worsening heart failure. Digoxin has a serious potential side effect: "digitoxicity".

## What is digitoxicity?

Digitoxicity is a dangerous excess of digoxin in the bloodstream. In some people, and particularly in people taking diuretics, the amount of digoxin in the bloodstream slowly builds up to toxic levels. The reason for this build-up relates to slowed metabolism of the drug or reduced excretion of the drug by the kidneys. When this happens and a person keeps taking digoxin, digoxin accumulates in the body and digitoxicity occurs.

## What are the symptoms of digitoxicity?

The most common symptoms are loss of appetite and nausea. The heart rhythm may become irregular and heart failure could worsen.

## How is the diagnosis of digitoxicity made?

The new symptoms which the person reports will raise the suspicion of digitoxicity. The electrocardiogram may show major abnormalities that strongly suggest digitoxicity. Blood tests that demonstrate the elevated level of digoxin in the bloodstream make the diagnosis of digitoxicity.

## What is the treatment of digitoxicity?

There is a biotechnology medicine called "Digibind" which specifically attaches to digoxin and clears it from the bloodstream. Digibind is a highly effective treatment of digitoxicity.

There usually is an improvement in the symptoms of digitoxicity within 30 minutes of administration of Digibind. Other medications to stabilize the heart rhythm as well as supplemental potassium may be required in conjunction with the Digibind.

## BIVENTRICULAR PACEMAKER AND IMPLANTABLE CARDIOVERTER DEFIBRILLATOR

### What is a biventricular pacemaker?

In the heart, the right ventricle pumps blood to the lungs where the blood receives oxygen, and the left ventricle pumps this oxygen-rich blood to the rest of the body. When a person is in good health, the right and the left ventricle pump at the same time, that is, in "synchrony". In heart failure, the right and the left ventricle may not be pumping in synchrony. This can interfere with the ability of the right and left ventricle to fill with blood as the heart relaxes and pump blood out as the heart contracts. This can seriously worsen heart failure and its symptoms.

A biventricular pacemaker is a device that can correct this. The pacemaker itself consists of a power source inserted under the skin, with wires from that power source implanted in the left and right sides of the heart. By providing the heart with electrical signals, the pacemaker can force the two ventricles to beat at the same time. This is "cardiac resynchronization therapy", sometimes abbreviated as "CRT".

## When is the cardiac resynchronization therapy useful?

A simple electrocardiogram can show evidence that the left and right ventricles are not beating in synchrony. When this lack of proper synchrony is present, and the person has mild to moderate symptoms of heart failure and an "ejection fraction", as described earlier in this chapter of less than 30%, cardiac resynchronization therapy can be very helpful. In this situation, cardiac resynchronization therapy combined with the internal defibrillator (see below) reduces symptoms as well as the risk of hospitalization from heart failure, and reduces the risk of sudden death.

## What is an implantable cardioverter defibrillator?

People with advancing heart failure are at a high risk of sudden death. "Ventricular fibrillation" in which the heart quivers instead of beating, stops blood from flowing to the body, and is the cause of sudden death. The internal defibrillator detects this ventricular fibrillation and, if it occurs, shocks the heart back to a normal rhythm. The implantable cardioverter defibrillator (sometimes abbreviated as "ICD") has proven to be a very important new development in the treatment of heart failure and has been highly effective in preventing sudden death.

Most of the time, the implantable cardioverter defibrillator is inserted along with the biventricular pacemaker.

## WORSENING HEART FAILURE

*What is the treatment if, despite these medicines and devices, and despite implanting a biventricular pacemaker and implantable cardioverter defibrillator, heart failure worsens?*

When heart failure worsens, it will be important to make certain that no new illness such as pneumonia or anemia is worsening the heart failure. If such an illness exists, it may be possible to treat the new illness, and lessen the heart failure.

If heart failure worsens, physicians will do their best to adjust the doses of ACE inhibitors, ARBs, digoxin, diuretics and other heart failure medications and try to improve the effectiveness of the medications.

Worsening heart failure despite medical therapy is a dangerous problem. It will be critical that the physician managing the person's medical care have extensive experience in the management of heart failure. Consultation with a highly experienced cardiologist and, perhaps, consultation with an academic cardiologist at a university or teaching hospital may be helpful.

*What can the academic cardiologist do that the local physician or cardiologist cannot do?*

Often, no further effective treatments are available. At times, however, a modification in the dosage or combinations of medications could be of real value to the person with heart failure.

463

The treatment of heart failure is an area of active investigation. There are many studies evaluating different and innovative methods of administering the currently available medications. Preliminary findings of these clinical studies may only be available at a few academic medical centers. Recent publications suggesting alternative treatments may not have come to the attention of a busy local or community physician.

At academic or teaching institutions, there may be new medications under evaluation which are not yet FDA approved and, therefore, locally unavailable. Some of these medications may be very useful or life saving if administered before heart failure has progressed too far.

## <u>SURGERY</u>

### *Can surgery be helpful?*

Surgery can be remarkably helpful for people with heart failure caused by disease of the heart valves. Replacement or repair of the damaged valve or valves may return heart function to normal or near normal.

Another cause of heart failure which surgery may help is removal of a ventricular aneurysm. A "ventricular aneurysm" is a damaged area of the heart (the damage usually caused by a myocardial infarction) in which the damaged, scarred area of the heart balloons outward and interferes with the pumping action of the heart. Removal ("resection") of the aneurysm can improve heart function.

For most other people with heart failure, the only remaining surgical procedures that can be helpful are implanting a "left ventricular assist device" or a heart transplant.

# LEFT VENTRICULAR ASSIST DEVICE

## *What is a left ventricular assist device and when is it useful?*

Despite great improvements in the medicines used to treat heart failure, and despite the development of the biventricular pacemaker, it is very common for heart failure to progress to the point where treatment is no longer working adequately and the heart failure is at a point that is barely compatible with continued life.

A left ventricular assist device assists a severely weakened left ventricle with driving blood through the body. In the past, these devices, which drew blood from the left ventricle into a pump from which it is was pumped into the aorta, intermittently drew the blood into and out of the pump and reproduced the pulsing nature of the normal blood flow in our arteries. The newer left ventricular assist devices work differently, creating a steady or continuous flow of blood into and out of the pump and to the aorta for delivery throughout the body. These newer devices are smaller, easier to use, quieter, and can be enormously effective in relieving symptoms, and improving and extending life.

# HEART TRANSPLANT

## *When is a heart transplant a consideration?*

A heart transplant is a consideration when a person has severe heart failure that is not under control with medication or any medical device and when survival, because of the severe heart failure, for more than a year is unlikely.

People with severe medical problems aside from heart disease, including advanced cancer, are not candidates for heart transplantation. Because powerful medicines to suppress the immune system are necessary to prevent rejection of the transplanted heart, people with serious viral infections such as hepatitis are not candidates for heart transplant.

## What are the problems associated with a heart transplant?

The surgery itself is difficult and risky and carries an immediate death risk of about one in ten.

After the transplant, there is the risk that the body's immune system will recognize the new heart as foreign, attack it, then reject it. Although powerful medicines to suppress the immune system are generally successful in preventing this, these medicines also impair the ability to fight serious infections. For this reason, a person who has had a heart transplant is at risk of developing infections that can rapidly become life threatening if not promptly recognized and treated. Further information about these infections is in the chapter entitled "Opportunistic Infections".

## How are signs of rejection identified after a heart transplant?

A biopsy device, introduced through a vein in the arm, and threaded all the way into the heart, can take a tiny snip out of the heart muscle for the hospital pathologist to examine under the microscope. This procedure, called an "endomyocardial biopsy", will identify early signs of rejection of the transplanted heart.

### What is the treatment if there are signs of rejection?

If there is evidence of rejection, the doses of the immunosuppressant medications may be increased. New or experimental immunosuppressant medicines may be used. In extreme cases, a new heart transplant, if possible, may be necessary.

### What is the outlook for a person who has had a heart transplant?

With recent improvements in surgical technique and the new and safer immune system suppressing medicines, the odds of surviving after a heart transplant are now about eight to one in favor of survival after one year and about four to one in favor of survival after five years.

## HEART FAILURE WHICH IS REFRACTORY TO MEDICATION

### What treatment is possible when heart failure is severe and worsening despite medication and heart transplantation is not an option?

In this situation, new doses of the medicines a person is already taking, or switching to or adding different medicines may be considered. A strict low salt diet and further limitations on physical activity may be considered.

### What if despite all measures, heart failure is still worsening?

At a certain point, heart failure can become refractory to further treatment. At this point, it may be appropriate to take some measures which pose some small risk to life, but which may provide very considerable relief from the severe discomforts associated with truly refractory heart failure.

Some people may not want to use treatments that may themselves endanger the life of people with refractory heart failure. People with truly refractory and severe heart failure generally survive for only a few months. Relief from the severe shortness of breath and anxiety associated with this shortness of breath will help improve the quality of a person's life in the short time left to them.

### How can this shortness of breath and anxiety be relieved?

Low doses of morphine may be very useful in somewhat relieving shortness of breath, and diminishing anxiety. Morphine may also relieve pain caused by the swelling in the legs and liver that is common in refractory heart failure. Use of morphine is not without some risk. Morphine can drop blood pressure too low and may suppress the reflex by which the brain drives respiration.

Higher doses of diuretics may get more fluid out of the lungs and legs. High doses of diuretics increase the risk of dangerous drops in blood pressure and may dangerously reduce blood flow to the kidneys and produce kidney failure. The benefits and the risks of higher dose diuretics are important considerations when attempting to relieve terribly distressing symptoms.

# SOME ADDITIONAL THOUGHTS ABOUT REDUCING THE RISK OF PREMATURE DEATH FROM HEART FAILURE

*What else can a person and their family do to reduce the risk of dying prematurely from heart failure?*

People with heart failure and their families should be particularly aware that sudden worsening of shortness of breath might mean acute severe heart failure, discussed in the chapter entitled "Cardiogenic Pulmonary Edema". If shortness of breath suddenly worsens, it is critical that the person immediately get to their doctor or hospital emergency room for prompt treatment. Every person with heart failure should have a specific plan of action of what to do in the event of rapidly worsening heart failure or sudden shortness of breath. Family members should know the plan and be ready to take action any time the need arises. This plan of action should include calling the physician, and if there is any delay at all in getting through, having a family member or, in a crisis, an ambulance, get the person to the local hospital emergency room.

Infections such as the flu or strep throat can suddenly worsen heart failure. Prompt treatment of these infections is important. A flu shot does not provide 100% protection against the flu but does have some protective effect.

Because a person with chronic heart failure has a significant risk of cardiac arrest and sudden death, it will be a good idea for family members to learn basic CPR techniques.

# FLUID COLLECTIONS

# MALIGNANT ASCITES

## DEFINITION

### What is ascites?

Ascites is an abnormal accumulation of fluid in the abdominal cavity in the space between the lining of the inside wall of the abdomen and the abdominal organs.

### What is malignant ascites?

Ascites caused by cancer is "malignant ascites".

## SYMPTOMS

### What are the symptoms of ascites?

The most obvious symptom is a gradual development of a sense of bloating and distension of the abdomen. As the amount of fluid increases, the skin over the abdomen becomes tense and the navel may bulge outward. The weight of the fluid in the abdomen can cause serious discomfort.

When a great deal of fluid collects, it may put upward pressure on the diaphragm. As we draw in a breath, our lungs expand and the diaphragm moves downward. As we exhale, the diaphragm moves upward. Fluid in the abdomen that is exerting an upward pressure on the diaphragm makes it difficult for the diaphragm to move downward, making it difficult to breathe in.

## MAKING THE DIAGNOSIS

### What tests confirm the presence of ascites?

A simple physical exam is usually sufficient to make the diagnosis of ascites. One commonly used test for ascites is to put the fingers of one hand on one side of the abdomen, and to give a sharp tap to the opposite side of the abdomen with the other hand. The fluid in the abdomen will quickly shift, and the opposite hand feels a sensation called "a fluid wave".

An ultrasound examination or a CT scan confirms the diagnosis of ascites.

## THE CAUSES OF ASCITES

### Which diseases cause ascites?

The most common cause of ascites in a person with cancer is the spread of the cancer inside the abdomen.

Several diseases other than cancer can cause ascites if a person apparently in remission with their cancer develops ascites. The most common cause of ascites that unrelated to cancer is cirrhosis. Ascites in a person who does not have cirrhosis or cancer is usually caused by a chronic medical problem such as heart failure (see chapter entitled "Heart Failure"), or chronic kidney failure.

## IDENTIFYING THE CAUSE OF THE ASCITES

### How is the cause of the ascites identified?

Based upon knowledge of a person's underlying illness, the cause of ascites may be obvious, and there may be no need to do extensive testing to determine the cause.

If cancer is the most likely cause, using local anesthesia, a small amount of the ascites fluid is withdrawn and sent to the laboratory for analysis. Based upon the chemical characteristics of the fluid and the appearance of the fluid under the microscope, the cause of the ascites can often be determined.

A CT scan or ultrasound examination may show clear evidence of metastatic cancer and make a definitive diagnosis.

Simple blood tests can show evidence of severe liver or kidney disease that could be responsible for ascites. Physical examination may show unequivocal signs of heart failure, or may show one of the several signs of chronic liver disease.

If the examination of the fluid and the radiologist's tests do not clarify the cause of the ascites, it may be appropriate to perform a "laparoscopy". Laparoscopy is a surgical technique that allows a surgeon to examine the inside of the abdomen without performing a major operation. The instrument used, a "laparoscope", is inserted into the abdomen through incisions of less than an inch in length. The surgeon directs the instrument through the various parts of the inside of the abdomen and examines it through images projected to a video monitor. Tissues that are abnormal can be biopsied and sent to the laboratory for analysis. Laparoscopic examination will often allow physicians to identify the cause of a person's ascites.

*What is the priority if the first evidence a person has cancer is the development of malignant ascites?*

When a person develops malignant ascites without a previous history of cancer, the immediate priority will be to determine the exact type of cancer that is causing the ascites. In women, the most common cause of malignant ascites is cancer of the ovary. In men, the most common causes of malignant ascites are cancer of the stomach or colon or pancreas. The source of the cancer can usually be found with CT or MRI scans, ultrasound, and if necessary, with surgery.

## TREATMENT OF MALIGNANT ASCITES

*How do physicians treat malignant ascites?*

The treatment of malignant ascites is to treat the malignant tumor itself with the anti-cancer treatment that is most effective. This could mean surgically removing as much cancer as is possible or attempting to shrink or control that specific type of cancer with chemotherapy or other anti-cancer therapies.

The cancers that are most likely to cause ascites may progress to the point where they are no longer responding to treatment. When cancer is no longer responding to treatment, the goal of therapy of ascites is "palliative", that is, to prevent serious and life-threatening complications such as infection, and to maintain as much comfort as possible.

### Are diuretics and salt restriction helpful in malignant ascites?

Diuretics can help a person urinate out ascites fluid. A commonly used diuretic treatment regimen will first use the medicine "spironolactone", and then, if this is not working adequately, add the medicine "furosemide". Although these medications are effective in reducing the fluid in the abdomen, they can have serious side effects. Diuretics help the person urinate out fluid from the abdomen but also cause a loss of fluid from the bloodstream. This can lead to low blood pressure, which, if excessive, can be dangerous. Contraction of a person's blood volume can reduce blood flow to the kidneys and cause kidney failure (see discussion of "pre-renal azotemia" in the chapter entitled "Acute Kidney Injury"). It is therefore appropriate to be cautious with the use of diuretics.

Although diuretics can have some beneficial effect in malignant ascites, salt restriction is not very effective and is not generally worthwhile, considering its effect on quality of life.

### What is diuretic resistant ascites?

The situation where diuretics are not working properly is "diuretic resistance ascites". When a great deal of fluid has accumulated such that the skin on the surface of the abdomen is pulled tight, and there is discomfort, pain, or shortness of breath related to the ascites, this is sometimes referred to as "tense ascites". Before concluding that a person has diuretic resistant tense ascites and should resort to other measures, a physician will generally want to confirm that the person is taking the diuretic medications properly. Sometimes, better medication compliance or alternate doses of medications can bring the ascites back under control.

## What is paracentesis?

Paracentesis is the removal of fluid from the abdomen with a needle.

## How effective is paracentesis?

Removal of fluid from the abdomen with a needle immediately relieves symptoms. This relief lasts until the fluid accumulates again, often within days or weeks. In order to relieve the distressing symptoms of recurring ascites, paracentesis as often as every two weeks or so may be needed. With each paracentesis, the physician may remove as much as several liters of fluid.

# SPONTANEOUS BACTERIAL PERITONITIS

## What is spontaneous bacterial peritonitis?

Spontaneous bacterial peritonitis is a spontaneous bacterial infection of the ascites fluid. Spontaneous bacterial peritonitis is a very dangerous complication of ascites.

## What are the symptoms of spontaneous bacterial peritonitis?

Symptoms of spontaneous bacterial peritonitis are pain in the abdomen, fever, and confusion. When a person with ascites develops some or all of these symptoms, immediate evaluation is critical.

## How is the diagnosis of spontaneous bacterial peritonitis made?

The diagnosis of spontaneous bacterial peritonitis requires a small amount of ascites fluid to be withdrawn with a needle from the abdomen for examination under the microscope. Samples of the ascites fluid as well as of the blood and urine sent to the laboratory will identify the presence of bacteria and the antibiotics most likely to kill the bacteria and cure the infection.

A high number of white blood cells and the presence of bacteria in the ascites fluid make the diagnosis.

## What is the treatment of spontaneous bacterial peritonitis?

If there is a high suspicion that a person has spontaneous bacterial peritonitis, physicians will begin treatment with powerful antibiotics on the assumption that bacteria that are normally inside the intestines, and are sensitive to these antibiotics, have gotten into the ascites fluid and are causing infection. Treatment with intravenous antibiotics is quite effective, if treatment begins before complications of the infection appear, such as acute kidney injury (see chapter entitled "Acute Kidney Injury") or sepsis and septic shock (see chapter entitled "Sepsis and Septic Shock").

## How is recurrence of spontaneous bacterial peritonitis prevented?

If spontaneous bacterial peritonitis is a recurrent problem physicians may advise a person to take an antibiotic pill every day to reduce the risk of a recurrent infection. The antibiotics commonly used to do this are "trimethoprim-sulfamethoxazole" (brand names "Septra" or "Bactrim") and norfloxacin (brand name is "Noroxin").

# PERICARDIAL EFFUSION

## DEFINITIONS

### What is the pericardium?

The pericardium is a membrane that surrounds the heart. This membrane forms a sac (the "pericardial sac") that contains a very small amount of slippery fluid. This fluid allows the heart to glide past neighboring structures without friction as it contracts and expands with each beat.

### What is a pericardial effusion?

A pericardial effusion is an abnormally large amount of fluid surrounding the heart inside the pericardial sac.

## COMPLICATIONS OF PERICARDIAL EFFUSION

### Why is pericardial effusion dangerous?

The heart pumps blood as the heart contracts (during "systole") and fills with blood when the heart relaxes (during "diastole"). Fluid build-up inside the pericardium puts pressure on the outside wall of the heart and interferes with the heart's ability to fill with blood during diastole. This "cardiac tamponade", that is, the high pressure exerted on the outside of the heart within the unyielding pericardial sac, will severely impair the heart's ability to pump blood around the body and will produce heart failure.

## THE CAUSES OF LIFE-THREATENING PERICARDIAL EFFUSION

### Who gets a life-threatening pericardial effusion?

When pericardial effusion is sufficient to cause "cardiac tamponade" and threaten life, cancer is the most common cause. The most common cancers that cause this are cancer of the lung or breast.

## SYMPTOMS

### What are the symptoms of pericardial effusion?

The major symptoms of pericardial effusion are low blood pressure, shortness of breath, and severe and obvious bulging of the veins in the neck.

## MAKING THE DIAGNOSIS

### How is the diagnosis of pericardial effusion made?

The initial evidence that a person has a pericardial effusion emerges from a person's medical history, symptoms, and physical examination.

The physical examination will often reveal one or more components of a "triad" of findings that point to the diagnosis: a low blood pressure, enlarged neck veins, and a reduced volume to the heart sounds heard with a stethoscope.

There is a unique finding, discovered almost 150 years ago, that when a person with a large pericardial effusion takes a very deep breath, the pulse in the wrist either disappears, or can barely be felt. A large drop in "systolic blood pressure" (the top number of the two in a blood pressure measurement) reflects this diminished pulse. This finding, called "pulsus paradoxus", raises a very high suspicion of the presence of a life-threatening pericardial effusion.

An echocardiogram, using harmless sound waves, can demonstrate the excessive fluid in the pericardial sac and make a definitive diagnosis. The echocardiogram will also give vital information about the extent to which the fluid is compromising heart function.

## TREATMENT

### What is the initial treatment when a pericardial effusion is causing severe symptoms?

When a person with a pericardial effusion has severe shortness of breath or low blood pressure, it will be important to withdraw fluid out of the pericardium by performing a procedure called a "pericardiocentesis".

A pericardiocentesis is performed under local anesthesia. The physician performing the pericardiocentesis will use a special needle to insert a thin, hollow plastic tube (a "catheter") just below the breastbone and into the pericardial sac. The physician (usually a cardiologist or a cardiothoracic surgeon) will often use an echocardiogram to guide the catheter into the fluid-containing area within the pericardial sac.

### How successful is the pericardiocentesis at treating pericardial effusion?

The pericardiocentesis is quite successful at getting fluid out of the pericardial sac. Unless, however, there is a remission or cure of the disease causing the pericardial effusion, the pericardial effusion will usually return.

### How is the cancer causing the pericardial effusion put into remission?

Specific treatment is necessary for whatever cancer is causing the pericardial effusion. Successful treatment of cancer-related pericardial effusion is usually dependent on the administration of chemotherapy that effectively treats the person's cancer wherever it may be in their body. Radiation therapy to the pericardium can sometimes control the accumulation of a pericardial effusion if the underlying cancer is sensitive to radiation.

### What is done for a person with recurring cancer-related pericardial effusion if there is no chemotherapy that can effectively treat the person's cancer?

Recurrent accumulation of fluid in the pericardium can be treated by "percutaneous catheter drainage". To establish "percutaneous catheter drainage", with the assistance of an echocardiogram, the physician will insert a needle into the chest just below the bone on the bottom end of the sternum called the "xiphoid bone". Once this needle reaches the pericardium, a guidewire is advanced through the needle, into the pericardial sac, and the needle removed. Using the guidewire, the physician can then guide a catheter into the pericardial sac, and connect the catheter to drainage tubing that will carry fluid from the pericardium into a drainage bag outside the body. The catheter and drainage apparatus remains in place for several days, by which time the drainage from the pericardium should have stopped or slowed very considerably.

An alternate way of draining a pericardial effusion is through an operation called a "subxiphoid pericardiotomy". To do this, under anesthesia, a surgeon will make an incision just below the end of the sternum and create a pathway to the pericardium. An incision in the pericardium permits insertion of a large tube into the pericardial sac. This can provide very rapid drainage of the fluid and relief of symptoms of cardiac tamponade.

If the pericardial effusion cannot be controlled by other means, a surgeon can remove some or all of the pericardium (this is called a "pericardiectomy"), and thereby prevent recurrent pericardial effusion. This is a complex operation and is associated with a prolonged and difficult recovery period. People with far advanced cancer and their families may choose not to have a pericardiectomy when life expectancy is already quite short.

## OUTLOOK

### What is the outlook for a person with pericardial effusion because of cancer?

The outlook depends upon the cancer and upon whether the cancer is responsive to treatment. People who have a pericardial effusion because of chemotherapy-resistant lung cancer usually have advanced cancer and a short life expectancy, surviving, on average, for only a few months. Women who develop a pericardial effusion because of advanced breast cancer have a better outlook and can survive for a year or longer after treatment of their pericardial effusion.

# PLEURAL EFFUSION

## DEFINITION

### What is a pleural effusion?

A pleural effusion is a collection of fluid in the space between the lung and the surrounding chest wall and diaphragm.

Normally, with breathing, the chest expands and the diaphragm moves downward. This action creates a negative pressure that sucks air into the lung when a person breathes in. Significant fluid between a lung, the chest wall and the diaphragm, compresses the lung and prevents it from expanding properly. If the volume of fluid is large enough, it may become impossible for the lung to expand. A large pleural effusion can cause the lung to partially or entirely collapse and become non-functional.

### How much fluid can there be in a pleural effusion?

Normally, each side of the chest contains only a few ounces of a clear, slippery fluid that allows the lung to slide smoothly and without friction against the inside wall of the chest as we breathe in and out. When a person has a significant pleural effusion, there can be several quarts of fluid in one or both sides of the chest.

## THE CAUSES OF PLEURAL EFFUSION

### Which diseases can cause a pleural effusion?

Although the list of diseases that can cause pleural effusion is a long one, the cause of most significant pleural effusions is cancer, heart failure, cirrhosis, pneumonia, or pulmonary embolism.

When an otherwise healthy person develops a pleural effusion, careful evaluation to determine the cause is necessary.

## SYMPTOMS

### What are the symptoms of pleural effusion?

The major symptom of pleural effusion is shortness of breath. This may, at first, be somewhat mild, and only noticeable with some exertion. As the effusion grows larger, the shortness of breath worsens. There may also be some vague pain in the chest that worsens when taking a deep breath. A person with a pleural effusion may also complain of an annoying and persistent cough.

## MAKING THE DIAGNOSIS

### How is the diagnosis of pleural effusion made?

A pleural effusion, if large enough to cause symptoms, is visible with a simple chest x-ray. With a relatively small pleural effusion, the x-ray shows that the usual sharply visible angle between the diaphragm and the left or right side of the chest wall is absent. When the pleural effusion is large, it has the appearance on the x-ray of a very white area where normal lung with air in it is supposed to be. When a person lies on their side, the fluid will shift in the same way that the fluid will shift in a half empty bottle of water laid on its side. The line of fluid seen when an x-ray is taken with a person lying on their side (this type of x-ray is called a "lateral decubitus film"), confirms the diagnosis of pleural effusion.

## DETERMINING THE CAUSE OF THE PLEURAL EFFUSION

*What tests determine the cause of the pleural effusion?*

The cause of the pleural effusion is often obvious, in the context of a person's other medical problems. For example, if a person has a cancer that is widespread and not responding to treatment, or severe heart failure or cirrhosis, the cause of the pleural effusion will generally be obvious and additional testing to find a cause may not be necessary.

When the cause is uncertain, a sample of the fluid in the chest can be removed under local anesthesia by using a needle on a large syringe. Based upon the chemical characteristics of the fluid as well as examination under the microscope for evidence of infection or cancer, the cause of the pleural effusion can often be determined.

At times, the person's medical history, physical examination, as well as examination of the fluid itself may not clarify the cause of the effusion. Additional testing will then be important.

A CT scan of the chest can give vital information regarding the presence of cancer or inflammation and may point toward the cause of the pleural effusion. If cancer or infection is not evident and pulmonary embolism (see chapter entitled "Deep Vein Thrombosis and Pulmonary Embolism") is a possibility, a "CT angiography" to look for a blood clot blocking an artery in the lung may be necessary. Along with the CT scan, some medical centers may perform a test called a "PET scan" which can identify areas of inflammation or cancer inside the chest with somewhat greater sensitivity.

A PET scan is a sensitive test that can often detect the presence of cancer before detection by CT scans. To do this test, a small amount of radioactive glucose is injected into the bloodstream. Cancer cells have a greater affinity for this radioactive glucose than other tissues. The PET scanner can then find "hot spots" inside the body that contain the cancer and transmit this information to a computer for the physician to evaluate. The identification of a "hot spot" suggests, but does not prove, the presence of cancer cells in the hot spot. Although a "hot spot" may indicate the presence of cancer, areas of inflammation without cancer can also produce "hot spots". A "hot spot" indicates a suspicious area that needs evaluation, often with a biopsy to confirm the presence or absence of local cancer.

If the CT or PET scan identifies areas that appear to contain cancer or infection along the membrane lining the inside wall of the chest (the "pleura") it may be important to take a biopsy of the pleura.

A pleural biopsy is done by injecting a local anesthetic into the skin and tissues around a rib, and then carefully introducing a small needle with a special cutting edge between the ribs and into the chest cavity. The biopsy needle will then clip out a small piece of pleura for examination under the microscope. Often, and especially when a CT scan has identified an area that appears to contain cancer or another abnormality requiring biopsy, the physician who is doing the pleural biopsy will be actively guided by the CT scan.

To perform a good examination of the pleura and, if necessary, take biopsies from many areas inside the chest, it may be important to have a "thoracoscopy" done. To perform a thoracoscopy, a physician will put a scope through a small incision between the ribs, look around the inside of the chest for the cause of the trouble, and take biopsies from suspicious looking areas.

## WHEN THE DIAGNOSIS IS CANCER

*What are the next steps if the biopsy indicates that the diagnosis is cancer?*

A pleural effusion caused by cancer is a "malignant pleural effusion". If the diagnosis is cancer, the critical issue will be to determine the organ from which the cancer originated. Sometimes, the answer to this is readily apparent. As an example, a woman who has recently been treated for metastatic breast cancer and who develops a new pleural effusion with cancer cells in the fluid or in the pleural biopsy, almost certainly has her pleural effusion as a result of metastatic breast cancer. When the first evidence of the cancer is the pleural effusion and the source of the cancer is unknown, it will be important to begin a search for the source of the cancer. Physicians refer to the source of the cancer as the "primary site".

## *How do physicians search for and identify the "primary site"?*

The variety of commonly available x-rays and CT and MRI scans of the chest and abdomen can often find the primary site. There are times when a source of the cancer is not clear, leading to the diagnosis of "cancer of unknown primary site". In the case of cancer of unknown primary site, the appearance of the malignant cells under the microscope as well as some blood tests and more sophisticated genetic testing can provide evidence as to where the cancer probably originated from and what the appropriate therapy should be.

## *Which cancers cause pleural effusion?*

The cancers that most commonly cause pleural effusion are lung cancer and breast cancer. Most cancers, however, can cause pleural effusion. It is very common for a person with any kind of metastatic cancer to be troubled, at some point in their illness, by a malignant pleural effusion.

## **TREATMENT**

## *What is the treatment of pleural effusion?*

The treatment of pleural effusion is to treat the disease that caused the pleural effusion. The malignant pleural effusions that people with metastatic cancer develop can become refractory to the anti-cancer treatments. "Palliative treatments" which diminish the size of the pleural effusion without effectively controlling the cancer are the only available treatments when the underlying cancer cannot be controlled or eradicated.

## *What palliative treatments are available?*

Fluid drained from the chest with a needle (this is a "thoracentesis"), with well over a quart of fluid removed from the chest at any point in time, provides major relief of symptoms. For some people, depending on the underlying disease, this can relieve symptoms for an extended period. For many others, however, the fluid in the chest and symptoms may return within days.

When fluid quickly returns, there are catheters that can be "tunneled"" beneath the skin and then between the ribs and into the chest cavity. These catheters, left in place for weeks or months, can repeatedly drain fluid from the chest. With a bit of training, family members or even the person with the pleural effusion can do this at home.

Putting the chemical "talc", which is actually "magnesium silicate", inside the chest, can cause a scarring of the tissues that surround the lung and slow or stop the re-accumulation of fluid. This scarring treatment, called by some "sclerotherapy" and by others "pleurodesis", involves inserting (under local anesthesia) a half-inch or so wide tube between the ribs and into the chest cavity. The tube (a "chest tube") is connected to a device that helps remove almost all of the fluid out of the chest. When the inside of the chest appears to be practically dry, the talc is inserted through the chest tube into the chest cavity. The chest tube is then clamped and the person with the pleural effusion is instructed to roll their body around in bed every fifteen minutes or so. This technique has a scarring effect inside the chest that is helpful in slowing or stopping the accumulation of fluid in the chest in many people with recurring pleural effusion.

## *Can surgery be a useful treatment of a malignant pleural effusion?*

The surgery necessary to treat pleural effusion requires a major operation to remove the inner lining of the chest wall. This operation (called a "pleurectomy" because it removes the pleura) is very difficult and has many, many complications. Pleurectomy is reserved for people with severe, refractory pleural effusion who have a disease which otherwise might allow them some reasonably long survival.

## <u>OUTLOOK</u>

### *What is the outlook for a person with pleural effusion?*

The outlook depends upon the disease causing the pleural effusion and the responsiveness of that disease to treatment. In the case of incurable cancer that is not responding to chemotherapy or other treatments, the outlook depends upon the rate of growth of the cancer and the extent to which the cancer involves other areas of the body.

# HEART AND MAJOR BLOOD VESSEL COMPLICATIONS

# HEART ATTACK: ACUTE MYOCARDIAL INFARCTION

## DEFINITIONS

### *What is an acute myocardial infarction?*

An acute myocardial infarction is sudden, irreversible heart muscle damage caused by inadequate blood flow to the wall of the heart. The muscular wall of the heart is the "myocardium". An "infarction" is an area of irreversible damage caused by lack of adequate blood supply.

## THE CORONARY ARTERIES AND WHAT CAN BLOCK THEM

### *Where does the myocardium's blood supply come from?*

The heart consists of four chambers surrounded by muscle and filled with blood. These chambers are the right atrium, right ventricle, left atrium and left ventricle. Contraction of the heart muscle (the "myocardium") surrounding the blood will abruptly compress blood in the heart's chambers. This will push blood from the right atrium to the right ventricle, from the right ventricle to the lungs, then, after the blood returns to the heart from the lungs,

497

from the left atrium to the left ventricle and from the left ventricle to the entire body.

Three large arteries (called "coronary arteries") supply blood to the myocardium. Each of these three arteries is responsible for providing blood supply to a specific region of the myocardium. The "left anterior descending artery" supplies the front (the "anterior wall") of the left ventricle and the wall between the left ventricle and the right ventricle ("the interventricular septum"). The "left circumflex artery" supplies the sidewall (the "lateral wall") of the heart. The "right coronary artery" supplies the right ventricle and the bottom wall (the "inferior wall") of the heart.

Most of the time, there is no absolute boundary between the region of myocardium supplied by one coronary artery and the region supplied by another. Coronary arteries share responsibility with each other for supplying blood flow to regions of the myocardium. This shared source of blood supply, called "collateral circulation", helps to preserve myocardium in the event there is a blockage of circulation through a coronary artery.

## What can block blood supply to the heart and cause an acute myocardial infarction?

The most common cause of acute myocardial infarction is a blood clot that forms in an area of a coronary artery damaged by atherosclerosis. Atherosclerosis, commonly known as "hardening of the arteries", is the accumulation of fatty deposits, calcium, and other substances in the wall of an artery. Blood clots have a tendency to form in the coronary arteries in an area of atherosclerosis.

This blood clot (called a "thrombus") can completely shut off blood flow through a coronary artery and cause irreversible damage to the area of heart muscle that depends on that coronary artery for blood supply.

### Why might a person with cancer develop an acute myocardial infarction?

In addition to the well-known risks for acute myocardial infarction such as diet, exercise, and family history, people who have received some forms of radiation to the chest area, for lymphoma or for breast, lung, or other cancers, are at a higher risk of developing coronary artery disease leading to an acute myocardial infarction.

People with metastatic cancer can develop "nonbacterial thrombotic endocarditis" in which small, fragile growths called "vegetations" develop on the heart valves. These vegetations can break off the valve and float into a coronary artery, blocking blood supply to an area of heart muscle, and triggering an acute myocardial infarction.

## SYMPTOMS

### What are the symptoms of acute myocardial infarction?

Most people who develop an acute myocardial infarction will experience sudden severe pain in the left side or in the center of their chest. The pain is often a terrible "constricting" pain or as though something large and heavy is pressing on the chest. Pain in the arms, neck, jaw, and the upper abdomen are common.

Nausea, severe weakness, and profuse sweating are other common symptoms.

## Are all acute myocardial infarctions dramatically symptomatic?

The symptoms of acute myocardial infarction can occasionally be so subtle as to pass virtually unnoticed. This serves to emphasize the importance of immediate medical evaluation of a new pain or discomfort in the chest, upper abdomen, left upper arm or shoulder for which no obvious cause (such as recent muscle strain) can be identified. Sometimes, an acute myocardial infarction may cause no pain at all, but rather cause sudden shortness of breath, or sudden severe weakness, confusion, loss of consciousness, or a general sense of impending medical danger.

## MAKING THE DIAGNOSIS

### How is the diagnosis of acute myocardial infarction made?

The diagnosis of acute myocardial infarction is usually be made with a simple electrocardiogram. The electrocardiogram can identify damage to heart muscle and determine the area of the heart that has sustained the damage.

When an acute myocardial infarction damages heart muscle, the heart muscle will release a substance called "cardiac specific troponin" into the blood stream. This is an indication of damage to the heart muscle and measurement of cardiac specific troponin is a critical blood test used to confirm a diagnosis of acute myocardial infarction.

An echocardiogram, using harmless sound waves, can detect a lack of normal motion of portions of the heart as it contracts and relaxes with each beat. This "regional wall motion dyskinesia" may indicate that a myocardial infarction has occurred although it cannot say if the abnormal motion of a portion of the heart wall represents a new myocardial infarction or the after-effects of an old myocardial infarction. The echocardiogram provides vital information about the magnitude of the damage to the heart and can help guide physicians' decisions regarding treatment.

## IMMEDIATE TREATMENT

### What first steps are taken after the diagnosis of an acute myocardial infarction has been made?

A first step after making the diagnosis of an acute myocardial infarction will be to insert an intravenous catheter in the arm so that rapid direct access to the bloodstream is available for necessary medicines. Supplemental oxygen, delivered by a mask over either the mouth or nose or by tiny plastic tubes in the nostrils ("nasal prongs"), is useful if there appears to be inadequate oxygen in the bloodstream. Severe pain can be relieved with intravenous morphine. A sedative such as "Valium" can help relieve anxiety.

## STEMI

### What is STEMI?

STEMI are the initials for "ST elevation myocardial infarction". This refers to the appearance on the electrocardiogram, which clearly indicates, in the context of the symptoms the person is experiencing, that sudden damage to heart muscle because of a blocked artery is taking place. It is a signal that emergency treatment is necessary to open the blocked artery so that blood can flow through it again to the heart muscle. The opening up of a blocked coronary artery to allow the resumption of blood supply to the heart is "reperfusion".

When blockage of a coronary artery is quickly relieved, areas of heart muscle injured by lack of blood supply ("ischemic") but not permanently damaged by lack of blood supply ("infarcted") are preserved. The preservation of ischemic heart muscle, that is, the prevention of having endangered ischemic myocardium evolve into irreversibly damaged infarcted myocardium, is critical to preventing heart failure both in the immediate aftermath of a myocardial infarction and after a person leaves the hospital.

How is the flow of blood through a blocked coronary artery restored in the setting of STEMI?

The two major methods that restore blood flow through a blocked coronary artery are with medical devices or with medicines.

A commonly used technique used to restore blood flow through a blocked artery is "percutaneous coronary intervention" or "PCI". To perform PCI, physicians will insert a catheter into a blood vessel in the arm and, using x-rays and a dye to track the tip of the catheter, will insert the tip of the catheter into the blood vessels feeding the heart. Once the catheter tip is located in these vessels feeding the heart, injection of a dye and sophisticated x-rays permit physicians to identify the blocked artery causing the myocardial infarction. With the blocked artery identified, a very thin wire passed through the catheter and across the area of the artery blocked by the thrombus will guide insertion of a catheter that has a balloon at its end. The physician will then expand the balloon inside the blockage in the artery and force open a channel inside the artery through which blood can flow. If it is possible to do so, the physician will usually insert a "stent" into the artery. A "stent" is a mechanical device that props the artery open and keeps it open so that blood can continue to flow through it.

The alternative to mechanical opening is to open the artery with an injected medicine that can possibly dissolve or break up the blood clot (this is called "thrombolytic therapy").

The choice of the method of reperfusion will depend upon whether the hospital has the proper equipment, skills, and experience to do one technique or the other, as well as upon many other medical considerations that might encourage the use of one technique or the other. In general, if the hospital treating the person with an acute myocardial infarction has the proper experts and equipment, PCI is the more effective method of opening a blocked coronary artery and produces the better medical outcome.

### Is transfer to another hospital followed by PCI helpful if a person first received thrombolytic therapy?

To answer this question, a clinical trial evaluated over a thousand people who had a STEMI and who had just received thrombolytic therapy. Half of these people received standard supportive treatment and transfer to another hospital for PCI only if worsening symptoms or events made it necessary, and the other half were urgently transferred to a hospital that had PCI capability where they received PCI within six hours of thrombolytic therapy. People who received PCI were less likely, within the following 30 days, to have recurrent chest pain and further heart muscle damage, and had less risk of developing heart failure. The combined analysis of development of a new myocardial infarction, new or worsening heart failure, worrisome new chest pain, and survival, indicated that people transferred to another hospital for PCI had the better outcome. Other studies have suggested that, for best results, the proper length of time that should have elapsed between the thrombolytic therapy and the PCI is somewhere between 2 and 24 hours.

*After PCI or thrombolytic therapy has been successful, what can prevent a thrombus from recurring in and blocking the coronary artery?*

Continued administration of aspirin along with another medicine called "clopidogrel" (brand name is "Plavix", manufacturer's product website is www.plavix.com) can reduce the risk of the blood clot forming again in the coronary artery. As an alternative to clopidogrel, some physicians prefer a newer medication called "prasugel" (brand name is "Effient", manufacturer's product website is www.effient. com). Both Plavix and Effient are medications that prevent platelets in the bloodstream from sticking together to form the clots that can be very dangerous after a stent has been inserted into a coronary artery.

*If PCI is not available, how successful is thrombolytic therapy in opening up a coronary artery blocked by thrombus?*

The effectiveness of thrombolytic therapy depends upon the length of time between the onset of symptoms of acute myocardial infarction and treatment. Treatment given within one hour of symptoms is most effective. With each passing hour, the treatment becomes less effective.

## What is the risk of thrombolytic therapy?

The major risk of thrombolytic therapy is an increased risk of serious bleeding. The most serious type of bleeding which can occur is intracerebral hemorrhage (see chapter entitled "Hemorrhagic Stroke: Intracerebral Hemorrhage"). The risk of intracerebral hemorrhage is small and is usually less than the high risk that a blocked coronary artery will cause serious permanent heart muscle damage after an acute myocardial infarction.

## What happens if a thrombus again blocks flow of blood through a coronary artery?

Recurrent blockage of the coronary artery by thrombus will produce recurrent symptoms of chest pain, a rise in the blood levels of cardiac specific troponin (see above) and changes on the electrocardiogram consistent with further heart muscle injury. When this occurs, the cardiologist may either make a second attempt at thrombolytic therapy or perform a PCI in an attempt to restore blood flow through the artery. In some circumstances, open-heart surgery may be necessary to restore blood flow through the coronary artery.

# OPEN HEART SURGERY

## What type of open-heart surgery opens up a blocked coronary artery?

The operation performed is a "coronary artery bypass graft", more commonly referred to as "CABG" which is pronounced like the word "cabbage"To perform a coronary artery bypass graft, the cardiac surgeon will make an incision down the center of the chest and surgically split the breastbone (the "sternum"). A solution injected into the arteries of the heart will temporarily stop the heartbeat and chill the heart muscle to approximately 55 degrees Fahrenheit. In order to supply oxygen to the blood during the heart operation, diversion of the blood flow through a "heart-lung machine" or "pump" will deliver oxygen to the bloodstream. This procedure, using the pump, is an "on-pump CABG". In some circumstances, the cardiac surgeon may prefer to operate on the beating heart without the pump ("off-pump CABG"), although there is recent evidence, which is disagreed with by many experienced cardiac surgeons, that the effectiveness of the bypass operation is somewhat improved by the on-pump version of CABG.

The goal of the surgery is to bypass the obstructed, narrowed areas of the coronary arteries by inserting pieces of blood vessels taken from elsewhere in the body. A vein in the ankle called the "saphenous vein" and an artery beneath the sternum called the "internal mammary artery" are the most common blood vessels used to bypass the areas of obstruction. Several areas of obstruction (occasionally, as many as ten areas) can be bypassed during the operation.

# CARDIOGENIC SHOCK

## *What is cardiogenic shock?*

Cardiogenic shock is a state of shock caused by heart failure. In this state of shock, blood pressure will be very low, and there is a dangerous reduction of blood flow to the brain, the kidneys, the intestines and other vital organs.

Most of the time, cardiogenic shock is a result of an acute myocardial infarction that has damaged a large portion of the heart's muscular wall. This major loss of muscle deprives the heart of the power it needs to pump blood throughout the body.

## *What is the treatment of cardiogenic shock?*

If cardiogenic shock develops within hours of the acute myocardial infarction, physicians may attempt PCI or thrombolytic therapy or, if necessary, open heart surgery with a coronary artery bypass graft in an attempt to promptly open the blocked coronary artery, restore blood flow to heart muscle, and preserve as much heart muscle as possible.

The goal of treatment of cardiogenic shock will be to increase the blood pressure, to increase the flow of blood to vital organs, and to encourage the heart to beat with greater force.

## *How is the drop in blood pressure in cardiogenic shock treated?*

A first step often taken in the treatment of cardiogenic shock is to insert a catheter called a "Swan-Ganz catheter" through a vein in the arm, shoulder, or groin. From there, physicians advance the catheter through the circulatory system until it reaches the right side of the heart. The Swan-Ganz catheter can then transmit signals to a bedside computer and give precise measurements of pressures in various areas of the heart. These pressures provide the medical staff with information that is essential to guiding treatment of cardiogenic shock.

Blood pressure monitoring with a catheter inserted in an artery (an "arterial line") also allows the medical staff to withdraw blood from the artery to see how well the lungs are providing oxygen to the bloodstream.

A reduction of the volume of blood circulating through the body can lower blood pressure. Determination of whether the blood volume is low (a low blood volume is called "hypovolemia") is made by assessment of the blood pressure and by measurements of pressures of the blood inside the heart that are provided by a Swan-Ganz catheter. The treatment of hypovolemia is to give more fluid by vein and then closely monitor the effect of this administered fluid therapy on the blood pressure, the Swan-Ganz catheter measurements of pressures in the heart, and by measuring a person's production of urine (the "urine output").

If blood pressure is still very low after fluid treatment, several different intravenous medicines can bring the blood pressure up. Intravenous medicines that bring blood pressure up are "pressors". "Dopamine" and "dobutamine" and "norepinephrine" are the most common pressors which physicians prescribe when they attempt to raise the blood pressure of a person with cardiogenic shock.

## What happens if the fluids and pressor medicines fail to bring the blood pressure up?

Physicians may attempt to use a device called an "intra-aortic balloon pump", which is often inserted through the artery in the groin (the "femoral artery") and into the aorta. The intra-aortic balloon pump inflates as the heart relaxes after each beat and helps drive blood through the coronary arteries. This may provide additional blood flow to jeopardized heart muscle and limit extension of heart muscle damage. The inflation of the balloon as the heart relaxes may also help to drive blood through the rest of the body so that vital organs such as the kidney have a better blood supply.

## BRADYCARDIA

### What is bradycardia?

Bradycardia means that the heart is beating too slowly. A heartbeat of approximately 60 per minute or less after a myocardial infarction is bradycardia and requires evaluation.

### What are the most common forms of bradycardia?

The most common forms of bradycardia are "sinus bradycardia" and "heart block".

### What is sinus bradycardia?

Sinus bradycardia means that the heart is beating in a very regular fashion, but at a rate of less than approximately 50 beats per minute. Sinus bradycardia is particularly common in people who have had a myocardial infarction involving the bottom wall of the heart (an "inferior wall myocardial infarction").

### *What is the treatment of sinus bradycardia?*

If the person's blood pressure is not dropping, sinus bradycardia may require no treatment and will usually resolve on its own. If blood pressure is dropping, a medicine called "atropine", given intravenously, will usually accelerate the heart rate to a normal or near-normal rate. If atropine fails to accelerate the heart rate, a pacemaker may be inserted which will electrically stimulate the heart to beat at a higher and more normal rate.

## **HEART BLOCK**

### *What is heart block?*

The stimulus for the heart to beat is an electrical signal generated in the top of the heart in the atria and transmitted down nerve fibers to the ventricles. These nerve fibers provide the impulses that cause the atria and then the ventricles to contract. A myocardial infarction that damages heart muscle, can also damage nerve fibers that conduct impulses through the heart. This can block transmission of electrical impulses down the heart's nerve fibers and produce "heart block".

Heart block is dangerous because it can cause a very dangerous, slow heartbeat.

## What is the treatment of heart block?

There are several different types of heart block caused by myocardial infarction.

A myocardial infarction involving the bottom of the heart (an "inferior wall myocardial infarction") can cause several different types of heart block. A "first degree heart block" is common after an inferior wall myocardial infarction and usually requires no treatment. A type of "second degree heart block" called a "Mobitz I" or "Wenckebach" may cause a slowing of the heartbeat which requires treatment with atropine or, if necessary, a temporary pacemaker. A "complete heart block" in which the conduction of electrical impulses to the ventricles is entirely disrupted can occur after an inferior wall myocardial infarction. A temporary pacemaker may be required if the complete heart block causes a drop in blood pressure.

Heart block associated with an anterior wall myocardial infarction can be quite dangerous. With anterior wall myocardial infarction, the heart block is commonly associated with extensive heart muscle damage and severe damage to the electrical system of the heart. The types of heart block associated with anterior wall myocardial infarction are most commonly the "Mobitz II" heart block or a "complete heart block" and urgently require insertion of a pacemaker. Abnormalities seen on the electrocardiogram that predict progression to complete heart block in people with anterior wall myocardial infarction such as "bundle branch block" or "bifascicular block" often require a temporary pacemaker to guard against a potential catastrophic heart block leading to severe slowing or stoppage of the heartbeat.

# ATRIAL FIBRILLATION

## *What is atrial fibrillation?*

Normally, an area of the atrium called the "SA node" generates an electrical impulse that travels down the heart and stimulates the heart muscle to beat with a regular rhythm. In atrial fibrillation, there is a chaotic firing of electrical impulses from many points of the atrium. These electrical impulses, transmitted to the ventricles, cause the heart to beat with an irregular rhythm. When atrial fibrillation occurs after an acute myocardial infarction, the atrial fibrillation often causes a very fast, irregular rhythm called "rapid atrial fibrillation".

## *Why is rapid atrial fibrillation dangerous?*

When the heart beats very rapidly, it works harder. This increased work increases the heart muscle's need for oxygen. If the arteries that supply oxygen-rich blood to heart muscle are narrow or blocked, extension of heart muscle damage can occur.

The heart pumps blood as it contracts and fills as it relaxes. When the heart is beating very quickly and irregularly, there may not be enough time for the heart to fill and then pump its blood outward. This can cause the blood pressure to drop and can send the person into shock.

## *In the setting of a myocardial infarction, what is the treatment of atrial fibrillation?*

The initial priority is to reduce the heart rate if the heart is beating too rapidly. Intravenous "propranolol", "digoxin" or "amiodarone" can be quite effective in slowing the heart rate down and can often stop the atrial fibrillation entirely. Other medicines including "propranolol", "diltiazem" and "verapamil" are also sometimes used to slow the heart rate.

If the heart rate is very rapid and the person's blood pressure is very low or unstable, it may be necessary to perform an "electrical cardioversion".

### What is electrical cardioversion?

Electrical cardioversion is the conversion of an abnormal heart rhythm to a normal rhythm by use of an electrical shock.

### How do medical professionals perform an electrical cardioversion?

Unless there is a sudden crisis, the person with the abnormal heart rhythm is first given a sedative such as "Valium". When a button is pressed, electrical paddles put in front of the breastbone and on the far left side of the chest send an electrical current through the chest.

The first electrical shock is often successful in converting atrial fibrillation into a normal rhythm. If the first electrical shock is not successful, additional shocks with gradually increasing current (up to a limit) are given.

## VENTRICULAR PREMATURE BEATS

### What are ventricular premature beats?

Ventricular premature beats are abnormal heartbeats caused by an independent electrical impulse in the ventricle.

513

### *Why are ventricular premature beats dangerous?*

Ventricular premature beats can lead to a very dangerous type of rhythm problem in which the ventricles begin to fire electrical impulses wildly. This can lead to "ventricular tachycardia" or to "ventricular fibrillation" in which the heart totally fails to pump.

### *In the setting of a myocardial infarction,*
### *what is the treatment of ventricular premature beats?*

The treatment of ventricular premature beats depends upon the frequency of the premature beats and the pattern with which they occur. Ventricular premature beats, which do not occur in a sequence or are not too close together or to the previous normal heartbeat, may not need treatment. In the past, an "anti-arrhythmic" medicine called "lidocaine" reduced these premature beats. It is now apparent that lidocaine or similar drugs can be harmful if routinely given. Medicines in the family of "beta blockers" are a common treatment when a person with STEMI has ventricular premature beats and can be quite effective in reducing or eliminating them.

## VENTRICULAR TACHYCARDIA

### *What is ventricular tachycardia?*

Ventricular tachycardia is a series of several ventricular premature beats in a row, during which the heart beats at a rate in excess of, and often far in excess of, 100 beats per minute. When this occurs in the setting of STEMI, blood pressure can drop and there is a major risk of progression to ventricular fibrillation (see below).

## *What is the treatment of ventricular tachycardia?*

People with acute myocardial infarction for a very short time, may maintain their blood pressure while having ventricular tachycardia. In this circumstance, the intravenous medications "amiodarone" or "procainamide" may convert the rhythm to normal. If, however, the person's blood pressure has dropped or if the ventricular tachycardia has not responded quickly to the intravenous medications, electrical cardioversion will often convert the rhythm back to normal.

## VENTRICULAR FIBRILLATION

### *What is ventricular fibrillation and what is the treatment of ventricular fibrillation?*

When a person has ventricular fibrillation, there is a complete cessation of the normal heartbeat and an immediate drop of the blood pressure to near zero. This requires immediate CPR and life-saving treatment.

A first step will be to attempt electrical cardioversion. If this first shock is unsuccessful at starting a heartbeat, CPR is continued and several more shocks are given. Injections of "epinephrine" or "amiodarone" followed by further electroshock are necessary if the electrical cardioversion initially administered fails to re-establish a normal heartbeat.

# NON-STEMI

## What is non-STEMI?

A non-STEMI is an abbreviation for "non-ST elevation myocardial infarction". This means that although the electrocardiogram does not show the characteristic appearance described earlier in this chapter of "ST elevation", there is clear evidence of some heart muscle damage as indicated by elevated blood levels of troponin. Although still dangerous as it can lead to a larger myocardial infarction or sudden death, non-STEMI is less dangerous than STEMI.

## What is the initial treatment of non-STEMI?

A person with non-STEMI has a lower acute risk than with STEMI. A first step in treatment is to try to improve circulation to the heart with nitroglycerin pills which, taken under the tongue, can dilate blood vessels in the heart and improve circulation to the heart muscle. A medicine in the category of "beta blockers" can reduce some of the work of the heart and some of the symptoms or consequences of inadequate circulation of blood to heart muscle.

## What medicine can relieve the blockage in the coronary arteries?

Medicines to relieve blood clots in the coronary arteries, including aspirin, clopidogrel, and some form of heparin, are given. In addition, potent drugs that inhibit blood clotting in the family of medicines called "GPIIb/IIIa inhibitors" may also be given.

## What is the role of PCI in the setting of non-STEMI?

It will be very common for a cardiologist to recommend that a person have a coronary angiogram to look for blocked arteries that a stent can open.

## UNCOMPLICATED MYOCARDIAL INFARCTION

### What is an "uncomplicated myocardial infarction"?

An uncomplicated myocardial infarction is an acute myocardial infarction that is not complicated by heart failure or by significant problems with heart rhythm.

### What is the treatment of an uncomplicated myocardial infarction?

A person with an uncomplicated myocardial infarction will initially be kept in bed, given supplemental oxygen, and have their pain controlled by pain medication. Within three or four days, the person can sit in a chair for about an hour twice a day. A day or so later, standing and a bit of walking will be good to do. If all goes well and the person is pain free, discharge from the hospital within a week of admission is likely.

# SUPERIOR VENA CAVA SYNDROME

## DEFINITIONS

### What is the superior vena cava?

The superior vena cava is the second largest vein in our body and carries blood from the head, neck, arms and upper chest back into the heart. The superior vena cava has a very thin wall and is easily compressed and obstructed by abnormal growths inside the chest.

### What is superior vena cava syndrome?

Superior vena cava syndrome is when there is an obstruction of the blood flow from the superior vena cava back into the heart. When this occurs, symptoms and medical problems develop that are very dangerous and life threatening.

## THE CAUSES OF SUPERIOR VENA CAVA OBSTRUCTION

### What can obstruct the superior vena cava?

By far, the most common cause of superior vena cava obstruction is a cancer that compresses the thin-walled superior vena cava, preventing blood from flowing through it properly. The most common cancers that can obstruct the superior vena cava are lung cancer and lymphoma, although other cancers can do this as well.

People with cancer sometimes have a surgically implanted intravenous catheter through which medicine is given and blood is drawn. The tip of this catheter runs through the superior vena cava. Sometimes, a large blood clot can form around this catheter and totally obstruct the superior vena cava.

## SYMPTOMS

### What are the symptoms of superior vena cava syndrome?

Because a cancer inside the chest which has not been controlled by treatment tends to grow slowly but steadily, development of symptoms of superior vena cava syndrome associated with cancer usually takes place over a period of days and weeks rather than all of a sudden.

Initially, the person may notice increasing shortness of breath associated with a cough. This is a result of swelling of veins and tissues in the neck and inside the chest that are compressing airway structures, that is, the "trachea" and the "bronchi", which carry air in and out of the lungs. As the obstruction of the superior vena cava worsens, the blockage of blood flow from the head and neck will cause the face to become very red and swollen and neck veins will bulge prominently. This is often associated with headaches and problems with vision. Since the superior vena cava also carries blood from the arms back into the heart, the arms can swell.

## MAKING THE DIAGNOSIS

### How is the diagnosis of superior vena cava syndrome made?

If a CT or MRI scan of the chest makes the diagnosis of superior vena cava syndrome. Most of the time, the cause is a cancer, which can be seen with the CT or MRI scan to be compressing the vena cava and obstructing its blood flow. If the CT or MRI does not show such a compression, a venogram, in which a dye put into the vein and tracked by x-ray as it makes its way back to the heart, can show the obstruction very clearly and give important information about its probable cause.

Superior vena cava syndrome may be the first evidence that a person has cancer. After making the diagnosis of superior vena cava syndrome, the priority is to identify the disease that is causing it.

## IDENTIFYING THE CAUSE OF SUPERIOR VENA CAVA SYNDROME

### How is the cause of superior vena cava syndrome identified?

If CT or MRI scan of the chest finds evidence of a cancer that is compressing the superior vena cava, determination of the exact nature of the cancer is critical to guiding appropriate treatment. Because lung cancer is such a strong possibility, a number of tests will seek to prove or disprove a lung cancer diagnosis. A pathologist, using the microscope, will examine sputum sent to the laboratory. If the person has a pleural effusion, (see chapter entitled "Pleural Effusion"), withdrawal of a sample of the fluid for laboratory analysis could produce important information. Other areas of the body suspected of harboring cancer, such as enlarged lymph nodes, may also be biopsied. Bronchoscopy (see the description of bronchoscopy in the chapter entitled "Lung Cancer") may show evidence of an obvious cancer involving the lung. When these tests fail to make the diagnosis, it may be necessary to perform a biopsy of the cancer that is compressing the vena cava using either a biopsy needle guided by a physician using a CT scanner, or occasionally by a surgeon using one of several other available techniques to do this.

## TREATMENT

*What is the treatment of superior vena cava syndrome?*

If the obstruction is very severe and a person's ability to breathe or to drain blood from their head is severely affected, death can result very quickly. Even before testing to determine the exact cause of the obstruction, emergency treatment may be necessary. The treatment used most commonly is to insert a rigid hollow tube called an "endovascular stent" into the superior vena cava to prop it open and allow blood to flow through it again. This will relieve the obstruction and associated symptoms very quickly. In this emergency, when life is in immediate danger and the diagnosis appears to be some form of cancer, physicians will commonly initiate radiation therapy immediately after the stent insertion in an attempt to shrink the cancer.

If the superior vena cava is causing symptoms but not immediately threatening life, the initial steps revolve around identifying the exact cause of the obstruction in order to enable proper treatment. As in the immediately life-threatening situation, placement of an endovascular stent can promptly relieve symptoms and reduce the immediate dangers and symptoms of the superior vena cava syndrome. When the exact nature of the cancer is determined, appropriate treatments, primarily radiation or chemotherapy, can attempt to control or cure the cancer.

### What is the treatment of superior vena cava syndrome caused by a clot around a catheter?

Placement of an endovascular stent can relieve obstruction of the superior vena cava by a blood clot. Following placement of the stent, medications will prevent recurrent clots in the superior vena cava. The outlook following successful placement of the stent for continued blood flow through the superior vena cava is very good.

### What is the outlook for a person who has developed the superior vena cava syndrome because of cancer?

With the placement of an endovascular stent, the obstruction to the superior vena cava can generally be relieved and the danger it poses to life diminished. The primary problem the person will face once the obstruction has been relieved is the cancer that caused the obstruction. If this cancer can be controlled or cured, the outcome will reflect the success of treatment. If cancer keeps growing despite treatment, the outlook for extended survival will reflect the complications caused by the unrestrained growth of the cancer.

# INFECTIONS

# BACTERIAL MENINGITIS

## DEFINITION

### What is meningitis?

Meningitis is a very dangerous medical condition in which the membranes surrounding the brain and the spinal cord are severely inflamed, usually by an infectious organism. Bacteria growing in the fluid surrounding the brain and spinal cord (this fluid is the "cerebrospinal fluid", abbreviated as "CSF") are the cause of the overwhelming majority of serious and life-threatening cases of meningitis. This chapter will focus on bacterial meningitis.

## HOW PEOPLE GET BACTERIAL MENINGITIS

### What is the blood brain barrier?

The "blood brain barrier" is the body's physical mechanism for keeping undesired substances, including bacteria, viruses, and toxins, from entering the brain and spinal fluid. The actual barrier exists at the level of the brain's capillaries, which are the smallest blood vessels in the brain. The cells lining these capillaries link together, forming a barrier that prevents toxic chemicals, bacteria, or viruses from passing through.

## *How do bacteria get through the blood brain barrier?*

Dangerous bacteria that get into the blood stream may have the ability to either anchor themselves onto the cells lining the brain's capillaries and swing into the brain, or push themselves through the tight junctions that exist between the cells lining the brain's capillaries. Through either method, they gain access into the cerebrospinal fluid where they can multiply and cause meningitis.

Serious infections, such as infections of the inner ear, or sinuses that are in close proximity to the brain and spinal fluid can spread directly into the cerebrospinal fluid. Neurosurgical procedures, such as operations to treat brain tumors, can create openings through which bacteria can travel and cause meningitis.

## SYMPTOMS

## *What are the symptoms of meningitis?*

The most typical symptoms of meningitis are a severe headache along with a stiff neck, fever, backache, and impairment of thinking ability or consciousness. When these symptoms develop over two days or less, there will be a high level of suspicion of the presence of bacterial meningitis.

In people with cancer, a suppressed immune system, either because of cancer treatment or of the cancer itself, can suppress inflammation and reduce or eliminate symptoms of headache and neck stiffness otherwise seen with meningitis. When changes in a person's state of alertness or thinking ability develop in a person with a suppressed immune system, it raises the suspicion of the presence of bacterial meningitis. Chemotherapy-induced neutropenia (see chapter entitled "Bone Marrow Suppression") is an important example of immune suppression that can predispose a person to serious bacterial infections, such as bacterial meningitis.

## MAKING THE DIAGNOSIS

### *How is the diagnosis of bacterial meningitis made?*

Based upon the symptoms and a rapid physical examination, it may be very clear that a person is suffering from bacterial meningitis. The most definitive diagnosis requires examination of cerebrospinal fluid obtained with a spinal tap.

### *How does the spinal tap obtain cerebrospinal fluid?*

The most common method that a physician will use is to have a person lie on either side with their knees curled up toward their chest. After injection of a local anesthetic, a special needle is inserted between the vertebral bones in the lower back until the physician feels a slight pop, which means that the needle has gone through the membrane containing the spinal fluid (the "dura"). At this point, spinal fluid will drip out of the physician's end of the needle and will be collected in plastic tubes for laboratory analysis.

### *When a person with cancer may have bacterial meningitis, why do physicians commonly recommend a CT or MRI scan before performing a spinal tap?*

When a person has cancer, brain metastases may have developed that are causing brain swelling and an increased pressure inside the skull. Similarly, if a person has a glioblastoma (see chapter entitled "Brain Cancer: Glioblastoma"), the tumor and associated swelling can greatly increase the pressure inside the skull. This increased pressure is "increased intracranial pressure".

With increased intracranial pressure, the withdrawal of cerebrospinal fluid from the area just beneath the spinal cord can create a pressure gradient that pulls the swollen brain downward toward the area of lower pressure. Catastrophically, if there is very high intracranial pressure, a spinal tap can pull a portion of a region of the brain called the "cerebellar tonsils" into the large opening at the base of skull called the "foramen magnum". When this happens, (this is "tonsillar herniation") the portion of the brainstem called the medulla, which controls respiration and heartbeat, is compressed, and may stop functioning. This can cause sudden death.

The CT or MRI scan can identify brain metastasis and associated swelling, and assess the risk of performing a spinal tap.

*What specific information does the spinal tap give?*
*How does the spinal tap help to guide therapy?*

The cerebrospinal fluid of a person with bacterial meningitis has an exceedingly high number of white blood cells. This high number of white blood cells makes the diagnosis.

Examination of the cerebrospinal fluid with special dyes may give essential information regarding the specific bacteria causing the infection. Not all bacteria are equally sensitive to all antibiotics. By identifying the probable bacteria causing the infection, treatment with the antibiotics most likely to cure the infection can begin.

When a person has symptoms consistent with meningitis along with a high number of white blood cells called "neutrophils" in the cerebrospinal fluid, it is clear that the person has bacterial meningitis whether bacteria are initially seen under the microscope or not. This high level of neutrophils in the spinal fluid may not be present if a person has "febrile neutropenia", as described in the chapter with that title.

By understanding a person's risk factors, such as presence of intravenous catheters, or existing ear or sinus infections, or a recent neurosurgical operation, along with the analyzed cerebrospinal fluid, the antibiotics most likely to treat the infection can be chosen.

### TREATMENT

*When the diagnosis of meningitis is a possibility,*
*when should antibiotic treatment begin?*

Meningitis is a medical emergency and needs prompt evaluation and treatment. If meningitis is likely, the sooner antibiotic treatment begins, the better the outlook for survival and recovery.

*What is the treatment if there is a delay*
*in the ability to perform the spinal tap?*

Meningitis is a medical emergency. If bacterial meningitis appears likely, and there is a delay in obtaining a CT or MRI or a spinal tap, physicians begin antibiotic treatment with antibiotics most likely treat the infection. Physicians will often draw "blood cultures" just prior to starting the antibiotic. The blood culture results that are available a day or two later will determine if bacteria are growing in the bloodstream and, if they are, determine the exact bacteria that is growing and its sensitivity to specific antibiotics.

## Who makes the decision about antibiotics?

Ideally, the physician will have had a good amount of experience treating people with meningitis. In major medical centers, this often will be a specialist in infectious diseases or critical care medicine, along with expert hospital pharmacists.

## What is the antibiotic treatment of meningitis?

The treatment of bacterial meningitis is to administer high doses of intravenous antibiotics. Generally, the antibiotic treatment regimen will consist of two or more antibiotics chosen based upon knowledge of a person's predisposing factors, symptoms, physical examination findings and examination of the cerebrospinal fluid under the microscope. The combined information derived from this will generally identify antibiotics that can effectively treat the infection.

## Are there medications given along with antibiotics that can improve the outlook of a person with bacterial meningitis?

A type of steroid medication called "dexamethasone" (brand name is "Decadron") can be helpful to people with a type of meningitis called "pneumococcal meningitis". If this is a possible cause of a person's meningitis, dexamethasone administration, along with antibiotics, may improve the chances of a full recovery.

# OUTLOOK

## *What is the outlook of bacterial meningitis?*

The outlook is enormously dependent on how rapidly treatment begins after the onset of symptoms. There is a great deal of variation in outlook, largely depending upon the time until initiation of treatment with antibiotics, the type of bacteria, and the age and underlying health of the person. Overall, about one in four people who develop bacterial meningitis do not survive their hospitalization. Of those who survive, about one in ten has some residual problem such as loss of memory or thinking ability, hearing loss or weakness on one side of the body. People at particularly high risk of dying of bacterial meningitis are people with severe immune system problems, people with diabetes, and the elderly.

Survivors of bacterial meningitis very commonly make a complete recovery. Because the illness was a severe one with quite a high degree of brain irritation, it may take a period of weeks or even months before a person's previous state of health returns.

# COMMUNITY-ACQUIRED PNEUMONIA

## *DEFINITIONS*

### *What is bacterial pneumonia?*

Bacterial pneumonia is a bacterial infection of the lung. Despite tremendous improvements in our ability to diagnose and treat bacterial pneumonia, it remains a major cause of death throughout the world and is a leading cause of death in people with cancer.

In considering the diagnosis, treatment, and outlook of bacterial pneumonia, it is helpful to separate the discussion of pneumonia into the categories of those people who develop pneumonia in a community setting, and those who develop pneumonia while in a hospital.

### *What is community-acquired pneumonia?*

Community-acquired pneumonia refers to pneumonia that develops while a person is not in the hospital or in a setting similar to a hospital such as a nursing home. Because it often takes a couple of days or so for an infection to take hold in the lung, physicians generally refer to pneumonia that is discovered within 48 hours of admission to a hospital as community-acquired pneumonia.

Because bacterial infections are the most common cause of community-acquired pneumonia, this chapter only covers pneumonia caused by bacterial infection.

## THE CAUSE OF COMMUNITY-ACQUIRED PNEUMONIA

*What causes community-acquired bacterial pneumonia?*

The atmosphere, in which we live, as well as the inside of our mouth and throat, contains a wide assortment of dangerous bacteria. The natural defense systems of our bodies must maintain barriers to prevent these bacteria from infecting our lungs. The anatomy of our nose, throat and lungs, our ability to cough, and the cells lining the air passages in our lungs, all play a role in defending us against these bacteria. Our intact immune system eliminates most bacteria that make their way past these barriers and down into our lungs. There are times, however, when our natural protection fails us. Exposure to aggressively virulent bacteria can overwhelm our natural defenses.

Weakened lung defenses against bacterial infection that are a result of cancer or of treatments such as chemotherapy, radiation, or steroid medications, can diminish a person's ability to prevent the growth of dangerous bacteria in the lungs, and increase a person's susceptibility to pneumonia.

## SYMPTOMS

*What are the symptoms of community-acquired bacterial pneumonia?*

Cough, fever, pain in the chest and production of deep yellow or greenish sputum, intense sweating, and shaking chills, are typical symptoms of pneumonia. As the bacterial pneumonia worsens, a person becomes short winded. The speed with which the symptoms develop can range from hours to weeks, and will depend upon the bacteria causing the infection and upon the state of the person's immune system.

The classic pneumonia symptoms of cough and production of yellow sputum can be diminished or absent in people with severe pneumonia and a much suppressed immune system. The primary symptom of pneumonia, with severe immune system suppression as is seen with "febrile neutropenia" (please see chapter with that title), may be fever and the very rapid development of severe difficulty breathing.

## MAKING THE DIAGNOSIS

*How do physicians or medical professionals make the diagnosis of community-acquired bacterial pneumonia?*

The history given by the ill person or family or friends can lead to a strong suspicion of bacterial pneumonia. Examination with a stethoscope can identify the abnormal breath sounds commonly heard in people with bacterial pneumonia. A chest x-ray can confirm the diagnosis of bacterial pneumonia and may give important clues as to the specific type of bacteria that is causing the infection.

## TREATMENT OF COMMUNITY-ACQUIRED PNEUMONIA

*What is the treatment for community-acquired pneumonia in people with cancer when hospitalization is not necessary?*

In people who do not have cancer, the bacteria that cause community-acquired pneumonia are generally very sensitive to antibiotics and respond promptly to antibiotics. In people with cancer, community-acquired pneumonia can worsen very quickly and may not respond as promptly to antibiotics.

Prior to beginning treatment with antibiotics, the physician may ask a person to cough up a sample of "sputum" from their lungs for examination under the microscope. There is a difference between "spit" and "sputum". Spit comes from the mouth, while sputum is what the lungs produce. Sputum is what is worth evaluating, and a person is encouraged to make their best effort to cough the material out of the lungs for proper evaluation.

The sputum coughed up by a person with bacterial pneumonia is usually loaded with the bacteria causing the infection and may be sent to a laboratory for examination. The laboratory receiving this sputum puts it on a glass slide, stains it with a sequence of chemicals, and examines it under the microscope in an attempt to identify the bacteria that is causing the pneumonia.

The physician's understanding of the factors that predisposed the person with bacterial pneumonia to infection will allow the physician to make a very good assessment of the antibiotic most likely to eliminate the infection. "Sputum cultures", performed in the laboratory, can determine whether bacteria are present and give a highly specific identification of the bacteria and of its sensitivities to the different available antibiotics.

Sometimes, people with cancer who have developed community-acquired bacterial pneumonia receive treatment outside of the hospital with oral antibiotics. Frequently used antibiotics include antibiotics in the family called "fluoroquinolones", or combination treatment with antibiotics in the "beta lactam" family (such as "amoxicillin") and in the "macrolide" family (such as "azithromycin"). These antibiotics will generally cure pneumonia caused by the most common types of bacteria.

If the person is very short of breath, is not responding properly to antibiotic therapy, has severe immune system weakness, or has other factors that raise a concern about a person's safety if treated at home, physicians will often recommend hospitalization.

### How is community-acquired pneumonia requiring hospitalization evaluated and treated?

In addition to examination of the person's sputum, people whose pneumonia is severe enough to require hospitalization may have bacteria growing in their bloodstream as well as in their lungs. Upon admission to the hospital, samples of blood may be drawn and sent to the laboratory for "culture", that is, to see if any bacteria are growing in the bloodstream. The relatively standard blood tests called the "complete blood count", abbreviated as "CBC", as well as the standard blood chemistry tests, will help determine if other problems, such as anemia, or liver or kidney problems exist and need medical attention. Blood drawn from the artery in the wrist (the "radial artery") measures the amount of oxygen and carbon dioxide in the arterial blood. This measurement, called an "arterial blood gas" provides very important information regarding the degree of impairment, if any, of the ability of the lungs to perform its essential function of delivering oxygen and removing carbon dioxide to and from the bloodstream.

In the hospital, the antibiotics used to treat the community-acquired pneumonia commonly include a powerful antibiotic, given intravenously, in the category of a "respiratory fluoroquinolone", such as "moxifloxacin" (brand name is "Avelox", manufacturer's product website is www.avelox.com) or "levofloxacin" (brand name is "Levaquin", manufacturer's product website is www.levaquin.com).

## How might a physician evaluate risk for a hospitalized person with community-acquired pneumonia?

A scoring system called the "Pneumonia Severity Index/ Pneumonia Patient Outcome Research Team" and better known by its initials "PSI/PORT score" has been developed that gives a very good assessment of the risk posed by a person's episode of community-acquired pneumonia. This score evaluates specific aspects of a person's medical history, physical examination, x-rays, and laboratory tests, and assigns higher numbers for unfavorable findings. The sum of the numbers is the PSI/PORT score.

The PSI/PORT score can help a physician make a decision as to whether hospitalization is required as well as assess the danger posed by the pneumonia. A higher PSI/PORT score indicates a higher risk of a longer hospitalization, development of complications requiring intensive care unit admission, and a higher risk of death in the hospital from community-acquired pneumonia.

## OUTLOOK

*What is the outlook for a person hospitalized for community-acquired pneumonia?*

Most of the time, the symptoms associated with a person's pneumonia, including their fever, improve within 2 to 3 days after the antibiotic treatment begins, and a person is discharged from the hospital soon after. Although fever and shortness of breath can resolve quickly with antibiotics, and the danger posed by the community-acquired pneumonia may have passed, cough, chest discomfort, as well as a general feeling of fatigue may persist for a month or longer.

Despite the very best medical care, including prompt treatment with antibiotics, some people hospitalized with community-acquired pneumonia fail to respond adequately to treatment, requiring transfer to the intensive care unit and a prolonged hospitalization. Depending upon how sick the person is at the time of hospitalization, a person may be at risk of a prolonged, complicated hospitalization as well as death from the episode of pneumonia.

Please see the chapters entitled "Sepsis and Septic Shock", "Acute Respiratory Distress Syndrome" and "Acute Disseminated Intravascular Coagulation" for a discussion of three very dangerous potential complications of community-acquired pneumonia.

# HOSPITAL-ACQUIRED PNEUMONIA

## DEFINITION

### What is hospital-acquired pneumonia?

Hospital-acquired pneumonia is a lung infection that develops 48 hours or more after admission to the hospital. Hospital-acquired pneumonia is one of the most common and dangerous infectious complications that afflict people who are in the hospital.

### Why is hospital-acquired pneumonia so dangerous?

The bacteria that cause hospital-acquired pneumonia tend to be more dangerous than bacteria acquired in the community and are more likely to be resistant to antibiotics. In addition, people who are in the hospital for serious illness are more likely to have difficulty using their body's own defense mechanisms help eliminate the bacteria causing the hospital-acquired pneumonia, and are susceptible to other complications, such as the complications discussed in the chapters entitled "Sepsis and Septic Shock", "Acute Respiratory Distress Syndrome", and "Disseminated Intravascular Coagulation".

## *What is ventilator-associated pneumonia and why does it develop?*

Ventilator-associated pneumonia is a pneumonia that develops while a person is connected to a mechanical ventilator that has been moving air in and out of the lungs for 48 hours or longer. The air produced by the ventilator itself is quite clean, but the delivery of the air to the lungs is through a series of tubes that start at the ventilator, and ultimately attach to a tube that is inside a person's windpipe ("trachea"). This tube in the windpipe can either be an "endotracheal tube" which is passed through the mouth or nose, or directly into the trachea (via a "tracheotomy") through an incision made in the front of the neck. Contamination of these tubes occurs through bacteria in the general hospital environment or in the course of routine medical care.

## SYMPTOMS

### *What are the signs that a person who is in the hospital is developing a hospital-acquired pneumonia?*

The development of a new fever, associated with shortness of breath and, sometimes, with production of deep yellow or yellow-green sputum, are important signs that suggest the diagnosis of hospital-acquired pneumonia. When pneumonia is present, a chest x-ray will often show a changed abnormal appearance within one or both lungs (a new "infiltrate"). A simple blood count will generally show that the number of white blood cells in the bloodstream is increasing. Measurement of the level of oxygen in the blood in the arteries (the "arterial blood gas") determines whether the lungs are delivering an adequate amount of oxygen into the bloodstream, providing evidence of pneumonia and an indication of its severity.

## TREATMENT

*What is the treatment of hospital-acquired pneumonia or ventilator-associated pneumonia?*

Hospital-acquired pneumonia, especially in people with cancer, can be extremely dangerous and may be somewhat resistant to antibiotics. Treatment with combinations of intravenous antibiotics that have the best possibility of destroying the bacteria will begin. Knowledge of the recent bacterial infections spreading in the hospital, and an understanding of the person's underlying medical problem and the bacterial infections to which the individual is most likely to be susceptible, will initially guide the choice of the antibiotics most likely to be effective.

There are many antibiotic regimens used to treat hospital-acquired or ventilator-associated pneumonia. "Respiratory fluoroquinolones", such as "moxifloxacin" (brand name is "Avelox", manufacturer's product website is www.avelox.com) or "levofloxacin" (brand name is "Levaquin", manufacturer's product website is www.levaquin.com) are commonly used. Ceftriaxone (brand name is "Rocephin", manufacturer's product website is www.rocephin.com), ertapenem (brand name Invanz, manufacturer's product website is www.invanz.com) or an intravenous antibiotic containing a combination of ampicillin and sulbactam (brand name is "Unisyn") are among the other commonly used antibiotics.

"Sputum cultures" and "blood cultures" are tests in which the hospital laboratory attempts to grow bacteria from the sputum or blood. Sputum and blood cultures can identify the bacteria causing the infection and determine the antibiotics to which the bacteria are susceptible. Based upon results of the sputum and blood cultures, and the response a person has had to initial antibiotics, changes may be required in the antibiotic regimen.

## INADEQUATE RESPONSE TO ANTIBIOTIC TREATMENT

### When is there a concern that bacterial pneumonia is not properly responding to treatment?

The symptoms associated with a person's pneumonia should begin to resolve within 3 days of starting antibiotics. If they do not, there will be a concern that the antibiotics that were initially chosen will be insufficient to treat and cure the pneumonia. Further attempts to identify the specific bacteria causing the infection, or to identify other reasons that the antibiotics are not working properly, will be made.

### What is bronchoscopy?

A bronchoscope is a flexible long tube used to examine the inside of the lungs assisted by images projected from the bronchoscope to a video monitor. To perform a bronchoscopy, a lung specialist will administer a mild sedative and will spray the throat with a light anesthetic. The physician then advances the bronchoscope down the windpipe and into the bronchial tree. The scope itself has a space inside of it, which allows the physician performing the bronchoscopy to put instruments down the scope which can suck fluid out of the bronchial tubes or which can snip off and retrieve tiny pieces of lung tissue. During the bronchoscopy, the physician may inject a bit of salt water into the bronchial tubes and then suck the fluid out to try to retrieve and identify bacteria. This test is "bronchoalveolar lavage". These samples of fluid, or lung tissue, are sent to a pathology laboratory for analysis.

Bronchoscopy is, at times, essential to the identification of the specific organism that is causing the pneumonia. The bronchoscopy itself, even in a person with a very severe pneumonia, carries a relatively low risk of complications.

### Why might a physician want to perform a CT scan?

The CT scan can provide additional information about areas of the lung affected by the pneumonia as well as detect complications of pneumonia that can be responsible for delayed recovery or failure to respond properly to antibiotics.

### What happens if despite these treatments, the pneumonia worsens and a person cannot breathe adequately?

Despite best efforts with antibiotics and other medications, some people with bacterial pneumonia will develop a worsening of their condition to the point where it is impossible for them to breathe on their own. At this stage, a person has developed "acute respiratory failure" and will need assistance, either in the form of "non-invasive positive pressure ventilation" or "mechanical ventilation".

As an initial step, to support a person's ability to breathe, a tight mask applied to the mouth and nose and attached to a machine can push air into the lungs and help a person to breathe. This "non-invasive positive pressure ventilation", abbreviated as

"NPPV", will greatly reduce a person's feeling of breathlessness, and may be sufficient to support a person's ability to breathe until the pneumonia resolves.

If NPPV fails to maintain an adequate level of oxygen in the bloodstream, mechanical ventilation may be necessary. Mechanical ventilation requires a tube in the trachea (an "endotracheal tube") attached to the machine called a "ventilator" which pushes air into the lungs. The insertion of the endotracheal tube, as well as maintaining the endotracheal tube in place, commonly causes anxiety and discomfort. To help relieve this, physicians may give sedatives before and after insertion of the endotracheal tube.

## How does a person get off the mechanical ventilator?

Getting off the mechanical ventilator, (called "weaning off the ventilator") can take several days. Physicians will try to decrease the person's dependence on the ventilator by gradually decreasing the work the mechanical ventilator does to support breathing. Once the person gets to the point where he or she can breathe independently and maintain their level of oxygen without the mechanical ventilator, the tube in the trachea can be removed (removal of the endotracheal tube is called "extubation") and support with the ventilator discontinued.

## ASPIRATION PNEUMONIA

### What is aspiration pneumonia?

Aspiration pneumonia is an inflammation of the lungs caused by inhalation of fluids from the mouth into the lungs. The fluid in the mouth may have originated in the mouth or throat, or may have been thrown up from the stomach into the mouth and then inhaled into the lungs.

### Why can a person with cancer be susceptible to aspiration pneumonia?

With advanced cancer, a person may be largely confined to bed and receiving a significant amount of narcotics to control their pain. This can make it difficult for a person to use their normal reflexes to keep liquid material from their mouth or throat from getting into their lungs.

Conditions that increase the amount of fluid burped into the mouth, such as cancers of the esophagus, in combination with lying in a flat position, can predispose a person to aspiration pneumonia.

### Why can aspiration pneumonia cause bacterial pneumonia?

The material inhaled into the lungs can contain a wide variety of bacteria. In the context of a person with a weakened immune defense from cancer, these bacteria can rapidly grow and cause life-threatening bacterial pneumonia.

### How is bacterial pneumonia from aspiration pneumonia treated?

The treatment of bacterial pneumonia from aspiration pneumonia involves powerful antibiotics given for a week or longer.

# LUNG ABSCESS

## What is a lung abscess?

A lung abscess is an area of pus in the lung. The pus itself is composed of totally destroyed ("necrotic") lung tissue mixed together with white blood cells and a high concentration of the responsible bacteria or fungus. Following the body's natural instinct to try to contain the pus, a wall of scar tissue develops around the pus. The result is a pus-filled cavity that can be very difficult to treat.

## Why is a lung abscess difficult to treat?

The wall of scar tissue around the abscess may keep antibiotics from reaching and killing the bacteria within the abscess. Another problem that can develop is rupture of the abscess and spilling of pus into the area between the lung and the chest wall ("the pleural space"). A collection of pus in the pleural space is an "empyema".

## How is a lung abscess or an empyema treated?

High doses of intravenous antibiotics given for three weeks or longer can cure most lung abscesses. When the abscess is very large and antibiotics are not working, it may be necessary for a surgeon to remove the area of lung with the abscess in it.

If an empyema develops, a tube inserted into the pleural space allows the pus fluid to drain out of the chest cavity. Antibiotics given before and after the drainage of empyema fluid assist with clearing the infection.

## OUTLOOK

### What is the outlook for a person with hospital-acquired pneumonia?

Although most people recover from hospital-acquired pneumonia and leave the hospital after several days, serious and life-threatening complications can develop. Bacteria that are resistant to some or all antibiotics can cause serious lung damage as well as other complications. Suppression of the immune system by cancer or its treatments increases the risk of a prolonged hospitalization or a fatal outcome.

Please see the chapters entitled "Sepsis and Septic Shock", "Acute Respiratory Distress Syndrome" and "Acute Disseminated Intravascular Coagulation" for a discussion of three very dangerous potential complications of hospital-acquired pneumonia.

The development of new antibiotics that can overcome the resistance of bacteria to treatment is an area of intense research. Although there has been considerable progress in developing new and potent antibiotics, bacteria are continually evolving and developing defenses against them. Although at this time, the balance of power between people and bacteria is generally in our favor, death from hospital-acquired pneumonia, despite the very best medical treatment, often occurs.

# CANDIDA INFECTIONS

## DEFINITIONS

### What is candida and who gets candida infections?

Candida is a common type of "yeast" that belongs to the larger "fungus" family of organisms. In good health, candida causes "yeast infections" of the vagina, which are itchy, uncomfortable, and easily treated with medications. In people with a weakened immune system, candida can cause infections of the mouth, throat, and esophagus, and can spread throughout the body and put life in great jeopardy. In addition, people who are using inhaled steroid medications such as "fluticasone" for COPD are at a higher risk of developing candida infections of the mouth, throat, and esophagus.

## THRUSH

### What is thrush?

Thrush is a candida infection of the mouth, tongue and throat.

### What are the symptoms of thrush?

The most common symptom of thrush is discomfort and burning in the mouth and throat. When looking at their mouth and throat in the mirror, a person will notice a whitish, cottage cheese-like material on the inside of their mouth.

## How is the diagnosis of thrush made?

The characteristic white cheesy material in the mouth and on the tongue, and the irritation and slight bleeding beneath this white material when gently scraped off, can be sufficient to make the diagnosis. Looking under the microscope at scrapings from the mouth can identify the yeast and confirm the diagnosis.

## What is the treatment of thrush?

"Troches" are medicated lozenges that dissolve slowly in the mouth and deliver medication to the inside of the mouth and throat. Antifungal medicines such as "clotrimazole" (brand name is "Mycelex"), available as "troches", are dissolved in the mouth over 30 minutes at evenly spaced intervals five times a day for two weeks, and will usually cure thrush. Because thrush has a tendency to recur if immunosuppression persists, it may be necessary to suck on an antifungal troche one or more times a day to prevent the thrush from recurring.

If, despite oral antifungal troches, recurrence is a problem, the medicine "fluconazole" (brand name is "Diflucan"), given as a pill swallowed once daily or every other day, can usually prevent recurrent thrush.

# CANDIDA ESOPHAGITIS

### What is candida esophagitis?

Candida esophagitis is an infection of the esophagus by candida.

### What is the major symptom of candida esophagitis?

The major symptom of candida esophagitis is difficulty and pain with swallowing. Pain just beneath the center of the chest is consistent with the location of the esophagus as it travels downward from the back of the throat to the stomach.

### How is candida esophagitis diagnosed?

The presence of thrush and typical symptoms of candida esophagitis in a person receiving intensive chemotherapy is often sufficient to make a diagnosis of candida esophagitis and begin treatment.

To confirm the diagnosis, a gastroenterologist can examine the interior of the esophagitis by "endoscopy". To do this, the gastroenterologist inserts the "endoscope", which is a flexible tube with a light and camera on its end, through the mouth into the esophagus. Through the endoscope, the gastroenterologist can view the characteristic white cheesy-appearing material on the inner lining of the esophagus, and will take a biopsy and cultures from the tissues lining the inside of the esophagus.

### How is candida esophagitis treated?

Candida esophagitis is a serious infection that is more difficult to treat than thrush. Treatment of candida esophagitis requires the use of medicines that deliver antifungal treatment into the bloodstream.

The common treatment of candida esophagitis is the oral antifungal medicine "fluconazole" (brand name is "Diflucan"). If symptoms do not resolve with fluconazole, the oral medicines "voriconazole" (brand name is "Vfend") or posaconazole (brand name is "Noxafil", manufacturer's product website is www.noxafil. com) are effective alternate treatments.

There are times when the candida esophagus is not responding adequately to the oral medications. A new type of highly effective antifungal drugs has become available which can destroy candida by destroying its cell wall. Destruction of the cell wall destroys the fungus because the cell wall, among other things, prevents water from getting into and exploding the cells of the fungus. These medicines, as a group, are the "echinocandins". Echinocandins, given intravenously, include "micafungin" (brand name is "Mycamine, manufacturer's product website is www.mycamine.com), "anidulafungin" (brand name is "Eraxis") and "caspofungin" (brand name is "Cancidas", manufacturer's product website is www.cancidas.com).

## CANDIDEMIA

### What is candidemia?

Candidemia is candida infection in the bloodstream.

### Who gets candidemia?

As with thrush and candida esophagus, candidemia can develop in people with immune systems suppressed by chemotherapy or medication.

Candidemia is a common problem in people who are in intensive care units. People with acute kidney injury, bacterial infections requiring powerful antibiotics, as well as people critically ill with more than one medical problem, are predisposed to developing candidemia. Approximately one in ten major bloodstream infections acquired in the hospital are candida infections.

## What are the symptoms of candidemia?

The symptoms of candidemia are very similar to the symptoms developed during bacterial sepsis (see chapter "Sepsis and Septic Shock"). Fever and chills, a rapid heartbeat, rapid breathing, a sense of lightheadedness, and dizziness or confusion can develop. Candida can involve major organs of the body, and symptoms related to the specific organs involved can be present.

## How is the diagnosis of candidemia made?

Candidemia can be difficult to diagnose since its symptoms are very difficult to separate from those of bacterial infections. Occasionally, a physician performing a careful physical examination will find things, such as a particular abnormality in the back of the eye or distinctive tiny areas of pus ("pustules") on the skin, that are characteristic of candidemia.

Blood cultures or other laboratory tests sometimes show evidence of the candidemia, but can fail to show evidence of candida in the bloodstream even though a person may have a severe case of candidemia. For this reason, an experienced physician may make a "presumptive diagnosis" of candidemia, based upon symptoms of sepsis not responding to antibiotics, or based upon findings of physical examination and an understanding of the person's overall medical condition and the risks it poses to development of candidemia.

## What is the treatment of candidemia?

The treatment of candidemia is similar to the treatment described above for candida esophagitis. When a person appears to be ill with candidemia but not in immediate danger, the medicine "fluconazole", which is generally well tolerated, may be sufficient to treat the infection. If the person with candidemia appears to be very ill or in danger of rapidly developing complications, physicians may begin therapy with one of the somewhat more potent "echinocandins" described above. If candida is present in blood cultures, treatment with antifungal medicine continues until blood cultures fail to show evidence of candida in the bloodstream for at least two weeks. If candidemia developed of "neutropenia" (please see the next chapter entitled "Febrile Neutropenia and Neutropenic Sepsis"), physicians may continue treating with the antifungal medicine until the person's neutrophils have recovered sufficiently to restrain recurrent infection.

# FEBRILE NEUTROPENIA AND NEUTROPENIC SEPSIS

## DEFINITIONS

*What is "febrile neutropenia" and "neutropenic sepsis"?*

Neutrophils are the major defense system our body has to destroy bacteria or fungal organisms that have gained access to the inside of the body. Neutropenia is a reduction of the number of neutrophils in the bloodstream.

Thresholds of "neutrophil count" in the bloodstream have been set, below which a person is at a low, moderate, or high risk of developing serious infections. Specifically, if the neutrophil count is "less than 500 cells per microliter", the person is at a high risk of developing very serious bacterial or fungal infections. If the laboratory determines the neutrophil count is "less than 100 cells per microliter", the person is at a very high risk of developing very serious bacterial or fungal infections.

"Febrile neutropenia" is development of a fever above 100.4 degrees Fahrenheit in a person with neutropenia. "Neutropenic sepsis" means that a microorganism, usually a bacteria or a fungus, is in the bloodstream, causing a life-threatening illness.

## SYMPTOMS

### What are the symptoms of neutropenic fever and neutropenic sepsis?

Symptoms result from the infectious problems caused by the febrile neutropenia, rather than the neutropenia itself. These symptoms may include fevers, chills, difficulty breathing, confusion, and dizziness and often reflect the serious infections discussed in the section of this book discussing infectious complications of cancer. Other symptoms can include local pain, redness, and swelling associated with infection of intravenous or "central venous catheters" used for administering chemotherapy.

People who are severely neutropenic can occasionally develop sepsis without a fever. This is most common in people who are elderly or who are receiving steroid medications such as "prednisone" or "Decadron".

## TREATMENT

### What is the significance of fever in a person with neutropenia?

The most common cause of fever in a person with neutropenia ("febrile neutropenia") is a bacterial infection. Without the protection of neutrophils, the infection can quickly spread throughout the body and become extremely dangerous. For this reason, febrile neutropenia is an emergency requiring prompt treatment with antibiotics.

## How do physicians evaluate a person with febrile neutropenia?

When a person who is neutropenic develops a fever, physicians will perform a thorough physical examination to identify, if possible, any area of the body containing infection, or any catheter, such as an intravenous catheter or a urinary catheter, that is the source of the infection. Several samples of blood will be withdrawn from peripheral veins and from intravenous catheters and sent to the microbiology laboratory for "blood cultures", looking for specific organisms causing infection and evaluating those organisms for their sensitivities to different antibiotics. A chest x-ray or CT scan of the chest will look for evidence of pneumonia. If symptoms suggestive of an infection inside the abdomen are present, a CT scan of the abdomen or pelvis may identify an abscess or another source of infection.

## What is the treatment of febrile neutropenia?

Treatment of febrile neutropenia involves the use of antibiotics that are most likely to destroy any member of the broad spectrum of bacteria that can cause life-threatening infections in a person who is neutropenic. The antibiotic treatment usually continues until there is no more fever and the neutropenia resolves to the point where a person has the ability to fight a bacterial or fungal infection.

Decisions regarding the choice of antibiotics, and whether the person requires hospitalization, will take into account the degree of neutropenia, the expected duration of the neutropenia, evidence of sepsis or septic shock (see chapter entitled "Sepsis and Septic Shock"), and a person's age and other medical conditions.

If it appears that a catheter infection has developed, depending on the bacteria causing the infection, removal of the catheter may be required.

*What is the significance of fever and neutropenia that persists for several days despite the antibiotics?*

When a person remains neutropenic, persistent fever could mean that the antibiotics are not affecting the organism that is infecting the person and causing the fever. After evaluation of new symptoms, findings of physical examination, and x-rays or other tests that may be required, a change of the antibiotic regimen may be required.

With severe neutropenia, "candidemia" and other "opportunistic" fungal infections (see chapters entitled "Candida Infections" and "Opportunistic Infections") may develop. Because of this, physicians consider adding antifungal medications when a severely neutropenic person has a fever that persists despite antibiotics.

# INFECTIVE ENDOCARDITIS

## DEFINITION

### What is infective endocarditis?

The "endocardium" is the inner lining of the heart. "Endocarditis" means that the endocardium is inflamed. "Infective endocarditis" means that the inside surface of the heart is infected.

Most of the time, this infection involves heart valves, and most of the time, the infection is caused by a bacteria. Infection of the inside of the heart caused by bacteria is "bacterial endocarditis".

## THE CAUSE OF INFECTIVE ENDOCARDITIS

### How does blood flow through the heart normally?

The heart consists of four chambers surrounded by muscle and filled with blood. These chambers are the right atrium, right ventricle, left atrium and left ventricle.

In a healthy heart, blood glides smoothly from the right atrium to the right ventricle, from the right ventricle to the lungs, then, after the blood returns to the heart from the lungs, from the left atrium to the left ventricle and from the left ventricle to the entire body. "Valves" protect the forward movement of blood during heart muscle contraction by snapping shut at appropriate split seconds and preventing blood from rushing backward in the wrong direction. These valves are located between the right atrium and right ventricle (the "tricuspid valve"), right ventricle and pulmonary artery ("pulmonary valve"), the left atrium and left ventricle (the "mitral valve") and the left ventricle and aorta (the "aortic valve").

### *What problems with the flow of blood through the heart put a person at risk of developing infective endocarditis?*

Heart problems that cause local areas of turbulence in the normal movement of blood through the heart predispose a person to infective endocarditis.

The most common cause of infective endocarditis is heart valves that have sustained previous damage. The valves in the heart normally flip open, allowing blood to flow forward and then snap shut, preventing blood from flowing backward (this is called "regurgitation"). A scarred narrowed valve opening is "stenosis". Regurgitation or stenosis will create a turbulence of blood flow on and around the abnormal valves. Infectious organisms can plant themselves and grow in these areas of turbulence.

In the past, when antibiotics were not yet available, rheumatic fever was the most common cause of scarring of the heart valves and of infective endocarditis. Today, other heart valve diseases such as "mitral valve prolapse", "calcification" of the aortic valve in the elderly and artificial ("prosthetic") valves are the more common risks for developing infective endocarditis.

Many other structural abnormalities of the heart can cause local areas of turbulence inside the heart and predispose a person to infective endocarditis. Many different forms of congenital heart disease pose a life-long risk of development of infective endocarditis. "Hypertrophic cardiomyopathy", a generally inherited disease in which thickened heart muscle can cause, among other problems, obstructed flow from the left ventricle into the aorta, can cause turbulence inside the heart and predispose someone to infective endocarditis.

**Are there conditions other than structural abnormalities that predispose a person to infective endocarditis?**

The sophisticated measures available to sustain the life of seriously ill people involve the use of catheters and pacemaker wires along which bacteria can travel and infect the heart. People with kidney failure who are receiving dialysis are at risk of having bacteria inadvertently introduced into the body through the catheters used to perform dialysis.

## THE ORGANISMS THAT MOST COMMONLY CAUSE ENDOCARDITIS

**What organisms cause infectious endocarditis?**

Most of the bacteria that cause infectious endocarditis are in the "streptococcus", "enterococcus", or "staphylococcus" families. Bacteria in the "gram negative" family can also infect the heart, and most commonly cause infective endocarditis in the elderly and in people with a seriously weakened immune system.

Uncommonly, the organism causing the infection is a fungus. The most common fungus organisms that cause infective endocarditis are "Candida" and "Aspergillus".

## *Where do these organisms come from?*

Staphylococcus infections (most commonly, the bacteria called "staph aureus"), can come from infection by staphylococcus organisms in the environment of a hospital. These hospital-acquired infections are "nosocomial infections". The most common source of nosocomial infections by staphylococcus is from infected intravenous catheters.

The bacteria causing infective endocarditis may also come from within the person's own body. Streptococcus is a normal inhabitant of the mouth and throat. Enterococcus is a normal inhabitant of the mouth and the gastrointestinal tract.

When a person has "fungal endocarditis", the organism usually comes from a catheter, such as an intravenous feeding catheter or a catheter used to provide access to the circulation through the vein ("venous access catheter") for giving chemotherapy. These catheters, which remain in a vein for weeks or months, can provide an entry point for dangerous bacteria or fungus organisms.

## SYMPTOMS

### *What are the symptoms of infective endocarditis?*

Most people with infective endocarditis will have a fever in the 101-104 degrees Fahrenheit range. A generalized ache in the joints along with a general sense of weakness and feeling ill are common. These symptoms, in conjunction with the knowledge of a person's predisposition to infective endocarditis, raise the suspicion of the presence of infective endocarditis.

## MAKING THE DIAGNOSIS

*How is the diagnosis of infective endocarditis made?*

In evaluating a person with infective endocarditis, it is critical to determine if bacteria are growing in the bloodstream. To do this, and to make sure the results are correct and not caused by skin bacteria that have contaminated the blood samples, three separate samples of blood will be obtained from three separate veins. Given the importance of making a prompt diagnosis, and because some unusual organisms can cause infective endocarditis, the laboratory will be notified of the suspected diagnosis. If all cultures grow the same bacteria, it is major evidence that a person has infective endocarditis.

When bacteria infect the heart valves, they form fragile lumps on the valves called "vegetations", which resemble, to some extent, natural vegetation. An echocardiogram, which generates images of the interior of the heart using harmless sound waves, can often spot the vegetations on heart valves and confirm the diagnosis of infective endocarditis.

When it is available, a "transesophageal echocardiogram" is a more sensitive and accurate test.

## *What is a transesophageal echocardiogram?*

A transesophageal echocardiogram is a test in which, through the mouth, a device that gives off sound waves is advanced through the mouth into the esophagus (the tube between the mouth and the stomach). Since the esophagus is located inside the chest next to the heart, these sound waves will bounce off the heart and back to the device, which transmits an image onto a screen. This is a highly specialized test and not every hospital has this device or the experts available who can accurately interpret the images shown by this test. If transesophageal echocardiogram is not available, the standard echocardiogram, called a "transthoracic echocardiogram" is another very effective test.

## COMPLICATIONS OF INFECTIVE ENDOCARDITIS

## *Why is infective endocarditis dangerous?*

Infection of heart valves can seriously impair their normal ability to prevent the backflow of blood from the aorta back into the left ventricle if there is aortic valve damage, or from the left ventricle into the left atrium if there is mitral valve damage. The infections can spread deep into the muscle of the heart. These problems can cause severe damage to the heart's ability to pump and cause sudden, severe heart failure (see chapter entitled "Heart Failure"). If the infection of the heart involves the nerve fibers controlling the rhythmic beating of the heart, dangerous irregular heart rhythms can result.

When bacteria infect the heart valves, they form the fragile lumps on the valves called "vegetations" that were discussed earlier in this chapter. The vegetations will often break free of the valve, float through the bloodstream, and lodge in an artery feeding the brain, liver, spleen, lung, kidney, or elsewhere. This blockage of arterial blood supply can cause major damage to the organ deprived of its blood supply.

The vegetations that break free from the heart are highly infectious and can carry bacteria throughout the body. Abscesses of the brain, lung, kidney, and other organs can develop.

The complications caused by infective endocarditis made it virtually 100% fatal in the era before the discovery of antibiotics. Now, prompt diagnosis and antibiotic treatment prevents complications and cures infective endocarditis.

## TREATMENT

### What is the treatment of infective endocarditis?

The treatment of infective endocarditis is with intravenous antibiotics. Because of the importance of choosing the correct antibiotic regimen, if a person appears medically stable, physicians may sometimes choose to delay initiation of antibiotics until the laboratory confirms the organism causing the infection and the antibiotics that are most likely to be effective. If, however, the person is medically unstable, physicians will initiate antibiotic therapy with a combination of antibiotics that are most likely to treat infective endocarditis. The choice of antibiotics prescribed will consider the underlying medical condition, whether the person is in an intensive care unit, and the types of intravenous catheters or other medical devices that a person may be attached to.

Because of the complexities involved with choosing the correct antibiotic regimen, a specialist in the field of "infectious diseases" often directs therapy. In general, the treatment will be to administer intravenous antibiotics in the hospital or, if appropriate, at home by specially trained medical professionals. Most commonly, the antibiotic regimens involve a combination of two or more medications given over a six-week period.

## How can the physician tell if the person is responding to antibiotics?

If a person's body temperature normalizes and many of their symptoms are relieved, it generally means that the antibiotic is having its desired effect. In some circumstances, such as when the bacteria nicknamed "staph aureus" causes a person's infective endocarditis, physicians may want to draw another set of blood cultures after several days to be sure the bacteria are not still growing in the bloodstream. There should not be any evidence of bacteria in the blood cultures within a few days after antibiotic treatment begins. If the blood cultures do not stop growing bacteria, a new antibiotic regimen may be necessary.

## What happens if the blood cultures continue to grow bacteria despite intensive antibiotic treatment?

When blood cultures show that the person is failing to respond to antibiotic treatment, it may mean that there is massive infection of the heart valves or that an abscess has formed in heart muscle. The effective treatment for these problems will be the surgical replacement of the infected valves or surgical drainage of the heart muscle abscess.

## *Does persistent or recurrent fever mean the infective endocarditis is not getting better?*

Fever may persist for several days after the antibiotic treatment begins. At some point, however, persistent fever will lead to evaluation to be sure that the vegetation in the heart is not growing, or that an abscess has not developed in the heart or in some other part of the body to which a piece of the infected vegetation may have traveled.

## *What evaluation might physicians prescribe if it appears that the infective endocarditis is not resolving with antibiotics?*

A transesophageal echocardiogram can be useful in assessing the heart valves and heart muscle for evidence that the infection is not properly responding. Because vegetations that break off from the infected heart valves can travel to abdominal organs or to the bones additional testing may be required. A CT of the abdomen will look for abscesses, a bone scan will look for infected bones and a urinalysis looks for evidence of kidney infection. Repeated blood cultures will reassess the organisms, if any, in the bloodstream and re-evaluate their likely responsiveness to the different available antibiotics.

## FUNGAL ENDOCARDITIS

### *What is the treatment of fungal endocarditis?*

Although there are antifungal medicines that can be given, fungal endocarditis tends be resistant to this treatment. In addition to the damage fungal endocarditis can rapidly cause to heart valves, fungal vegetations from the heart valves tend to break loose and float into distant organs and cause major problems.

Successful treatment of fungal endocarditis generally requires a combination of surgery and antifungal medicines. A treatment regimen used may involve administration of a powerful antifungal medication such as "Amphotericin", followed by surgery to remove areas of fungal infection called "vegetations" from the heart valves, or replacement of the involved heart valves entirely. Six weeks or more of treatment with Amphotericin follows the surgery. After treatment with Amphotericin, further treatment with an oral antifungal medicine such as "Ketoconazole" is often necessary.

Treatment of fungal endocarditis can be very complicated and great skill and attention from the medical team including a cardiologist, cardiac surgeon, infectious disease expert, the family physician or general internist, as well as a wide range of medical professionals, is important for achieving a good outcome.

## WHEN INFECTIVE ENDOCARDITIS HAS DAMAGED HEART VALVES

*What happens if the infective endocarditis has caused significant damage to heart valves?*

Heart valves damaged by infective endocarditis can cause relatively sudden and life threatening heart failure. Depending on the details of a person's individual situation, severe damage to the mitral or aortic valve, especially in the presence of heart failure, requires prompt surgical repair. This involves open-heart surgery, often with replacement of the person's infected valve with an artificial one.

*Are there other reasons for urgent surgery when a person has infective endocarditis?*

If a person 's blood cultures fail to clear, and there is continued evidence of an inadequately functioning heart valve despite a week or more of antibiotics, and it appears that the infection is coming from the heart, surgery to identify and remove vegetations or infected areas inside the heart will commonly be prescribed. In addition, surgery is important if, despite antibiotics, a person continues to show evidence of vegetations breaking off the heart and traveling to distant organs. Infected artificial ("prosthetic") heart valves may need replacement.

## OUTLOOK

*What is the outlook for a person with infective endocarditis?*

The outlook depends upon the person's pre-existing health, the promptness with which the diagnosis was made and treatment begun, and on the type of bacteria infecting the heart.

With prompt diagnosis and treatment of infective endocarditis, a person can make a very good recovery. The person will always, however, remain susceptible to new episodes of infective endocarditis and will have to take antibiotics as a precaution before dental work, or before any medical procedures which involve manipulation of their gastrointestinal or urinary tract.

# INFLUENZA

## DEFINITION

### *What is influenza?*

Influenza is a viral infectious disease, more commonly known as "the flu", which is transmitted from person to person because of coughs and sneezes that send infected droplets of fluid into the air. Although most people who develop influenza will have a relatively brief, but uncomfortable illness, people who are elderly or have a chronic illness are at risk of developing serious and life-threatening complications.

## SYMPTOMS

### *What are the symptoms of influenza?*

The major symptoms of influenza are fever, chills, headache, a sore throat, severe fatigue, and a general aching feeling that is most prominent in the legs and back.

## MAKING THE DIAGNOSIS

### *How is the diagnosis of influenza made?*

Influenza commonly occurs in the winter months as an outbreak affecting many people in the community. In this context, and with the typical symptoms of influenza, the diagnosis is often obvious and additional testing to make the diagnosis is not necessary. If testing is necessary, laboratory tests are available that can identify the virus from the sputum (which is the material a person may be coughing up out of their lungs), or from a swab of the throat.

## COMPLICATIONS OF INFLUENZA

### What is the usual course of influenza?

Most of the time, the symptoms of influenza, such as fever and chills, resolve over a few days and are largely gone at the end of the week. This course of the illness is "uncomplicated influenza".

People who are elderly or who have a serious chronic illness may not recover quickly from influenza. Symptoms may persist and worsen and can be associated with serious and life-threatening complications. The remainder of this chapter will discuss the diagnosis and treatment of these complications.

### What is the most common life-threatening complication of influenza?

The most common complication of influenza is pneumonia, either caused by the influenza virus, by a bacterial infection on top of the influenza infection, or by a combination of viral and bacterial pneumonia. This pneumonia can worsen to the point of serious danger to life, and admission to an intensive care unit may be necessary.

*How can physicians determine if someone
with influenza has developed pneumonia?*

If pneumonia develops, the person often will have a persistent fever, which is associated with difficulty breathing or a feeling of being out of breath. The chest x-ray may show distinctive shadows called "infiltrates" which are consistent with the presence of pneumonia. If the pneumonia is severe, and the level of oxygen in the bloodstream drops to dangerous levels, the skin can take on a slightly bluish tinge called "cyanosis".

*How can physicians determine whether the pneumonia is
caused by the influenza virus, or by a bacterial
infection on top of the influenza infection?*

In general, although not always, pneumonia that is caused by the influenza virus itself worsens without interruption, and is associated with the production, upon coughing, of very little sputum. When a person develops bacterial infection on top of the influenza, there often has been a period when the symptoms of influenza seemed to have been lessening, followed a couple of days later by recurrent fever, difficulty breathing, and production of quite a bit of greenish or yellow sputum.

## TREATMENT OF VIRAL PNEUMONIA
## ASSOCIATED WITH INFLUENZA

*What is the treatment for viral pneumonia
associated with influenza?*

Medicine that can suppress the growth of the virus can shorten the illness and accelerate recovery when a person has pneumonia that is associated with infection with influenza. The antiviral medicines that are used are "zanamivir", which is an inhaled powder that is marketed under the brand name is "Relenza" (manufacturer's product website is www.relenza.com), and "oseltamivir", which is a liquid or capsule that is marketed under the brand name is "Tamiflu" (manufacturer's product website is www.tamiflu.com). The United States agency called the "Centers for Disease Control" (abbreviated as "CDC" and with the website www.cdc.gov) closely monitors every influenza season and will issue recommendations regarding the antiviral medications most likely to be effective.

## TREATMENT OF BACTERIAL PNEUMONIA ASSOCIATED WITH INFLUENZA

*What is the treatment for bacterial infection that develops on top of the influenza?*

The treatment of bacterial pneumonia that develops on top of influenza is with antibiotics. The choice of antibiotics is often made after examining a sample of the sputum under the microscope using a special stain called the "gram stain" that may allow identification of the likely bacteria causing the infection. The choice of the antibiotic administered is based upon examination of the sputum gram stain, and based upon the knowledge of the bacteria in the local community that are most likely to infect a person with influenza.

Antibiotics used to treat the bacterial pneumonia that develops in a person with influenza commonly include a powerful antibiotic, given intravenously, in the category of a "respiratory fluoroquinolone", such as "moxifloxacin" (brand name is "Avelox", manufacturer's product website is www.avelox.com) or "levofloxacin" (brand name is "Levaquin", manufacturer's product website is www.levaquin.com). Dangerous bacteria called "staph aureus" can cause bacterial pneumonia in a person with influenza, and for this reason, antibiotics that can specifically kill these bacteria, such as "oxacillin", "nafcillin", or "vancomycin", often are included in the antibiotic regimen. Additional information about the treatment of life-threatening bacterial pneumonia in people in the hospital is in the chapter entitled "Hospital-Acquired Pneumonia".

# OPPORTUNISTIC INFECTIONS

## DEFINITIONS

### What is an opportunistic infection?

An opportunistic infection is an infection that develops in a person with a severely suppressed immune system. Opportunistic infections occur in people who have a suppressed immune system because of cancer chemotherapy, medicines that suppress the immune system after an organ or bone marrow transplant or because of suppression of the immune system by the cancer itself or another underlying disease. People who have a suppressed immune system are "immunosuppressed" and medicines that suppress the immune system are "immunosuppressive medications".

### Which opportunistic infections commonly occur in people whose immune system has been impaired by chemotherapy or immunosuppressive medications?

Serious opportunistic infections in people who have received strong immunosuppressive medications include "candida" (discussed in the chapter entitled "Candida Infections"), "shingles", "pneumocystis pneumonia", "cytomegalovirus", and "cryptococcal meningitis",

# SHINGLES: HERPES ZOSTER

## What is shingles?

Before the chickenpox vaccine was available, most children had the unpleasant but transient illness "chickenpox". Although the chickenpox resolves, the virus that causes it, the "varicella zoster virus", can survive for decades, without causing any symptoms, in a portion of nerves called the "dorsal root ganglion". If there is suppression of a person's immune system, the virus can become active, travel back down the nerve to the skin, and produce the painful problem called "shingles".

## What are the symptoms of shingles in people with severely depressed immune systems?

Shingles, in the context of a severely suppressed immune system, causes a very painful blistering rash in the area of skin receiving nerve fibers from the nerve infected by the virus. Fever commonly accompanies the rash, and breathing difficulties related to infection of the lung with the varicella zoster virus can develop.

## How is the diagnosis of shingles made?

The diagnosis of shingles only requires visual examination of the skin lesions.

## What is the treatment of shingles?

Antiviral medicines called "valganciclovir" (brand name is "Valtrex", manufacturer's product website is www.valtrex.com), famciclovir (brand name is "Famvir", manufacturer's product website is www.famvir.com) and "acyclovir" (brand name is "Zovirax", manufacturer's product website is www.zovirax.com) are quite effective in suppressing varicella zoster virus and making symptoms of the viral infection disappear more quickly.

Because the pain associated with shingles can be quite severe, narcotic medications may be required.

## PNEUMOCYSTIS PNEUMONIA

### What is pneumocystis pneumonia?

Pneumocystis pneumonia is a pneumonia caused by an organism called "pneumocystis jirovecii". Pneumocystis jirovecii is a common inhabitant of the lungs of a healthy person. Pneumocystis jirovecii can produce a serious and life-threatening form of pneumonia in people with a seriously weakened immune system.

Pneumocystis pneumonia became an important problem in the 1980s when it was a very common first major sign that a person had AIDS. Since then, it has become apparent that pneumocystis pneumonia can develop in people who have a severely suppressed immune system because of treatments used to treat cancer or blood malignancies. Medications used to prevent rejection of transplanted organs or bone marrow can also make a person susceptible to pneumocystis pneumonia.

The discussion that follows only relates to people who are not HIV-infected who develop pneumocystis pneumonia.

## What are the symptoms of pneumocystis pneumonia?

As with most forms of pneumonia, the major symptoms of pneumocystis pneumonia are fever, discomfort in the chest, and a feeling of being short of breath. Coughing is common and usually does not bring up a significant amount of sputum. These symptoms can develop very rapidly, causing severe difficulty with breathing and requiring intensive care unit support shortly after the onset of symptoms.

## How is the diagnosis of pneumocystis pneumonia made?

The rapid onset of symptoms of fever and shortness of breath in a person with suppressed immune system along with a characteristic appearance of the chest x-rays will raise the suspicion of pneumocystis pneumonia. Other infections can cause identical symptoms and require completely different treatment than would be necessary for pneumocystis pneumonia. For this reason, physicians will do their best to confirm the diagnosis of pneumocystis pneumonia before treatment begins.

The pneumocystis jirovecii fungus is quite abundant in the lungs of people with pneumocystis pneumonia. The key to making the diagnosis of pneumocystis pneumonia is to try to get some fluid out of the bronchial tubes for examination in the microbiology laboratory. This fluid can be obtained by having the person breathe in a fine mist of salt water, and then by having the person do their best to cough up some sputum. Most of the time, this will produce clear evidence of pneumocystis pneumonia.

If a sputum sample fails to make the diagnosis of pneumocystis pneumonia, it may be necessary to put a "bronchoscope" into the lungs, spray the bronchial tubes with salt water, and withdraw the fluid for analysis. This medical procedure, called "bronchoalveolar lavage", can establish the diagnosis of pneumocystis pneumonia.

### What is the treatment of pneumocystis pneumonia?

Several medicines are quite effective as treatment of pneumocystis pneumonia. "Trimethoprim/sulfamethoxasole" (which is sold under the brand names "Bactrim" or "Septra") is the most commonly used treatment. If a person has very severe pneumocystis pneumonia and is allergic to trimethoprim/sulfamethoxasole or for other reasons cannot take it, the somewhat more toxic but equally effective alternative is "pentamidine". Other medication used for people allergic to trimethoprim/sulfamethoxasole but less severely ill include "atovaquone" (brand name is "Mepron"), or the generic medications "clindamycin" combined with "primaquine".

People with pneumocystis pneumonia are extremely ill and the outlook for recovery is uncertain. When the antibiotic treatment is successful, there is an improvement in lung function within several days after beginning treatment. Treatment with the antibiotics continues for approximately three weeks.

### Is there a way to prevent recurrent pneumocystis pneumonia in a person with a weakened immune system?

Medicines given to prevent pneumocystis pneumonia are "PCP prophylaxis". "Trimethoprim/sulfamethoxasole" (also known as "Septra" or "Bactrim"), taken by mouth every day, reduces the risk of developing pneumocystis pneumonia. If a person cannot tolerate trimethoprim/sulfamethoxasole, "atovaquone" (brand name is "Mepron"), is an effective alternative.

## CYTOMEGALOVIRUS INFECTION

### What is cytomegalovirus?

Cytomegalovirus is a virus that can cause life-threatening illness in people with a severely weakened immune system. In the absence of HIV infection, serious cytomegalovirus infection is most common in people who have had heart, lung, kidney, liver, or bone marrow transplants. Severe and life-threatening cytomegalovirus infections in people who are not HIV-infected primarily involves the lung (causing "cytomegalovirus pneumonia"), and the gastrointestinal system (causing "cytomegalovirus gastroenteritis").

### What are the symptoms of cytomegalovirus pneumonia?

The symptoms of cytomegalovirus pneumonia are fever, cough and shortness of breath that can progress very rapidly.

### How is the diagnosis of cytomegalovirus pneumonia made?

A wide variety of organisms can cause pneumonia in people with severely weakened immune systems. The evaluation of pneumonia in a person with immune system suppression will include a chest x-ray, and sputum stains and cultures. If these tests fail to identify the organism that is causing the pneumonia, it may be necessary to perform a bronchoscopy (see description of bronchoscopy in the chapter entitled "Lung Cancer") during which fluid or tissue from inside the lung is obtained with "bronchoalveolar lavage" and a "transbronchial biopsy". Using this material taken during bronchoscopy, the laboratory can sometimes make the diagnosis of cytomegalovirus pneumonia.

## What are the symptoms of cytomegalovirus gastroenteritis?

The symptoms of cytomegalovirus gastroenteritis depend upon the area or areas of the gastrointestinal system infected and damaged by cytomegalovirus. Cytomegalovirus esophagitis causes painful swallowing and pain beneath the breastbone or in the upper abdomen. Cytomegalovirus colitis causes diarrhea, fever, abdominal pain, and bloody stool.

## How is the diagnosis of cytomegalovirus gastroenteritis made?

The diagnosis of cytomegalovirus gastroenteritis is made by having a physician visually inspect the esophagus and stomach with an "endoscope", or visually inspect the colon and rectum with "sigmoidoscopy" or a "colonoscopy". Biopsies from inflamed areas can establish the diagnosis of cytomegalovirus infection.

## What is the treatment of cytomegalovirus infections?

The most commonly used antiviral medicine is "ganciclovir" (brand name is "Cytovene"). Other antiviral medications that can suppress the cytomegalovirus include "foscarnet" (brand name is "Foscavir) and "valganciclovir" (brand name is "Valcyte", manufacturer's product website is www.valcyte.com).

*How effective are antiviral treatments of cytomegalovirus?*

Ganciclovir can suppress cytomegalovirus and put cytomegalovirus infections of the bowel or lung into remission. Because cytomegalovirus commonly recurs in people with severely suppressed immune systems, initial, intensive treatment with ganciclovir followed by long-term lower dose treatment with oral ganciclovir or oral valganciclovir will usually be required.

## CRYPTOCOCCAL MENINGITIS

*What is cryptococcal meningitis?*

Cryptococcal meningitis is an infection of the surface of the brain and of the brain itself with a fungus called "cryptococcus". Cryptococcal meningitis can develop in people with a suppressed immune system because of chemotherapy, steroids, and medicines to suppress the immune system after an organ or bone marrow transplant.

*What are the symptoms of cryptococcal meningitis?*

The most common symptoms of cryptococcal meningitis are fever, headache, and confusion. A change of behavior is occasionally the first symptom of cryptococcal meningitis.

*How is the diagnosis of cryptococcal meningitis made?*

The diagnosis of cryptococcal meningitis requires examination of spinal fluid obtained by a "spinal tap" (see description of spinal tap in the chapter entitled "Bacterial Meningitis"). About half of the time, the actual cryptococcus organism is evident under the microscope. It may also be possible to find a fragment of the cryptococcus called "cryptococcal antigen" in the spinal fluid.

The diagnosis of cryptococcal meningitis is confirmed when the laboratory reports that cultures of the person's spinal fluid are growing cryptococcus.

## What is the treatment of cryptococcal meningitis?

Several anti-fungal medicines are quite effective in treating cryptococcal meningitis.

Treatment begins with a combination of two powerful antifungal medications. "Lipid-based" formulations of amphotericin with the brand names "Abelcet", manufacturer's product website is www.abelcet.com), "Amphotec" (manufacturer's product website is www.amphotec.com), and "AmBisome" (manufacturer's product website is www.ambisome.com), are given along with the medication "flucytosine" until the spinal fluid no longer shows evidence of the presence of cryptococcus. After clearing of the spinal fluid, in order to prevent recurrent infections, antifungal treatment with the medication "fluconazole" (brand name is "Diflucan") continues for approximately a year.

# SEPSIS AND SEPTIC SHOCK

## DEFINITIONS

### *What is sepsis?*

Sepsis is a severe and life-threatening illness caused by an infection.

### *What is the "systemic inflammatory response syndrome"?*

When confronted by serious infection, our body's natural defense will trigger an "inflammatory response" which seeks to rid the body of the microscopic invader. This inflammatory response can become excessive and extremely dangerous, triggering a life threatening "systemic inflammatory response syndrome". When systemic inflammatory response syndrome develops, inflammation involves the entire body, possibly causing a serious drop of blood pressure and damage to the lungs, kidneys and other major organs.

### *What are the key signs that a person with an infection is developing systemic inflammatory response syndrome?*

The key signs that a person has systemic inflammatory response syndrome are a very high or very low body temperature, rapid breathing, and an elevated number of white blood cells in the blood stream, including the mature and immature versions of infection-fighting white blood cells called "neutrophils".

When a person has an infection such as pneumonia, the degree of the person's signs of systemic inflammatory response syndrome determines the danger posed by the illness. If a person with an infection has the signs of systemic inflammatory response syndrome described above, but the blood pressure is not abnormally low and there is no evidence of lung, kidney, or other organ damage, the person has "sepsis". If there is evidence of damage or injury to organs at a distance from the infection, and the blood pressure, although low, increases when giving intravenous fluids, the person has "severe sepsis". If blood pressure is low and difficult to elevate with intravenous fluid, the person has "septic shock".

## *THE CAUSE OF SEPSIS*

### *Who gets sepsis?*

Many people who develop sepsis are already suffering from a serious illness. A weakened immune system is common in people with cancer, diabetes, in alcoholics, and in the elderly. The more severely weakened the immune system, the greater the likelihood that bacteria normally cleared by a healthy immune system will cause sepsis.

Bacteria find catheters very comfortable places to live and grow. Intravenous catheters can provide bacteria with a home to live on and a base from which to quickly seed the bloodstream and cause sepsis. Bacteria can grow on catheters that drain urine from the bladder (Foley catheters), and, particularly in the elderly, can cause sepsis.

Not everyone with sepsis has a seriously weakened immune system. Sepsis can follow an injury or an operation if the area affected by the injury or operation is infected. Any infected area of the body, whether involving the skin, the lung, the kidney, or elsewhere, can release bacteria into the circulation and produce sepsis.

## SYMPTOMS

### What are the symptoms of sepsis?

The most common symptoms of sepsis are fever, a feeling of severe chilliness, a rapid heartbeat, rapid breathing, a sense of lightheadedness, and dizziness or confusion associated with low blood pressure. These symptoms may be absent or very subtle in the early stages of sepsis. When a person has a severe underlying disease such as leukemia or kidney failure, or is very elderly or alcoholic, there may be fewer symptoms despite having sepsis.

An early symptom that can raise the suspicion of sepsis is a rather abrupt change in a person's ability to think clearly. The person may develop a personality change or may have a lack of a clear idea of exactly where they are or to whom they are talking. This change in ability to think clearly is particularly worrisome in a person who is in the hospital for a serious illness or when a person has an intravenous or urinary catheter in place.

## MAKING THE DIAGNOSIS

### How is the diagnosis of sepsis made?

The finding of bacteria in laboratory cultures of the person's blood can make a diagnosis of sepsis. The problem with this method of making the definitive diagnosis is that it may take two or three days for bacteria to grow and be identified as the cause of the illness. In addition, the blood cultures do not always grow the bugs, whether they are bacteria, fungus or other organisms, that are causing the infection. Because of this, physicians must rely very heavily on the person's symptoms, physical examination, and on identification of an area of the body or of a catheter, tube or other foreign object that they suspect harbors an infection.

Based upon the physician's experience, and the experience of other medical professionals such as intensive care unit nurses, in caring for sick people and on the person's symptoms and physical examination, a diagnosis of probable sepsis is made and treatment started promptly. The sooner treatment begins, the more likely it is that a person will avoid serious complications of sepsis and survive the illness.

## **TREATMENT OF SEPSIS**

### *What is the treatment of sepsis?*

Upon making the diagnosis of sepsis, the major goal is to destroy the organism, which is usually a type of bacteria, which is causing the infection. Since blood culture results are generally not yet available at the time of diagnosis of sepsis, the physician will have to make a judgment about the likely source of the infection and the antibiotics most likely to destroy the bacteria.

Based upon whether bacteria take up or reject a staining material called "gram's stain", bacteria are classified as "gram positive" or "gram negative". These bacteria have different sensitivities to antibiotics. Because there generally is uncertainty as to whether the bacteria causing the sepsis is gram positive or gram negative, antibiotics which can destroy both types of bacteria are usually given at the maximum doses that can be administered safely. Nevertheless, in the minutes just prior to beginning antibiotics, it is important for the medical professionals to draw blood samples for testing in the laboratory to see if bacteria or other organisms grow, and if they do grow, to test their sensitivity to the different available antibiotics. Changes in the antibiotic treatment may be necessary, based upon results available a day or more after these blood samples are drawn.

Catheters or a urinary catheter or any other foreign object or medical device on which bacteria may be growing may need removal or replacement. If the person has an abscess, drainage of the abscess may remove a large source of bacteria and help the antibiotics to work more effectively.

## SEVERE SEPSIS AND SEPTIC SHOCK

*What is the difference between severe sepsis and septic shock?*

When sepsis is severe, blood pressure can drop significantly and serious damage can occur to body organs such as the kidney, liver, and lung. If there is evidence of damage or injury to organs at a distance from the infection, and the blood pressure, though low, increases with intravenous fluids, the person has "severe sepsis". If the blood pressure is low and is difficult to make higher with intravenous fluid, the person has "septic shock".

# TREATMENT OF SEVERE SEPSIS AND SEPTIC SHOCK

*What immediate steps will physicians take when
a person has developed severe sepsis or septic shock?*

"ABC" is the abbreviation for airway, breathing, and circulation. In every medical crisis, and severe sepsis or septic shock is definitely a medical crisis, proper movement of air in and out of the lungs and proper blood circulation must be maintained.

The "A" is the airway and the "B" is for breathing. In the context of sepsis or septic shock, the airway is clear and the person is breathing rapidly, but an insufficient amount of oxygen may be getting into the bloodstream because of excessive fluid or infection in the lungs. Supplemental oxygen, along with medications to treat the excessive fluid or infection in or around the lungs, can improve delivery of oxygen to the bloodstream. "Acute respiratory distress syndrome", which is discussed in its own chapter, is a dangerous complication of severe sepsis and septic shock and may require mechanical ventilation, as described in the "Adult Respiratory Distress Syndrome" chapter.

The "C" stands for circulation that must be maintained for life to continue. If the blood pressure is far too low, fluids can be administered which can help to bring the blood pressure up to a much safer level. If intravenous fluid alone does not do an adequate job, it may be necessary to administer intravenous medications (nicknamed "pressors") which can constrict blood vessels and help bring blood pressure up. The pressors that are commonly used include "norepinephrine", "dopamine" and "vasopressin".

### What happens if the fluid and the pressors fail to bring the blood pressure up?

If the blood pressure remains low despite fluid and pressors, a type of medicine called "inotropic therapy" can help the heart to beat more forcefully. The most commonly used inotropic therapy in a person with septic shock is an intravenous infusion of the medicine "dobutamine".

### What is the "APACHE II" score and how does it influence treatment of severe sepsis and septic shock?

"APACHE II" is an abbreviation for "Acute Physiology and Chronic Health Evaluation II". This score assesses the severity of disease of critically ill people, and especially those who are in an intensive care unit. The score derives from evaluating approximately a dozen different factors, such as body temperature, heart rate, blood pressure, kidney function, and age, and assigning points to each factor that add or subtract from the score. The higher the point value, the higher the risk to life. Determination of the APACHE II score provides a framework for understanding the severity of a person's clinical condition.

### Are steroids useful in the treatment of septic shock?

Several very large clinical trials have evaluated the effectiveness of high doses of steroids given intravenously in the situation of septic shock where pressors are necessary to maintain an adequate blood pressure. Some of these trials have indicated benefit, while others have indicated little or no benefit. Some physicians advocate the use of steroids for their possible, although marginal benefit.

# OUTLOOK FOR A PERSON WITH SEVERE SEPSIS OR SEPTIC SHOCK

*What is the outlook for a person with severe sepsis or septic shock?*

In general, a person with severe sepsis has an approximately three in four chance of surviving the episode, whereas a person with septic shock has an approximately 50-50 chance of survival. The outlook, however, largely depends upon the medical problem that caused the sepsis, the person's age and underlying health, and on the speed of identification and treatment of severe sepsis or septic shock.

# INTERNAL BLEEDING

# BRAIN HEMORRHAGE

## DEFINITION

*What is a brain hemorrhage?*

Brain hemorrhage is sudden bleeding into the brain.

## BRAIN HEMORRHAGE IN PEOPLE WITH CANCER

*What are the most common causes of
brain hemorrhage in people with cancer?*

Brain hemorrhage, in people with cancer, usually is a result of bleeding into an area of the brain containing cancer, which is, bleeding into a "brain metastasis".

A second and somewhat less common cause is a "coagulopathy", which means an abnormality in the blood's ability to clot. Among the coagulopathies a person with cancer can have that might predispose to a brain hemorrhage are "acute disseminated intravascular coagulation" (see chapter discussing this), a low number of platelets in the bloodstream ("thrombocytopenia") because of cancer in the bone marrow or chemotherapy, and anticoagulant medications, such as heparin, used to treat blood-clotting disorders.

## SYMPTOMS

### What happens when a person with cancer has a brain hemorrhage?

The major symptom of a brain hemorrhage is a sudden, excruciating headache followed shortly by vomiting. Very commonly, a person who has had a brain hemorrhage will develop weakness or paralysis on the left or right side of the body. Other common symptoms are severe dizziness and difficulty speaking.

If the hemorrhage is large or is located in a critical area of the brain, a person may become confused, then drowsy, and then fall into a deep coma. Following a brain hemorrhage, coma may develop extremely rapidly, or over several hours.

## MAKING THE DIAGNOSIS

### How is the diagnosis of brain hemorrhage made?

Based upon the history of the sequence of events and a quick, neurologic examination it will be clear that a sudden and serious brain disorder has developed and a CT scan of the brain is urgently necessary. The CT scan of the brain makes the definitive diagnosis of a brain hemorrhage.

## THE DAMAGE THE BLEEDING CAN CAUSE

### What makes a brain hemorrhage dangerous?

The mass of blood that quickly flows out of small, torn blood vessels pushes its way through the brain and damages brain tissue in its direct path. As the mass of blood inside the brain grows, areas of the brain compress against sharp ridges inside the skull. This pressure against the inside surface of the skull can lead to severe brain damage.

In addition to the damage caused by increased pressure in the brain, the blood itself releases toxic proteins that cause the brain to swell. This swelling, called "cerebral edema", aggravates the damage caused by the tearing and compression of the brain from the brain hemorrhage.

## TREATMENT

*What is the treatment of a brain hemorrhage in a person with cancer?*

A first priority whenever someone has a sudden life-threatening illness is to make sure the airway is secure, that is, that there is no risk to breathing. After a cerebral hemorrhage, there commonly is a decrease in the level of consciousness, and a person may fall into a coma. Even if the person is still able to breathe, the reflexes that normally prevent "aspiration", that is, inhaling secretions or regurgitated stomach contents, are inhibited. For this reason, if a person is unconscious, the emergency or critical care doctors first evaluating the person may insert a tube ("an endotracheal tube") into the windpipe (the "trachea"). If the person has lapsed into a deep coma, it will be necessary to maintain breathing with a mechanical ventilator.

A critical early decision made is whether to perform an emergency operation to remove the blood clot from the brain.

## When is an emergency operation to remove the blood clot appropriate?

When a person has bled into a metastatic brain tumor, removal of the blood clot can reduce or prevent some of the damage that the clot can cause through compression or toxic effects on surrounding brain tissue.

## How do surgeons remove the clotted blood in the brain?

In many medical centers, a neurosurgeon will make a large hole in the skull called a "craniotomy" and will expose the area of the brain involved, and using specialized surgical instruments remove the clotted blood from the brain.

## Are there better ways of removing the clot than through a craniotomy?

Some newer techniques involve making a very small hole in the skull and using a small instrument called an "endoscope" to remove the blood clot. The effectiveness and safety of this technique, which is more often available at major medical centers with neurosurgeons specially trained to do this, is under evaluation.

## What is the treatment for dangerous or worsening swelling in the brain?

Bleeding in the brain is damaging to the brain. Damaged brain swells, swelling causes damage, damage causes swelling. A circle of destruction is set up which must be interrupted to prevent death. In the event of very serious brain swelling, a technique called mechanical hyperventilation may be helpful. Mechanical ventilation requires insertion of an endotracheal tube as discussed earlier in this chapter, attaching the endotracheal tube to a mechanical ventilator and programming the ventilator to force a person to breathe in and out quickly.

A medicine called "mannitol", given intravenously, also has the effect of drawing fluid out of the brain and reducing brain swelling. If mannitol does not control the pressure and swelling in the brain, high doses of barbiturates to the point of inducing a coma can sometimes lower the pressure in the brain by reducing the brain's metabolism.

A simple measure to reduce some of the pressure in the brain is to raise the head of the bed somewhat.

The steroid medication "Dexamethasone", commonly known as "Decadron", can reduce some of the brain swelling and improve outcome when a person had a brain hemorrhage because of bleeding into a brain metastasis.

## TREATMENT OF BLEEDING CAUSED BY BLOOD CLOTTING DISORDERS

*What medications can cause blood-clotting disorders that predispose a person to brain hemorrhage?*

Medications that interfere with the blood's clotting ability are some of the most important and life-saving medications available. "Thrombolytic agents" used to treat myocardial infarction, ischemic stroke, and pulmonary embolism (see chapters), heparin and

Coumadin to prevent blood clots, and medicines to interfere with platelet function such as "Plavix", all carry some risk of causing serious internal bleeding including brain hemorrhage.

Intensive chemotherapy causing "bone marrow suppression" (see chapter entitled "Bone Marrow Suppression") can severely lower the number of platelets in the bloodstream and expose a person to the risk of brain hemorrhage.

### What is the treatment when these medications cause a brain hemorrhage?

Products derived from donated blood called "fresh frozen plasma" or "prothrombin complex concentrates" can replace the coagulation factors depleted or inhibited by medications and restore blood clotting ability.

If anticoagulation with a form of heparin called "unfractionated heparin" caused the bleeding, the abnormal blood clotting is reversible with a medication called "protamine", which is an antidote for heparin.

If the number of platelets in the bloodstream is extremely low, a transfusion of donated platelets can add sufficient platelets to the bloodstream to restore blood-clotting ability and prevent recurrent bleeding. If platelets are not functioning properly because of a medication such as Plavix or aspirin, it is not clear that platelet transfusions are helpful.

## <u>OUTLOOK</u>

*What is the outlook for a person with
cancer after a brain hemorrhage?*

Most people with cancer who develop a brain hemorrhage survive their illness and leave the hospital either completely or largely capable of self-care. The outlook for survival, for people who have survived the initial danger of a brain hemorrhage, will reflect the outlook associated with the extent of a person's cancer, in both the brain and elsewhere in the body.

# UPPER GI BLEEDING

## DEFINITION

### What is upper GI bleeding?

Upper GI bleeding is bleeding from the esophagus, stomach or duodenum. The severity of the bleeding can range from a minor trickle of blood that goes unnoticed to sudden massive bleeding which very quickly puts a person into shock. Serious upper GI bleeding can be rapidly fatal if not promptly and correctly treated. This chapter will focus on identifying and treating life threatening upper GI bleeding.

## SYMPTOMS

### What are the symptoms of serious upper GI bleeding?

The most common symptom is the vomiting of bright red blood. Vomiting of bright red blood is, of course, a very dramatic symptom and leaves no doubt to anyone as to what the problem is. When the bleeding is somewhat less severe and vomiting does not occur immediately, the vomit may look something like coffee grounds. With significant bleeding, the stool will often appear to be black like tar, and have a foul smell. If a person has lost a lot of blood, the blood pressure may drop such that the person feels dizzy and may faint when standing up.

## MAKING THE DIAGNOSIS

### How is the diagnosis of upper GI bleeding made?

The diagnosis of upper GI bleeding is usually obvious based upon a history of vomiting bright red blood or "coffee ground" appearing fluid. If such vomiting has not occurred, the diagnosis is often obvious by confirming the presence of tar-colored stool containing blood. If the diagnosis is in doubt, a thin tube (called a "nasogastric tube") can be inserted through the nose and down into the stomach, and a sample of the fluid in the stomach can be taken. If there has been significant bleeding, there will usually be blood in the fluid. An exception to this is when bleeding has occurred in the duodenum, and the blood has passed downward into the small intestine and beyond the reach of the nasogastric tube.

## SUPPORTING THE CIRCULATORY SYSTEM

### What is the initial treatment of upper GI bleeding?

A first step in the evaluation of any person who has significant bleeding is to determine whether the volume of blood in their bloodstream is sufficient to supply the body's vital organs. Loss of large amounts of blood can dramatically drop the blood pressure and endanger the adequate flow of blood to the brain and kidney and other vital organs.

When a person is having major upper gastrointestinal bleeding, medical staff will quickly put in intravenous lines. It may be necessary to insert more than one intravenous line to give fluid very rapidly. When blood pressure drops because of major bleeding, fluid replacement, usually with a solution called "Ringer's lactate", can often bring the blood pressure back up to somewhere close to, or within the normal range. The blood bank will receive a sample of the person's blood so that the blood bank can prepare to deliver several pints of compatible blood if needed. The greater the degree of blood loss, the greater the amount of fluid which will be needed and the greater the likelihood that blood which has been lost will have to be replaced with a blood transfusion.

## IDENTIFYING THE SOURCE OF THE BLEEDING

*With upper gastrointestinal bleeding, where is the bleeding coming from?*

The most common source of upper gastrointestinal bleeding is a bleeding ulcer in the stomach or duodenum.

Bleeding from multiple very shallow stomach ulcers can develop in people who have a major illness that transiently dropped their blood pressure. When blood pressure drops, blood flow and oxygen delivery to the lining of the stomach is impaired and shallow ulcers in the stomach can develop. These "stress ulcers" are particularly common in people who have had major body trauma or major burns. People with cancer taking "non-steroidal anti-inflammatory drugs" (abbreviated "NSAIDS") for pain relief, such as from bone metastases, can develop this type of shallow bleeding ulcers.

"Esophageal varices", which are discussed later in this chapter, can rupture and cause massive upper gastrointestinal bleeding.

When a person has severe retching and vomiting, such as can occur as a side effect of chemotherapy, a tear, called a "Mallory-Weiss tear", can form toward the bottom of the esophagus and bleed very rapidly.

## How is the source of bleeding identified?

When a person has had significant bleeding and their blood pressure is unstable, it is of critical importance to find the source of the bleeding and stop the bleeding. To do this, a physician specializing in gastrointestinal diseases (a "gastroenterologist") will perform an "endoscopy" by looking down into the stomach with an instrument called an "endoscope".

## What will the gastroenterologist try to accomplish with the endoscopy?

The gastroenterologist will try to identify the area that is bleeding or the area that has recently bled. If active bleeding is present, or of it appears likely that active bleeding will start again, treatment administered through the endoscope can stop the bleeding or prevent recurrent bleeding.

## What does the gastroenterologist see with the endoscope?

If the person is still bleeding, the gastroenterologist can often spot an area of the stomach or duodenum that is spurting or oozing blood. The appearance of the area or areas that are bleeding may allow the gastroenterologist to determine the exact problem that is causing the bleeding. This information enables the selection of the treatment that is most likely to stop the bleeding.

If the person has stopped bleeding, it may be possible for the gastroenterologist to diagnose the problem in the esophagus, stomach or duodenum that caused the bleeding and assess the risk of recurrent bleeding. Identification of the cause of the bleeding provides critical information that guides treatment that is most likely to reduce the risk of recurrence of the bleeding.

### What happens if the gastroenterologist cannot identify the source of the bleeding?

When bleeding is especially brisk, there may be so much blood in the stomach that it is not possible to identify the area of bleeding. At other times, the area of bleeding may be below the area that the endoscope can reach. An angiogram, in which a radiologist's dye permits examination of the arteries feeding the stomach, may identify the bleeding artery.

## TREATMENT OF UPPER GI BLEEDING FROM ULCERS

### What is the treatment of upper GI bleeding from ulcers?

When the blood pressure is stable and the source of bleeding identified, appropriate treatment stops the bleeding and prevents the bleeding from recurring.

Stomach acid may interfere with a person's own ability to form a good clot that can plug broken blood vessels at the area that is bleeding. Intravenous administration of a type of medicine called a "proton pump inhibitor", blocks the production of stomach acid, and provides some help with controlling the bleeding.

When the gastroenterologist spots the area of bleeding with the endoscope, and, if the source is an ulcer, instruments are available, called "contact thermal devices", which can be put through the endoscope and which can zap the bleeding vessel with highly focused heat and can often stop the bleeding. At times, the gastroenterologist may inject "epinephrine" into the area of bleeding to constrict the blood vessels and slow the bleeding before the contact thermal device is applied to the bleeding vessels. Other instruments called "endoscopic hemoclips" are available which can be closed and locked around the bleeding vessel in the stomach or duodenal wall, and which will stop the bleeding.

If bleeding is uncontrolled by endoscopy, a radiologist, using sophisticated x-ray guidance, can advance a catheter directly into the artery feeding the area that is bleeding. The artery responsible for the bleeding is sealed, and bleeding stopped, by injection of a surgical gelatin called "Gelfoam", or by the use of surgical glue or other similar materials.

If these techniques fail to stop the bleeding, surgery may be necessary.

### When is surgery necessary?

Surgery may be necessary when bleeding is severe and not stopped by the gastroenterologist and the radiologist. After transfusion of several pints of blood and when more transfusions are necessary, or when, despite administration of fluid and blood the person is still bleeding and remains in shock or hovers on the brink of shock, surgical intervention may be the safest way to quickly get control of the bleeding.

## How does the surgeon stop the bleeding?

The surgeon performs an operation through an incision made from just below the breastbone to just below the navel. The surgeon will identify the bleeding area and tie or obliterate blood vessels that are the source of bleeding. In some circumstances, it may be necessary to remove the general area of the stomach or duodenum in which there is bleeding. At the time of surgery, some surgeons will believe it important to sever the nerves that control acid production by the stomach, thereby reducing the risk of recurrent ulcers and bleeding.

## PORTAL HYPERTENSION

### What is portal hypertension?

Extensive involvement of the liver with cancer, or extensive scarring in the liver from cirrhosis, can steadily squeeze the liver's blood vessels and narrow them down or shut them off. This will cause a tremendous impediment to the normal flow of blood through the liver. When blood flow through the liver is blocked, pressure will build up in the main inflow vein into the liver (the "portal vein") and cause "portal hypertension".

The liver is one of the main channels through which blood flows as it travels around the body. When blood flow through the liver is impaired, the body will compensate by opening up vascular detours that allow the blood to take alternative circulatory channels. New veins that bypass the liver will open up and wind their way around the inside of the stomach and esophagus. These veins grow bigger and bigger as the circulation in the liver becomes more and more obstructed. These large veins (they are "varices") become very fragile as they grow and can burst and cause extremely dangerous internal bleeding.

## What treatment can reduce the high pressure in the portal vein?

The ideal way to reduce pressure in the portal vein would be to break up or dissolve the scarring in the liver associated with cirrhosis, or shrink areas of liver metastasis and, by doing this, relieve the obstruction of blood flow through the liver. Unfortunately, although chemotherapy may shrink large areas of liver metastasis, available medications cannot relieve the scarring in the liver that is associated with cirrhosis.

Available medications that can somewhat reduce the high pressure in the portal vein are in the family of medicines called "beta blockers". Two beta-blockers used to accomplish this are "propranolol" and "nadolol".

There is some recent information suggesting that eating dark chocolate can slightly reduce high pressure in the portal vein. This information is not yet well developed, but it has generated some interest as a pleasant way to reduce portal hypertension.

### What is the significance of the large new veins that develop because of portal hypertension?

The large new veins become "varicose veins", and grow and bulge in the top part of the stomach and in the esophagus. These veins are highly fragile. Rupture of varicose veins in the esophagus ("esophageal varices") is a particularly common problem in people with cirrhosis and can cause rapid, life threatening bleeding. Bleeding from esophageal varices is a catastrophic complication that requires immediate emergency medical treatment.

## BLEEDING ESOPHAGEAL VARICES

### What are the symptoms of bleeding esophageal varices?

The most common symptom is the vomiting of bright red blood.

The degree of symptoms will depend on the severity of the bleeding. If bleeding is brisk, a person can faint and rapidly go into shock. If blood is just oozing instead of flowing briskly, a person may feel weak from the blood loss and notice black or reddish black stool.

### What is the immediate treatment when a person with liver involvement with cancer and portal hypertension vomits bright red blood?

Vomiting bright red blood is a major medical emergency. In a person with portal hypertension, the cause of the bleeding is often esophageal varices, which can bleed extremely briskly and rapidly prove fatal.

The first step taken will be to assure that the person is "hemodynamically stable", which means that there is sufficient blood and fluid in the person's circulatory system to maintain blood pressure and provide blood flow to all the major organs of the body. A large intravenous line or sometimes two intravenous lines provide fluid and blood transfusions as needed.

Once the circulatory system is stable, attention will turn to finding the exact source of the bleeding and treating it appropriately.

## How is the source of the bleeding identified?

To find the source of the bleeding, a specialist called a "gastroenterologist" will put a tube called an "endoscope" down the mouth and into the esophagus and stomach and, if necessary, lower into the duodenum (which is the first part of the small intestine). Through this scope, the physician should be able to find the bleeding area and confirm whether the cause is bleeding esophageal varices.

## How do physicians stop bleeding from esophageal varices?

A first step in controlling the bleeding will be to give a medicine that can constrict some of the blood vessels that are feeding the ruptured esophageal varices. The medicines used to do this are "somatostatin" and "octreotide". Although these medicines can sometimes stop the bleeding on their own, they commonly do not, and physicians will often believe that a more direct approach is immediately necessary.

The most common direct approach taken is "endoscopic variceal ligation". In order to perform "endoscopic variceal ligation", the gastroenterologist will first put a scope down into the esophagus and identify the area of bleeding varices. The gastroenterologist will then use the scope to guide elastic bands to the bleeding varices, binding the bleeding vessels until bleeding stops.

A related approach sometimes used with very severe variceal bleeding is to have a gastroenterologist put a scope down the esophagus, find the bleeding veins and inject the bleeding veins with chemicals that scar and obliterate them. This procedure is "sclerotherapy".

There are times, especially in smaller hospitals, when a skilled gastroenterologist is not available, or, when despite a gastroenterologist's best attempts, bleeding continues. In this circumstance, bleeding may be controlled by pressure put on veins in the top of the stomach or in the esophagus, using a specially shaped balloon (called a "Sengstaken-Blakemore" tube) passed from the mouth down the esophagus and into the stomach. The balloon is then inflated and pulled up tightly into the top of the stomach and esophagus. This inflated balloon has the proper shape and size to fit snugly against the top of the stomach and the lower esophagus to put pressure on the bleeding veins. This balloon generally stops the bleeding temporarily and is useful as a short-term emergency measure.

Medications that can somewhat reduce the high pressure in the portal vein may also be given. A medicine given for this purpose is an intravenous infusion of "octreotide".

Because people with bleeding esophageal varices are prone to developing bacterial infections while in the hospital, intravenous antibiotics such as "norfloxacin" (brand name is "Noroxin", manufacturer's product website is www.noroxin.com) or "ceftriaxone" (brand name is "Rocephin", manufacturer's product website is www.rocephin.com) or "ciprofloxacin" (brand name is "Cipro", manufacturer's product website is www.cipro.com) are often prescribed as a precaution.

> **What is the treatment, if despite all these measures, a person is still bleeding or the bleeding rapidly recurs?**

Treatment must stop the bleeding and prevent its recurrence. As an additional measure, physicians can create a "portosystemic shunt" in which the high-pressure portal vein that is feeding the bleeding varices is connected to lower pressure veins. The most commonly used way of doing this has the abbreviation "TIPS" which stands for "transjugular intrahepatic portosystemic shunt". To do this, a radiologist, will use x-ray guidance and an entry point of the large vein in the neck called the "jugular vein". Through the jugular vein, a tube called a "shunt" is put into a position in the circulatory system that bypasses the compressed circulation in the liver and establishes a direct connection between the portal vein that carries blood from the intestines to the liver, and the hepatic vein that carries blood from the liver back to the heart. This decompresses the portal vein and the esophageal varices that derive from the portal vein and generally stops the bleeding.

> **After the bleeding stops, what can prevent rebleeding?**

After the bleeding is under control, the gastroenterologist can look down the esophagus with the endoscope, identify, and put a clip or tie a knot around, any visible varices. Medications which can somewhat reduce the pressure in the portal vein may also be given in an attempt to prevent rebleeding.

## <u>OUTLOOK</u>

*What is the outcome of upper gastrointestinal bleeding?*

Most of the time, bleeding can be brought under control. After the episode, the person's health will return to what it was before the episode of upper gastrointestinal bleeding.

Medicine that helps prevent and heal ulcers, such as the "proton pump inhibitors", along with modification of diet and smoking cessation may help prevent recurrent bleeding.

# LUNG COMPLICATIONS

# ACUTE RESPIRATORY DISTRESS SYNDROME

## DEFINITION

### What is acute respiratory distress syndrome?

In Vietnam, battlefield surgeons saw many soldiers with severe injuries who quickly and without explanation developed acute lung failure. It was puzzling to the surgeons that many of these young men developed this lung failure with major injuries, such as leg injuries, that did not at all involve the chest. What the military surgeons nicknamed "Da Nang lung", we now call "acute respiratory distress syndrome" or "acute lung injury".

Many sudden serious medical problems such as major trauma, sepsis, pneumonia, pancreatitis, drug overdose, and shock, can cause the lungs to suddenly accumulate excessive fluid and fail to carry out their essential function of delivery of oxygen to the bloodstream. Acute respiratory distress syndrome is a major problem in intensive care medicine and is fatal in about half of people who develop it.

## SYMPTOMS

### What are the symptoms of acute respiratory distress syndrome?

The person who develops acute respiratory distress syndrome is usually already in a hospital and quite sick. The problem begins with rapidly worsening difficulty with breathing which quickly progresses to the point where the assistance of a mechanical ventilator is necessary to keep the person alive.

## THE PROBLEM IN THE LUNGS

*What is the problem in the lungs that is causing difficulty breathing and inadequate delivery of oxygen to the bloodstream?*

To understand the problem, it is good to understand a bit of the anatomy of the airways. Air enters the mouth or nose and travels down the trachea into the large bronchial tubes. The bronchial tubes send off smaller and smaller branches (called "bronchioles") which eventually stop branching at the "terminal bronchiole" beyond which are the microscopic airspaces called "alveoli". Oxygen transfer to the bloodstream occurs in the alveoli. The lung expands and deflates with each breath, pulling air in and out of the alveoli.

In acute respiratory distress syndrome, damage to the cells lining the inside of the alveoli allows fluid and protein to leak into the alveoli and surrounding tissues. This flooding of the alveoli with fluid prevents delivery of oxygen into the bloodstream from the areas of the lung that are most affected.

If a person does not recover in the early stages of acute respiratory distress syndrome, a scarring or "fibrosis" can occur which can dramatically, and sometimes fatally, impair lung function.

## MAKING THE DIAGNOSIS

*How is the diagnosis of acute respiratory distress syndrome made?*

No specific test or classical finding on physical examination immediately establishes the diagnosis of acute respiratory distress syndrome. This can lead to some difficulties with rapidly making the diagnosis.

A person who develops acute respiratory distress syndrome usually has a number of medical problems that could lead to sudden lung failure. Because of the lack of specific tests for acute respiratory distress syndrome, the way to a diagnosis is to exclude the other diseases that might have caused the seriously sick or injured person to develop lung failure. Acute respiratory distress syndrome is one of those diseases where physicians make the diagnosis by excluding other major causes of the problem, so that the remaining cause, for which there is no perfect diagnostic test, is the only possibility that remains. Physicians refer to this as "making the diagnosis by exclusion".

The clinical picture of acute respiratory distress syndrome can initially be almost identical to the clinical picture of congestive heart failure and pulmonary edema (see chapter entitled "Heart Failure") or the clinical picture of rapidly progressing bacterial pneumonia (see chapter entitled "Hospital-Acquired Pneumonia"). Through the use of an echocardiogram and, occasionally, a Swan-Ganz catheter (see chapters entitled "Heart Failure" and "Heart Attack: Acute Myocardial Infarction"), and by the skill and insight of a physician experienced in pulmonary and intensive care medicine, other causes of lung failure can be excluded and the diagnosis of acute respiratory distress syndrome can be made.

## TREATMENT

### What is the treatment of acute respiratory distress syndrome?

The treatment of acute respiratory distress syndrome is to support respiration, and therefore, life, and hope that the acute respiratory distress syndrome will resolve on its own. The major treatment that is necessary to sustain life is mechanical ventilation

## MECHANICAL VENTILATION

### How do physicians provide mechanical ventilation?

A person with acute respiratory distress syndrome and respiratory failure will generally need to have a flexible plastic tube inserted through the mouth and into their trachea. The procedure to put that tube in is "intubation" and the tube in the trachea is an "endotracheal tube". Connection of the endotracheal tube to a machine called a "mechanical ventilator" will allow the medical professionals in an intensive care unit to control the delivery of oxygen and air into the lungs. Because the lungs contain excess fluid and tend to be a bit stiff, extra pressure will be required from the mechanical ventilator in order to blow air into the lungs and expand them properly. This extra pressure is "positive end expiratory pressure" or "PEEP".

### Is mechanical ventilation always necessary?

People with acute respiratory distress syndrome have extraordinary difficulty maintaining the proper level of oxygen in their bloodstream and generally cannot survive without some form of mechanical ventilation.

### What are the risks of mechanical ventilation?

Although the mechanical ventilation is necessary to sustain life, the artificial nature of blowing air into the lung at high volumes and high pressure can itself damage the lung, causing "ventilator-induced lung injury".

### What is the "tidal volume"?

The tidal volume refers to the amount of air a person breathes in and out with each breathing cycle. In the context of an intensive care unit with a person receiving mechanical life support, tidal volume refers to the amount of air the ventilator is delivering with each ventilator-driven breath cycle. The tidal volume that is programmed into the ventilator is designed to deliver as much volume of air as possible without causing "barotrauma", which is lung trauma caused by the pressure of too much air volume.

### How can physicians reduce the risk of ventilator induced lung injury?

Physicians caring for critically ill people with acute respiratory distress syndrome have to balance the need to adequately expand the lung with each breath and get oxygen into the bloodstream, against the risk that the volume and pressure of the air delivered by the mechanical ventilator can cause lung damage.

"Low tidal volume ventilation", in which the ventilator delivers sufficient but not excessive air volumes, reduces the risk of ventilator-induced injury. By measuring the level of oxygen in the bloodstream, the effectiveness of the "low tidal volume ventilation" can be determined. As required, intensive care unit professionals adjust the tidal volume, the "PEEP" (as described earlier in this chapter), and the amount of oxygen delivered by the ventilator.

## REDUCING THE AMOUNT OF FLUID IN THE LUNGS

### What treatment reduces the fluid in the lungs?

The amount of fluid in the lungs can be somewhat reduced by the use of diuretics and by restriction of the amount of fluid administered intravenously. Although diuretics and fluid restriction are helpful, physicians will have to monitor the person's blood pressure very closely and be sure that diuretics and fluid restriction are not dangerously reducing blood flow to vital organs such as the brain and the kidney.

### VENTILATOR-ASSOCIATED PNEUMONIA

### What is ventilator-associated pneumonia?

The "endotracheal tube" in the lung, which is attached to the ventilator, can serve as a conduit for bacteria to travel deep into the lung and cause life-threatening pneumonia. The longer a person remains on a ventilator in an intensive care unit, the higher the risk that a dangerous bacterial lung infection will develop. Lung infection that develops after two or more days on a ventilator is "ventilator-associated pneumonia". Infections acquired in the hospital environment are "nosocomial infections".

### Does everyone with an endotracheal tube receive antibiotics to prevent infection?

There are many different types of bacteria with a large variety of sensitivities to antibiotics. It is difficult to choose the right antibiotic combination that will always prevent pneumonia. More importantly, the frequent use of antibiotics in intensive care units with its many patients on ventilators, allows bacteria in the intensive care unit environment to become resistant to antibiotics. As a result, infections acquired in intensive care units, can become difficult to treat and potentially lethal. For these reasons, in most hospitals, use of antibiotics to prevent pneumonia in the absence of signs of infection may not be routine, while use of antibiotics to treat pneumonia is the standard of care.

### What are the signs that a person is developing ventilator-associated pneumonia?

When a person on a ventilator, who was previously stable or improving, suddenly starts having difficulty maintaining blood oxygen levels, develops a fever, or has a thick yellow or greenish material sucked out of their endotracheal tube by intensive care unit professionals, it raises the suspicion of ventilator-associated pneumonia.

## What is the treatment of ventilator-associated pneumonia?

Microscopic examination and culturing of the material from a person's endotracheal tube, as well as knowing the bacteria that seem to be causing a problem in a specific hospital, will guide the choice of antibiotic or combination of antibiotics prescribed to treat the pneumonia.

For additional information about ventilator-associated pneumonia, please see the chapter entitled "Hospital-Acquired Pneumonia".

## <u>OUTLOOK</u>

## What is the outlook for a person with acute respiratory distress syndrome?

In the early stages of acute respiratory distress syndrome, the outlook generally depends upon recovery from the underlying problem that caused the acute respiratory distress syndrome. People who do not recover quickly and who remain dependent upon the ventilator over an extended period can develop ventilator-associated pneumonia and are more likely to develop a scarring of their lungs that can have fatal consequences.

Recovery from acute respiratory distress syndrome can leave a person with some decrease in lung function, which is primarily noticeable with exertion.

# ACUTE PULMONARY EDEMA

## DEFINITION

### What is acute pulmonary edema?

Acute pulmonary edema is the sudden accumulation of fluid in the lungs. The most common causes of acute pulmonary edema are inadequate pumping ability of the heart and excessive fluid in the bloodstream.

## SYMPTOMS

### What are the symptoms of acute pulmonary edema?

The pumping action of the heart pushes blood from the right atrium to the right ventricle, from the right ventricle to the lungs, then, after the blood returns to the heart from the lungs, from the left atrium to the left ventricle and from the left ventricle to the entire body.

If the ability of the heart to pump blood forward is suddenly impaired, increased pressure transmits backward from the left ventricle, to the left atrium, and to the lungs. The lungs become stiff because of this increased pressure and leak a clear fluid into the air spaces ("the alveoli") in the lung. This leakage of fluid into the air spaces of the lung is "pulmonary edema".

When a person develops pulmonary edema, he or she will be tremendously short of breath and may feel as though they are suffocating. The observation of an anxious person gasping for air and the wet crackly sound of fluid heard in the lungs with a stethoscope makes the rapid diagnosis of pulmonary edema.

Worsening leg swelling and severe fatigue are other very common symptoms of acute pulmonary edema.

## THE CAUSE OF ACUTE PULMONARY EDEMA

*What can cause acute pulmonary edema?*

Many medical problems can trigger acute pulmonary edema. A heart attack (the medical term for a heart attack is "acute myocardial infarction") may have occurred. Medical problems such as pneumonia, anemia, or high blood pressure can put a strain on an already weakened heart and suddenly worsen heart failure. Administration of excessive intravenous fluid can cause pulmonary edema in people with impaired heart or kidney function.

## TREATMENT OF ACUTE PULMONARY EDEMA

*What is the treatment of acute pulmonary edema?*

People with acute pulmonary edema generally require admission to the hospital, since very serious and life-threatening complications can rapidly develop.

The most important and distressing symptom of acute pulmonary edema is the severe shortness of breath associated with pulmonary edema. The treatment of pulmonary edema consists of three key components: get oxygen into the blood, get the excess fluid out of the lungs, and reduce the pressure of blood in the lungs.

A mask over the mouth and nose, or nasal prongs, provides supplemental oxygen, if it appears that the shortness of breath is reducing the amount of oxygen in a person' bloodstream.

The head of the person's hospital bed will be elevated so that the person is in a sitting position. This will allow gravity to pull blood away from the lungs, thereby reducing the pressure of blood in the lungs.

Powerful diuretics called "loop diuretics", given intravenously, will allow excess fluid to move from the person's lungs into their urine, thereby decreasing fluid in the lungs. Restriction of sodium and fluid intake may help further diminish the fluid in the lungs.

Intravenous morphine can reduce the pressure in arteries and veins of the body, reduce pressure of blood in the lungs, and relieve shortness of breath.

Intravenous medications called "nitrates", such as "nitroglycerin" and "nitroprusside", can also help drop the pressure of the blood in the lungs. This reduction in blood pressure in the lungs will make the lungs less stiff and make it much easier for the person to breathe in and out.

If the heart rhythm is abnormal, treatment may be necessary to normalize the rhythm. The exact type of treatment used to normalize the heart rhythm will depend upon the type of rhythm abnormality that the person has.

If heart failure is very severe, transfer to the intensive care unit may be necessary. Mechanical breathing support, may be given with a method called "CPAP", which is the abbreviation for "Continuous Positive Airway Pressure" in which a tight mask is put over the mouth and nose, and air is forced into the lungs. Alternatively, in severe situations, it may be necessary to put a tube directly into the windpipe (the medical word for the windpipe is the "trachea" and the tube in the trachea is an "endotracheal tube") and blow air directly into the lungs. If the heart is severely failing and blood pressure is dropping, an intravenous medicine called "dobutamine", given with very careful monitoring, may help the heart to beat more forcefully.

Any other disease (such as pneumonia) which has apparently triggered the episode of sudden heart failure will require appropriate specific therapy.

## What other problems can develop when a person has acute pulmonary edema?

When a person develops acute pulmonary edema, their ability to move around is limited and they spend the overwhelming majority of their day in bed. Because of this immobility, the person is at risk of developing blood clots in the leg that can travel to the lung as a pulmonary embolism (see chapter entitled "Deep Vein Thrombosis and Pulmonary Embolism"). "Anticoagulant medications" can prevent these blood clots from developing. The administration of antibiotics to prevent deep vein thrombosis is "DVT prophylaxis".

The anticoagulant medications most commonly prescribed are one of the available forms of heparin.

The high doses of diuretics used to draw fluid out of the lungs can drop the blood pressure and compromise the flow of blood to the kidneys. This can cause a condition called "pre-renal azotemia" that is discussed in the chapter entitled "Acute Kidney Injury".

> ### What is the outlook for a person hospitalized for acute pulmonary edema?

Although most people respond very quickly to treatment with rapid reduction of their symptoms, acute pulmonary edema is a dangerous condition that can fail to respond adequately to treatment. Prolonged hospitalization, as well as failure to survive the episode can occur. Recurrence of acute pulmonary edema requiring another hospitalization is a common occurrence shortly after discharge.

# MASSIVE HEMOPTYSIS: COUGHING UP BLOOD

## DEFINITIONS

### What is hemoptysis and what is massive hemoptysis?

Hemoptysis means coughing up blood that originated in the lungs or in the airway leading to the lungs. Hemoptysis can range from very mild, with just a few streaks of blood in sputum, to massive, meaning eight ounces or more per day of bright red blood. Massive hemoptysis, although uncommon, is one of the most frightening complications of cancer.

## THE DANGER OF HEMOPTYSIS

### How does air normally flow into the lungs?

Air enters the mouth or nose and travels down the trachea that divides into the large bronchial tubes that deliver air to each lung. The bronchial tubes send off smaller and smaller branches that eventually stop branching at the "terminal bronchioles" and "respiratory bronchioles". These bronchioles deliver air to microscopic airspaces called "alveoli" that transfer oxygen to the bloodstream.

## Why is hemoptysis dangerous?

Extensive bleeding from the lungs causes blood to move in two directions. Coughing the blood up and out removes some blood from the lungs. "Aspiration", that is, breathing in the blood, moves the blood downward deep into the lungs. The aspiration of blood deep into the lungs can choke off the flow of oxygen to the alveoli and cause asphyxiation.

Rapid loss of a massive amount of blood exposes a person to a risk of a severe drop of blood pressure with inadequate flow of blood to the major organs of the body.

## What are the most common reasons a person with cancer can develop massive hemoptysis?

Cancer that is growing inside a bronchus is "endobronchial". Lung cancer most often originates inside the bronchus and is the most common "endobronchial" cancer. Cancer can spread to the inside wall of the bronchus from breast cancer, colon cancer, melanoma, and other cancers. These areas of cancer inside the bronchus are "endobronchial metastases".

The blood vessels that feed the wall of the bronchial tubes are the "bronchial arteries". When cancer grows inside a bronchus, it can burrow its way into the adjacent bronchial arteries, and pop a hole in an arterial wall. The communication between an open bleeding bronchial artery and the bronchus is the most common cause of massive hemoptysis.

The medication "bevacizumab" (brand name is "Avastin"), for reasons that are not clear, can occasionally cause massive hemoptysis.

Long time smokers with COPD (see chapter) can develop a chronic, destructive disease of the bronchial tubes called "bronchiectasis". The damaged bronchi in bronchiectasis can cause enlargement and occasional rupture of adjacent bronchial arteries, producing massive hemoptysis.

## **TREATMENT**

### *What is the initial treatment of massive hemoptysis?*

Massive bleeding in a bronchus can obstruct the movement of air into both lungs and rapidly prove fatal. The first steps, therefore, will be to protect the airways from obstruction and prevent asphyxiation.

When a person has lung cancer, it is very likely that the bleeding is coming from the lung from which the cancer originated. A simple immediate step is to take advantage of gravity and have the person lie on their side, with side from which the lung cancer originated facing downward. For example, if the cancer began in the right lung, it is helpful for the person to lie on their right side. This will encourage blood that is coming from the bleeding lung to remain in that lung, without bleeding into the opposite lung, obstructing the flow of air into that lung as well.

Upon arrival at the hospital, the first priority of the physician will be to make sure that major problems with breathing and circulation are immediately treated

## SUPPORTING BREATHING

*What will physician do to support breathing
when a person has massive hemoptysis?*

The emergency physician will check to make sure the mouth and throat are clear blood is not blocking the person's airway. Suction removes this obstruction.

Because of the extreme danger of asphyxiation from a blockage of the airways by blood, a physician will insert an "endotracheal tube". The endotracheal tube is a tube put directly into the windpipe (the "trachea") through the mouth. Special endotracheal tubes are available that can inserted all the way down into the lung that is not bleeding, so that the non-bleeding lung gets the air and oxygen needed to sustain life.

## SUPPORTING CIRCULATION WHEN THERE HAS BEEN MAJOR BLEEDING

*What does the hospital physician do to support
circulation when a person has lost a great
deal of blood and is in shock?*

When major blood loss has occurred, the physician will immediately begin the process of inserting large diameter intravenous lines through which fluid and blood transfusions are given. If large veins in the arm are difficult to find, an easily accessible vein in which to insert a catheter is the "saphenous vein", which is the vein just in front of the inside anklebone. This vein is easy to put a large intravenous line into quickly. Other veins into which the hospital physician may put intravenous lines are the veins in the groin (the "femoral vein"), the vein beneath the collarbone (the "subclavian vein"), and the largest vein in the neck (the "internal jugular vein").

> ### What kind of fluid will the hospital physician put in the intravenous lines?

The fluid is a sodium-containing solution. If there has been major bleeding, whole blood may be necessary.

> ### What if there has been massive bleeding and blood that matches the person's blood type is not immediately available?

In this circumstance, it may be necessary to give "Type O" blood, which, although not a perfect match, is likely tolerated without major complications.

> ### What will the hospital physician do after the airway has been somewhat protected by the endotracheal tube, the intravenous lines are established, and appropriate fluid is running in?

At this point, the priority will be to find the exact source of bleeding in the lung and to stop the bleeding. Once the airway is reasonably secure, and the blood pressure is stable, an emergency CT scan of the chest can provide critical information about the likely sources of the bleeding and the treatment with the best potential to stop the bleeding.

# EMERGENCY BRONCHOSCOPY

## What is bronchoscopy?

Bronchoscopy is a medical test in which a physician looks directly into the lungs by putting a scope through the mouth, down the windpipe (the "trachea"), and into the bronchial tubes which provide air to the lungs. The device used to perform this test (called a "bronchoscope") is a flexible long tube that projects images from inside the bronchial tubes in the lungs to a video monitor.

To perform the bronchoscopy, a lung specialist will administer mild sedation, spray the throat with a light anesthetic, and then advance the bronchoscope down the windpipe into the bronchial tree. Bleeding may be brisk and may obscure the view of a physician looking down the bronchoscope. Combined with the information available from the CT scan, however, it usually is possible to determine the exact area of the lung that is bleeding. Having found the source of bleeding, the physician has several options to attempt to control the bleeding by treatments administered through the bronchoscope.

## What can the physician do through the bronchoscope to stop the bleeding?

The bronchoscope has a hollow space inside of it that allow physicians to insert instruments or medications into the lung that can stop the bleeding.

Through the bronchoscope, the physician may insert one of several instruments that can either freeze, burn, or otherwise zap the bleeding vessels and stop their bleeding. At times, the physician may inject "epinephrine" into the area of bleeding, or bathe the area with iced saline, to constrict the blood vessels and slow or stop their bleeding. Balloon-like devices are available, that, if inflated inside a bleeding bronchus will compress the bleeding vessels and frequently stop their bleeding.

## BRONCHIAL ARTERY EMBOLIZATION

### What is bronchial artery embolization?

As described earlier in this chapter, the bleeding arteries are most commonly the "bronchial arteries". The bronchial arteries usually originate from the aorta, which is the major artery of the body. In order to find the bleeding arteries, highly specialized physicians will inject a radiologists dye (called "contrast material") into the aorta, allowing physicians to see, with x-rays, detailed images of the aorta as well as arteries, such as the bronchial arteries, the originate from the aorta. The x-ray images taken after injection of contrast material into the bronchial arteries, along with the findings of the CT scan and bronchoscopy, can often determine, with a high level of accuracy, where the bleeding is coming from. Tiny particles usually made of a synthetic resin called "polyvinyl alcohol", injected into the bleeding artery, will usually plug the artery and stop the bleeding. The injection of these tiny particles into the bronchial arteries is bronchial artery embolization.

## SURGERY

### Can surgery control massive hemoptysis?

Surgery can control massive hemoptysis, although the risk of complications from surgery is very significant. For this reason, physicians may initially attempt to control the bleeding through bronchoscopy and bronchial artery embolization, provided appropriately physicians and equipment necessary to perform these difficult procedures are available at the hospital in which the person is treated. In centers equipped to perform bronchoscopy and pulmonary artery embolization, surgery for massive hemoptysis caused by cancer is generally reserved for bleeding that does not respond to bronchoscopy or bronchial artery embolization, or for very massive bleeding where immediate control of the bleeding is necessary to preserve life.

# MALIGNANT AIRWAY OBSTRUCTION

## DEFINITION

### What is malignant airway obstruction?

Normally, air enters the mouth or nose and travels down the trachea into the large bronchial tubes that deliver air to the left and right lung. With malignant airway obstruction, a cancer causes a blockage to the normal flow of air, usually somewhere between the bottom of the trachea and the branches of the bronchial tubes that deliver air to each lung.

### Why is malignant airway obstruction dangerous?

The dangers associated with malignant airway obstruction reflect the region of the airway that is blocked and the speed with which the blockage developed.

A blockage in the trachea or in the region where the trachea divides into the right and left "mainstem bronchus" feeding each lung can cause a severe drop in the oxygen delivered to the lungs and put life in great danger.

If a bronchus feeding a portion of the lung is completely blocked, air will not be able to get in or out of that portion of the lung. Air that was present in the lung before the obstruction developed will get absorbed, and the portion of the lung fed by the obstructed bronchus will collapse and cease to function. This is "atelectasis".

Bacteria trapped inside the lung beyond the obstructed bronchus can infect the lung and cause a form of bacterial pneumonia called "post-obstructive pneumonia".

## SYMPTOMS

### What are the symptoms of malignant airway obstruction?

The first evidence of a malignant airway obstruction may be when a person notices a high-pitched sound when breathing in. This high-pitched sound, known as "stridor", reflects the turbulence of air getting past the area of obstruction into the lung.

As the malignant airway obstruction worsens, a person can develop a cough, shortness of breath, and may begin to cough up blood.

## MAKING THE DIAGNOSIS

### What is obstructing the airway?

The malignant airway obstruction can be either "intrinsic", meaning the something inside the trachea or bronchus is obstructing the airway, or "extrinsic", meaning that something in the chest is compressing the trachea or bronchial tubes and blocking airflow.

Lung cancer growing within the bronchus is the most common cause of intrinsic obstruction. Extrinsic obstructions can result from cancers that arise in the chest, such as esophageal cancer or lymphoma, or from cancers that spread from outside the chest such as breast cancer or melanoma.

## How do physicians confirm the presence of malignant airway obstruction?

Malignant airway obstruction is usually very evident with a CT scan of the chest. By looking directly into the lung with a "bronchoscope", a physician can gain a better understanding of the location and degree of obstruction, and determine the treatment most likely to relieve the obstruction.

## TREATMENT

### What treatment can relieve malignant airway obstruction?

An effective and rapid method to relieve malignant airway obstruction is for the physician, through the bronchoscope, to place a metallic or silicone tube called a "stent" across the area of obstruction. This can prop open the trachea or the bronchus, and allow air to easily flow past the area of obstruction.

If a stent cannot easily be passed across the obstruction, lasers are available that can either destroy or vaporize the cancerous tissue. This laser treatment of malignant airway obstruction is usually safe, although serious complications, such as bleeding or perforation of the wall of the airway, can occur.

Radiation or chemotherapy after stent placement or laser treatment can prevent recurrent or persistent growth of the cancer in the region inside or outside the airway, provided the cancer is sensitive to radiation or chemotherapy.

# PNEUMOTHORAX

## DEFINITION

### What is a pneumothorax?

Pneumothorax means that air is trapped between the lung and the inside wall of the chest. The trapped air puts pressure on the lung and does not allow the lung to expand normally. If a large enough amount of air gets into the chest cavity, the pressure on the lung can cause the lung to totally collapse.

## THE CAUSE OF PNEUMOTHORAX

### Where does the trapped air come from?

The trapped air can come from sources either inside the chest or outside the chest.

Inside the chest, the source is an air leak from the surface of the lung. A number of lung diseases can cause this leak, although most commonly, the leak occurs in people with COPD (see chapter entitled "COPD: Chronic Obstructive Pulmonary Disease") because of the breakage of abnormal balloon-like areas called "blebs" on the surface of the lung. Pneumothorax that occurs in a person with known lung disease is "secondary spontaneous pneumothorax".

When pneumothorax occurs in a person without known lung disease, it is "primary spontaneous pneumothorax".

When a physician's needle penetrates the chest wall, air can follow the needle into the chest cavity and cause a pneumothorax. A bronchoscopy, in which a physician puts a scope into the lung to look for disease, can sometimes accidentally pop through a bronchial tube and let air loose into the chest cavity. This can cause a pneumothorax.

## SYMPTOMS

### What are the symptoms of pneumothorax?

The symptoms of pneumothorax begin when there is a sudden introduction of loose air into the chest cavity. At that moment, there is sudden pain in the chest and a sense of breathlessness. Most people with normal lungs can tolerate a pneumothorax on one side of the chest reasonably well. People with serious pre-existing lung disease may not tolerate the further reduction in lung function, and may develop acute respiratory failure (see the discussion of acute respiratory failure in the chapter entitled "COPD: Chronic Obstructive Pulmonary Disease").

## MAKING THE DIAGNOSIS

### How is the diagnosis of pneumothorax made?

The diagnosis of pneumothorax is usually easy to make with a plain chest x-ray. Occasionally, in a person with severe COPD, the chest x-ray can leave the diagnosis in doubt. A CT scan may be necessary in this and other uncommon circumstances to confirm the diagnosis.

## TREATMENT

### What is the immediate treatment of pneumothorax?

If the pneumothorax is relatively small, and the person has minimal symptoms and no underlying lung diseases (that is, has a "primary spontaneous pneumothorax"), physicians may observe the person closely in the hospital, perhaps administer oxygen, and not initiate any additional treatment.

Pneumothorax that is causing significant shortness of breath needs treatment. If the person has not had previous lung disease and does not appear to be in acute danger, a physician may insert a needle into the chest cavity and pull out as much of the air as possible. When a person is having difficulty breathing, or if pneumothorax occurs in a person with previous lung disease, insertion of a chest tube will get the air out of the chest cavity with greater speed and certainty.

### How is the chest tube inserted?

The chest tube is inserted between the ribs into the chest cavity. A local anesthetic (usually "lidocaine") is injected into the area through which the chest tube will be inserted. Through a half-inch or so incision, the chest tube is inserted into the chest. In skilled hands, the procedure is quick and easy. An apparatus that can remove the abnormal air out of the chest will be connected to the chest tube.

### How long is the chest tube kept in place?

The chest tube has to remain in place until the source of the air leak has sealed. This usually takes several days.

### What is a "tension pneumothorax"?

A tension pneumothorax occurs when air is leaking from a break in the lung's surface into the chest cavity and, without any place for this air to go, the pressure from the air in the chest is increasing with every breath. Tension pneumothorax can occur because of being on a mechanical ventilator, where artificial inflation of a diseased and fragile lung tears the surface of the lung with escape of air into the chest cavity as the lung is inflated.

### What is the treatment of a tension pneumothorax?

With each breath, a person with a tension pneumothorax has a further compromise of the ability of their lungs to expand because of the increasing amount of trapped air inside the chest. In addition, the trapped air in the chest exerts pressure on the veins returning blood to the heart, resulting in dangerous heart failure. A tension pneumothorax is a medical emergency requiring immediate treatment with a chest tube to remove the air from the chest and permit proper expansion of the lungs and return of blood to the heart.

### What happens if an air leak from a damaged lung continues?

If the lung continues to leak air, it may be necessary for a thoracic surgeon to perform an operation in which the tear in the surface of the leaking lung is sewn shut. In some people with very severe lung disease and a hole in the surface of the lung which is leaking air into the space between the lung and the inside wall of the chest, it may be necessary to remove the segment of the lung that is leaking.

# METASTASIS

# BONE METASTASIS

## DEFINITION

### *What is a bone metastasis?*

A bone metastasis is an area of the bone to which cancer has spread. Most commonly, areas of bone metastasis involve the bones of the spine, the pelvis, the ribs, and the bones of the upper arm (the "humerus") or the upper leg (the "femur"). Bone metastasis is a very common, painful, and disabling problem for people with cancer.

## CANCERS THAT SPREAD TO BONE

### *Who gets bone metastasis?*

Cancers of the breast, prostate, lung, and kidney, as well as other cancers, can spread to the bone. Bone metastasis is often the first evidence that a cancer has spread from the area in which it originated. In the great majority of people, bone metastasis is a sign that the cancer, though possibly controllable, is incurable with the medicines that are currently available.

## Can bone metastasis be the first sign that a person has cancer?

Pain associated with a bone metastasis can appear as the first sign that a person has cancer. This is most common when the cancer, from which the bone metastasis originated, that is, the "primary site", only harbors a relatively small cancer, or when the primary site of cancer is not close to areas that are likely to cause obvious symptoms.

## SYMPTOMS

### What are the symptoms of bone metastasis?

Bone metastasis causes pain that is usually right at the spot in the bone which is affected and which worsens with movement. When the first symptoms of bone metastasis appear, the pain generally increases over a period of weeks or months and tends to be worse during the night than during the day. When bone metastasis involves the spine, there may also be pain similar to the pain of "sciatica" which starts in the back and radiates into the legs or buttocks. If the weakened bone fractures, there will be pain that is similar to the pain which any person will feel when they break a bone.

## THE DANGERS OF BONE METASTASIS

### Why is bone metastasis dangerous?

Bone metastasis is painful and can seriously interfere with a person's ability to enjoy day-to-day life and fight their disease

In addition to the problems associated with the pain of bone metastasis, damage to the bones can weaken them, and cause them to fracture with very slight stress. When a bone weakened by cancer fractures, it is called a "pathological fracture". Pathologic fractures in the spine can press on the spinal cord and cause a very dangerous condition called "malignant spinal cord compression" which is discussed in its own chapter later in this book. Destruction of bones in the hips, thighs or upper arms can cause terrible, disabling fractures that do not heal properly.

When a significant portion of the person's skeleton contains areas of bone metastasis, the bones can release calcium into the bloodstream that causes a problem called "malignant hypercalcemia". Malignant hypercalcemia is discussed later in this book in its own chapter.

The center of the bone contains the "bone marrow" which is responsible for making our white and red blood cells and platelets. When the bones are very extensively involved with metastasis, bone marrow replacement by cancer cells causes anemia and a loss of the white blood cells and platelets needed to properly fight infection and prevent abnormal bleeding.

## MAKING THE DIAGNOSIS

### How is the diagnosis of bone metastasis made?

The first evidence of bone metastasis may arise through a blood test that shows an elevation of a substance called "alkaline phosphatase" in the bloodstream. Many other conditions can cause the level of alkaline phosphatase in the bloodstream to be elevated, but in the context of new and increasing bone pain, raises the suspicion of bone metastasis.

When a person has a bone metastasis, an x-ray of the area will often show an area of "lucency" in which normal dense bone has been damaged by the cancer. A bone scan, which uses a radioactive material to spotlight cancer in bones, can show evidence of cancer in bones. If there is any doubt about the diagnosis, a biopsy of the bone can be done (under local anesthesia) by taking a piece of tissue from the bone, and having a pathologist examine the tissue under a microscope.

At times, and especially when there is a suspicion of bone metastasis in the spine, physicians may suggest a CT or MRI scan of the area in which bone metastasis is suspected. A CT or MRI of the spine can give a more precise image and might identify otherwise unseen areas of bone metastasis. Early identification of bone metastasis in the spine is important, because metastasis to the spine has the potential to compress the spinal cord and cause paralysis.

## What if a bone metastasis appears but the "primary site" from which it is originated is unknown?

Each cancer responds in a different way to the different available forms of treatment. It is important to determine, if possible, the area from which the cancer originated.

The primary site from which the cancer originated can usually be determined with blood tests, as well as CT scans of the chest, abdomen, and pelvis, and biopsies of areas that appear to show signs of cancer.

## THE CAUSE OF THE BONE DAMAGE

*What is it that is damaging the bone in*
*an area of bone metastasis?*

The bones in our skeletons are in a constant state of "remodeling" in which new bone is formed by cells called "osteoblasts" and old bone removed by cells called "osteoclasts". When cancer invades the bone, it abnormally activates both the "osteoblasts" and the "osteoclasts". When some types of cancer invade the bone, they can trigger osteoblasts to build up abnormal bone (called "osteoblastic metastasis") which are prone to fracture. Osteoclasts, on the other hand, which are also stimulated by cancer cells, break down bone faster than it can heal, and, combined with the damaging effects of chemicals released by the cancer cells, create "osteolytic metastases". "Metastases" is the plural of "metastasis" and is the word used to describe more than one area of metastasis. These osteolytic metastases can break down bone such that only a shell of what was present before remains. Bones harboring osteolytic metastases, especially in weight bearing bones such as the hips and spine, are prone to fracture.

## IMMEDIATE TREATMENT

*What is the greatest short-term risk of a bone*
*metastasis and what can reduce this risk?*

When a physician evaluates a bone metastasis, an immediate question is whether the bone damage has created an imminent danger of fracture. When a bone breaks because of weakening by cancer, it is a "pathological fracture". If pathologic fracture is an immediate risk, or if it has already occurred, immediate treatment to strengthen the bone is necessary. Once the short-term risk of fracture has averted, treatments to shrink the cancer in the bone, or prevent a worsening of the damage caused by bone metastasis, can be the focus of attention.

Because the pelvis and the femur, which is the bone in the upper leg, bear the full weight of the body when walking, these bones, if weakened, may be especially susceptible to pathologic fractures. When an x-ray of a bone shows a seriously weakened bone, it sometimes helps to have an orthopedic surgeon strengthen the bone with surgical cement or other surgical material in order to prevent a disabling fracture.

The uppermost portion of the femur contains the "femoral head" that fits into a socket in the pelvis, and the "femoral neck" that connects to the remainder of the femur at the "intertrochanteric region". Extensive involvement of this area by metastasis can seriously weaken the femur and expose a person to a high risk of fracture. The most practical way of immediately strengthening this area and relieving the risk of a dangerous fracture may be a partial hip replacement with a device that replaces the damaged area of the femur.

Radiation therapy, directed at a bone metastasis, shrinks the cancer in the bone, relieves pain, and reduces the risk that the bone metastasis will cause a pathologic fracture.

## PAIN MEDICATION

### What types of pain medication can be help relieve the pain of bone metastasis?

When pain is mild, non-steroidal anti-inflammatory medications such as "Naproxen" (commonly sold under the brand name is "Aleve", manufacturer's product website is www.aleve.com) and the different brands of ibuprofen such as "Advil" (manufacturer's product website is www.advil.com), can be helpful. If the pain is more intense, narcotic medications of varying degrees of strength may be required. Steroid medications, such as prednisone, can sometimes diminish the inflammation associated with bone metastasis and provide pain relief.

## TREATMENT THAT CAN PREVENT A METASTASIS FROM FURTHER DAMAGING BONE

### What medication slows or stops metastases from damaging the bones?

A family of medicines called "bisphosphonates", can slow, or stop the damage of a bone metastasis and considerably relieve bone pain. They do this primarily by inhibiting the bone damaging osteoclasts. Common bisphosphonates used by cancer specialists are "zoledronic acid" (brand name is "Zometa", manufacturer's product website is www.zometa.com) and "pamidronate" (brand name is "Aredia"). Zometa or Aredia, along with dietary supplementation with calcium and Vitamin D, can add minerals and strength to the bone.

A biotechnology-derived medication called "denosumab" (brand name is "Xgeva", manufacturer's product website is www.xgeva.com) reduces the risk of "skeletal related events", defined as a broken bone, pain in a bone needing radiation, or malignant spinal cord compression (see chapter entitled "Malignant Spinal Cord Compression"). Xgeva inhibits the development of the bone damaging "osteoclasts", and prevents them from damaging bone. Xgeva is given by an injection under the skin (a "subcutaneous injection") in the arm, abdomen, or thigh, every 4 weeks. Because Xgeva can lower the amount of calcium in the bloodstream, physicians usually prescribe calcium supplements and Vitamin D as well when prescribing Xgeva.

Comparing the effectiveness of Zometa with Xgeva, Xgeva appears to be more effective in preventing or delaying "skeletal related events" in people who have bone metastases. Xgeva is, however, roughly twice as expensive as Zometa, and some physicians question whether the superiority of Xgeva over Zometa is sufficient to make a universal recommendation to use Xgeva instead of Zometa in treating bone metastasis

Both Zometa and Xgeva can have side effects, including a destructive disease of the jawbone called "osteonecrosis of the jaw", which occurs in 1-2% of people receiving these medications. This risk of developing osteonecrosis of the jaw can be somewhat reduced by having preventive dentistry before starting treatment, and by maintaining good oral hygiene and avoiding dental procedures that can injure the jawbone. Zometa, which is given intravenously, can cause infusion reactions (see chapter entitled "Infusion Reactions"), and can be toxic to the kidneys. Xgeva can lower the blood calcium levels to dangerous levels. Physicians monitor a person receiving

Zometa or Xgeva for side effects, and give appropriate treatments if side effects develop.

With the availability of these new, effective treatments, many physicians believe that the best way to prevent the "skeletal-related events", as described above, is by initiating treatment at the first sign of the presence of bone metastases.

## TREATMENT THAT CAN SHRINK CANCER IN THE BONES

### *What kind of treatment can shrink a bone metastasis?*

The two kinds of treatments that shrink a bone metastasis are systemic anti-cancer therapy, or radiation therapy.

### *What systemic anti-cancer therapy is given and when is it useful?*

Systemic anti-cancer therapy that is used will take the form of chemotherapy, hormonal medicines, immune system enhancing therapy, or any other systemic treatments that are known to shrink or suppress the growth of the particular cancer, wherever it is in a person's body.

For most forms of cancer that have spread into the bone, systemic anti-cancer treatments only rarely induce a "complete remission", that is complete eradication of cancer everywhere in the body. Most commonly, cancer that responds to systemic therapy produces a "partial remission", in which the cancer shrinks in size, and symptoms may be relieved, but the cancer does not entirely disappear. Cancers that have shrunk, but not entirely disappeared, usually, at some point, become resistant to treatment. Resumption of growth of cancer in the bones and elsewhere will usually produce symptoms and complications.

## RADIATION THERAPY

### How is radiation therapy given?

Radiation therapy is focused on the specific area of the bone which is causing pain, or undermining the strength and stability of a bone. If, however, the painful bone is a weight bearing bone such as the bone of the upper leg (the "femur"), an orthopedic surgeon can advise whether it would be safer to put surgical cement, or a metal rod, in the hip to stabilize it prior to radiation. With regard to metastasis in the spine, surgical reinforcement of dangerously weakened vertebrae may also be appropriate prior to radiation.

There are many different ways of giving the radiation therapy ranging from one intense day of radiation therapy to three weeks of 5 days of treatment each week. In many circumstances, a single day of radiation may be as effective as the three-week treatment and a lot more convenient.

Radioactive medicines called "samarium-153", and "strontium 89", injected intravenously, can concentrate in bones which contain cancer. The concentration of the radioactive medicine in areas of metastatic cancer in bone can somewhat shrink cancers in bone and relieve some of the pain caused by bone metastases. These radioactive medications suppress the bone marrow's production of white blood cells and platelets, and can be dangerous if a person's ability to produce white blood cells and platelets has been limited by previous treatments or by extensive involvement of bone marrow with cancer.

## What are the side effects of radiation therapy of areas of bone metastasis?

When a bone is irradiated, the bone marrow (which produces the body's white blood cells, red blood cells, and platelets) inside that bone is also irradiated. When a person has extensive cancer, or has recently received chemotherapy or other radiation treatments, he or she is at risk of developing bone marrow suppression and a weakened immune system after radiation therapy. The risk of bone marrow suppression often limits the ability to irradiate too many different areas of bone involved with metastasis.

## OUTLOOK

## How effective is treatment of areas of bone metastasis?

The best treatment of areas of areas of bone metastasis is to administer treatment that can cure a person's cancer. Because this is rarely accomplished, the most effective therapy is generally limited to treatment directed at areas of bone metastasis, and which can give pain relief and prevent pathological fractures.

About half of the people who receive focused radiation therapy to an area of bone metastasis can have complete relief of pain in the area where the bone is irradiated. Most of the remainder of people with bone metastasis will have some significant, though not complete pain relief. Pain starts diminishing within about two weeks of beginning radiation therapy and continues to diminish over the next month or so. After radiation therapy has eradicated an area of cancer in the bone, the bone can heal and become strong again.

Surgical procedures to stabilize bones in the hip, pelvis, vertebrae, or elsewhere are quite effective in preventing fractures and in relieving pain, once the area operated on has healed.

> ### What effect does bone metastasis have on a person's longevity?

With the exception of a few cancers (metastatic testicular cancer, for example) bone metastasis usually means incurable cancer. However, many people with bone metastasis, especially people with metastatic breast cancer or metastatic prostate cancer, can live for many years after the diagnosis of bone metastasis. With some of the newer forms of cancer treatment currently under development, we can hope and expect that people with bone metastasis will soon have longer survival with therapy and, occasionally, have a cure of their disease.

# BRAIN METASTASIS

## DEFINITION

### *What is brain metastasis?*

Brain metastasis (also called "metastatic brain tumor") is cancer that has spread from elsewhere in the body to the brain.

### *From which cancers is brain metastasis most likely to originate?*

Most commonly, cancer that has spread to the brain originated in the lung, breast or kidney, or from a melanoma, although a brain metastasis can originate from almost any form of cancer.

## SYMPTOMS

### *What are the symptoms of brain metastasis?*

The first symptoms a person has because of a brain metastasis will vary depending on where in the brain the metastasis is located.

Headache is the most common early symptom. The headache can be most severe in the morning, more in the front of the head than the back, and more on one side of the head than on the other. A sense of nausea accompanying the headache can be present.

Neurologic function, which reflects the area of the brain where the tumor is located, may be affected. For example, if the tumor involves an area of the brain that controls movement of one side of the body, there may be weakness of that side of the body. If the tumor involves the area of the brain that controls vision, there may be visual disturbances.

Seizures can be a first sign of the presence of brain metastasis (please see chapter entitled "Seizures"). The ability to move, to sense, to think, to speak, or any of the countless functions performed continually by the normal brain can be severely affected.

## MAKING THE DIAGNOSIS

### How is the diagnosis of brain metastasis made?

When a person has symptoms suggestive of brain metastasis, a CT or MRI scan of the brain will generally be the key test that a physician will recommend. These scans will show a tumor, or in medical language, a "mass lesion" wherever it is located in the brain. The scans cannot define the precise nature of the "mass lesion", although the location and appearance of the mass lesion, especially if there are multiple lesions, can raise a high suspicion of the presence of brain metastasis.

A medical history, physical examination, routine blood chemistry panels, a chest x-ray, and a CT scan of the chest, can identify, or raise the suspicion of, the presence of a new cancer outside of the brain. If this work-up fails to identify a cancer outside of the brain, consideration will be given to having a surgeon remove a piece of the tumor for examination under the microscope, that is, of obtaining a "brain biopsy".

There are important differences in the way the different types of malignant brain tumors are treated. A biopsy of the brain lesion makes the precise diagnosis.

## Is a brain biopsy always necessary?

When a single "mass lesion" develops in a person with a history of cancer, physicians may recommend a brain biopsy to be sure that the mass lesion is a brain metastasis. Although brain metastasis may be the more likely diagnosis, other causes of the "mass lesion", such as benign or malignant brain tumors, or inflammation or infection, can give an appearance on MRI that is similar to a brain metastasis. Because these other conditions have very different treatment, and because the outlook for these conditions is so vastly different from the outlook with brain metastasis, the biopsy may be critical and necessary.

People with cancer of the lung, breast or other organs who have already had a confirmed spread of their cancer into other body organs and who develop a "mass lesion" in the brain usually have a brain metastasis. If many mass lesions are present in the brain, and especially in a person who has had lung cancer or melanoma, the great likelihood is that these lesions are brain metastases ("metastases" is the plural of "metastasis" and is the word used to describe more than one area of metastasis). In these circumstances, a biopsy is often not necessary to make a reasonably definitive diagnosis.

### *How does a neurosurgeon obtain a brain biopsy?*

Depending on the location and size of the lesion or lesions, as well as the probability, based upon the MRI scan, that the lesions can be completely removed, the goal of the neurosurgeon may not only be to perform the biopsy, but to remove each of the tumors. In order to perform this procedure, a "craniotomy" (in which the neurosurgeon makes a hole in the skull and operates on the brain) may be performed with the goal of making the diagnosis and removing as many of the lesions as possible in the same operation.

There are circumstances where the neurosurgeon believes that removal of the metastasis or multiple metastases is too dangerous or where it is not clear that removal of the metastasis or metastases is possible. A procedure called a "stereotactic biopsy" may be done in which a very tiny hole is made in the skull and a fine needle is passed deep into the brain with the guidance of a CT or MRI scan. Using this technique, the neurosurgeon is usually able to remove enough tumor tissue to allow a pathologist to examine the tissue under a microscope and make a precise diagnosis.

## TREATMENT OF BRAIN METASTASIS

### *When is surgery a useful treatment of brain metastasis?*

If the cancer is under control elsewhere in the body, and if, aside from the brain metastasis, the person's general state of health is good, surgical removal of one or more brain metastases may be very helpful in relieving symptoms and extending life. The ability to perform the surgery safely and without an unacceptable risk of the surgery causing brain damage depends upon the size and location of the brain metastases.

## What is radiosurgery and when is it useful?

Radiosurgery, sometimes referred to as the "gamma knife", involves the use of intense and highly focused radiation to destroy a dangerous abnormality, such as a metastatic brain tumor. For this to be an effective option, the one or several areas of brain metastasis targeted by radiosurgery must be small enough for the beam of radiation to entirely destroy the area of cancer without causing damage to surrounding normal brain. In many circumstances, radiosurgery is an important alternative to surgical removal of one or more areas of brain metastasis.

## What can be done to prevent recurrence of the brain metastasis after surgery or radiosurgery?

Radiation delivered to the entire brain (called "whole brain irradiation") can reduce the risk of recurrence of brain metastasis. This reduced risk of brain recurrence does not, however, appear to improve the likelihood of longer survival or lengthen the time until a person with cancer is not capable of self-care (called "functional independence"). Whole brain radiation can cause memory loss and learning disabilities. With the questionable benefit and possible side effects from the whole brain radiation, physicians may recommend following a person with frequent CT or MRI scans, treating localized recurrences, should they occur, with further surgery or radiosurgery, and reserving whole brain irradiation for situations in which local control with surgery or radiosurgery is not possible.

### What is the treatment of metastatic brain tumors when surgery is not appropriate?

Whole brain irradiation can transiently shrink areas of cancer in the brain and relieve some symptoms of the metastatic brain tumors.

Commonly, a person with brain metastasis has cancer elsewhere in the body that is not adequately controlled. Optimal treatment would consist of a therapy, such as chemotherapy, that effectively controls the cancer wherever it may be in the body, including the brain. Unfortunately, this effective treatment may not be available.

### If treatment is not available to control the growth of the cancer in the brain, what treatment can diminish or control symptoms of brain metastasis?

If the cancer is not controlled, it will be important to take whatever measures are possible to increase a person's comfort and to reduce the effects of the cancer in the brain.

Two major problems caused by a metastatic brain tumor that can benefit from available treatments are the swelling of the brain ("cerebral edema") near the cancer and the incidence of seizures. A steroid medication called "dexamethasone", which is more commonly called "Decadron", reduces some of the brain swelling. Many commonly used antiepileptic medications can prevent, or reduce the frequency of, seizures associated with the metastatic brain tumors.

## What is the outlook for a person with a metastatic brain tumor?

If the neurosurgeon can entirely remove the areas of brain metastasis, and if the cancer outside of the brain is well controlled, the outlook for survival can be quite good. Otherwise, a person with brain metastasis that is not treatable or not responding to treatment generally has a short survival time, with the length of survival reflecting the size and location of the cancers in the brain, and the extent to which the cancer has spread elsewhere in the body.

# LEPTOMENINGEAL METASTASIS

## DEFINITIONS

### *What are the leptomeninges?*

Three layers of membranes, called the "meninges", surround the brain and the spinal cord. The innermost layer is the "pia mater", which is Latin for "tender mother", reflecting the delicacy with which the pia mater adheres to the brain and spinal cord, encloses the nourishing and protective cerebrospinal fluid, and allows blood vessels and nerves to pass in and out. The second layer is the arachnoid mater, whose spidery connections (hence the name "arachnoid") connect the pia mater to the outer most layer, the dura mater. Together the pia mater and the arachnoid mater are the "leptomeninges". The "subarachnoid space" is between the pia mater and the arachnoid mater, and contains the cerebrospinal fluid.

### *What is leptomeningeal metastasis?*

Leptomeningeal metastasis is the spread of cancer from elsewhere in the body to the leptomeninges. Although breast cancer, lung cancer, lymphoma, and melanoma are the most likely cancers to spread to the leptomeninges, almost any form of cancer can spread to the leptomeninges.

## How does cerebrospinal fluid flow in and around the brain?

Cerebrospinal fluid forms in cavities in the brain called "ventricles". The largest of these cavities are the lateral ventricles, which are inside the right and left side of the brain. Cerebrospinal fluid formed there flows down into the third ventricle and then into the fourth ventricle, from which, through openings called "foramina", the cerebrospinal fluid flows into the subarachnoid space. Cerebrospinal fluid in the subarachnoid space will then bathe the entire surface of the brain and spinal cord.

## SYMPTOMS AND COMPLICATIONS OF LEPTOMENINGEAL METASTASIS

### Why is leptomeningeal metastasis dangerous?

When cancer grows in the leptomeninges and subarachnoid space, it can obstruct the pathways by which cerebrospinal fluid flows. When this happens, continued production of cerebrospinal fluid in the ventricles, and obstruction of the flow of cerebrospinal fluid out of the ventricles, can cause pressure inside the ventricles to rise. This increased pressure is "hydrocephalus" and can seriously damage the brain.

Cranial nerves that emerge from the brainstem, which is the lowest area of brain, control the ability to see, smell, hear, swallow, and move the face. Spinal nerves enter or exit the spinal cord and control sensation and the ability to move every portion of the body below the neck. Leptomeningeal metastasis can damage these nerves and severely impair their function.

Because blood vessels enter and exit the brain through the subarachnoid space, leptomeningeal metastasis can interfere with the normal movement of blood to and from the brain, causing damage to vital structures inside the brain.

When a leptomeningeal metastasis adheres to the surface of the brain, it can grow inward and compress or directly injure the brain, impairing its functions.

## What are the symptoms of leptomeningeal metastasis?

The symptoms of leptomeningeal metastasis reflect the dangerous problems it can cause to normal brain functioning.

Obstruction of cerebrospinal fluid flow and hydrocephalus can cause severe headache, as well as nausea and vomiting. As the pressure increases, the person can become very confused and ultimately comatose.

When leptomeningeal metastasis affects the cranial nerves, weakness of the muscles that move the eyes or control the movements of the face can develop. A common symptom of cranial nerve involvement with leptomeningeal metastasis is double vision. If leptomeningeal metastasis involves the nerves entering or exiting the spinal cord, there may be pain associated with the nerve irritation as well as inability to move the areas of the body controlled by those nerves. Normal bladder functioning may be seriously impaired. Pain associated with spinal nerve irritation is a very common symptom of leptomeningeal metastasis.

Invasion of the brain by the cancer or blockage of arteries entering the brain can cause local areas of damage that may produce associated symptoms such as weakness on one side of the body or visual disturbances.

## DIAGNOSIS OF LEPTOMENINGEAL METASTASIS

### What tests confirm the diagnosis of leptomeningeal metastasis?

A MRI scan of the brain and spinal cord will usually provide strong evidence of the presence of leptomeningeal metastasis. The diagnosis is confirmed when cancer cells are identified in cerebrospinal fluid obtained by a spinal tap.

## TREATMENT OF LEPTOMENINGEAL METASTASIS

### What is the common treatment of leptomeningeal metastasis?

Leptomeningeal metastasis usually develops in the context of cancer that already has spread elsewhere in the body. Treatment decisions for a person with leptomeningeal metastasis must assess the likelihood that treatment can extend life and improve life without causing difficult side effects.

If cancer elsewhere in the body is not advanced, treatment may relieve symptoms and extend life. This treatment can include radiation to regions of the brain in which cerebrospinal fluid flow appears to be blocked, radiation to areas of the spinal cord causing painful symptoms, and, occasionally, injection of chemotherapy directly into the cerebrospinal fluid. A steroid medication called "Decadron" can relieve increased pressure in the brain caused by hydrocephalus or brain swelling. If a person has developed hydrocephalus, as described earlier in this chapter, and symptoms are not relieved by this treatment, a plastic tube called a "ventriculoperitoneal shunt" can be inserted that carries spinal fluid from the ventricles of the brain into the abdomen, thereby relieving pressure in the brain. This shunt can have many side effects and is generally reserved for situations in which radiation and chemotherapy are ineffective, or in which a medical emergency requires placement of this shunt.

If the cancer is very far advanced, and survival because of cancer outside of the brain is very limited, treatment will focus upon relief of discomfort without subjecting a person to aggressive treatments.

## OUTLOOK FOR PEOPLE WITH LEPTOMENINGEAL METASTASIS

*What is the outlook for people with leptomeningeal metastasis?*

The outlook depends upon the extent to which cancer has spread elsewhere in the body and the responsiveness of the cancer to radiation or chemotherapy. If the cancer elsewhere in the body is not extensive and the cancer responds to radiation and chemotherapy, survival for months or longer is possible. If, however, the cancer is very advanced and unresponsive to treatment, the expected survival is most often only a few weeks.

# LIVER METASTASIS

## DEFINITION

*What is liver metastasis?*

Liver metastasis is the spread of cancer from elsewhere in the body to the liver. Although liver metastasis can arise from almost any form of cancer, the most common cancer that produces liver metastasis is colon cancer.

## SYMPTOMS

*What are the symptoms of liver metastasis?*

The extent to which a person with liver metastasis has symptoms is very variable. Many people with liver metastasis have no symptoms at all, or have vague abdominal discomfort that can be consistent with a wide range of other medical problems. When liver metastasis is advanced, a person can develop weight loss, fatigue, or a sense of bloating and discomfort in the abdomen. With very extensive liver metastasis, the yellowish eyes and skin that are the characteristics of jaundice can develop.

## <u>MAKING THE DIAGNOSIS</u>

### *What tests confirm the presence of liver metastasis?*

The routine blood chemistry panel used to assess a person's general health includes "liver function tests", often abbreviated as "LFT's", that assess the normal functions of the liver and that can identify early evidence of liver damage. When cancer involves the liver, damaged liver cells, or blockage of the flow of bile from the liver into the intestine, can cause release of "liver enzymes" from the liver into the bloodstream. Elevated levels of "liver enzymes", found with a routine blood test, are often the first sign of liver metastasis.

When liver metastasis is suspected, physicians will often suggest further evaluation with a CT or MRI scan of the abdomen, which can determine the presence and extent of metastasis in the liver, and identify evidence of spread of the cancer elsewhere in the abdomen.

## <u>WHEN LIVER METASTASIS IS THE FIRST SIGN A PERSON HAS CANCER</u>

### *Can liver metastasis be the first sign that a person has cancer?*

Liver metastasis, especially from a previously undetected colon cancer, can be the first sign a person has cancer.

### *Does it make a difference where the liver metastasis has come from?*

There are major differences in treatments given for cancer that has spread to the liver from the different areas of the body. For example, the treatment of liver metastasis from colon cancer is different from the treatment of liver metastasis from lung cancer. When liver metastasis develops in the absence of a previous history of a cancer from which the metastasis is likely to have originated, a critical next step will be to discover the origin of the metastasis.

## What does it mean when physicians refer to the "primary site"?

The primary site refers to the area from which the cancer originated. For example, if the cancer originated in the lung, the primary site would be the lung. The liver and any other organs to which the cancer has spread are "secondary sites".

## What tests can identify the primary site?

The most common source of liver metastasis is from a cancer of the colon. Because of this, an initial test performed may be "colonoscopy" in which an instrument, inserted from the anus into the colon, enables the physician to examine the inside of the colon either directly through the instrument or through images projected onto a video monitor. With colonoscopy, the physician can examine the inside of the colon and, if necessary, take out snips of abnormal appearing tissue for examination under the microscope. These "biopsies" can give conclusive evidence of the presence of a cancer of the colon.

CT or MRI scans of the chest or abdomen can identify cancers in the lung, pancreas, or other organs from which the cancer may have originated. Examination of the breasts can identify previously undetected breast cancer, although it is very unusual for a breast cancer to make its initial presence known as a liver metastasis. Examination of the skin may detect a previously unnoticed melanoma. Blood tests can show elevations of substances in the bloodstream that may be more likely to be associated with one cancer or another.

If, despite these tests, the primary site is still unknown, a liver biopsy may be necessary. The liver biopsy is done by putting a biopsy needle through the skin (under local anesthesia) and into the liver and pulling out a tiny piece of liver tissue. Examination of the tissue under the microscope can confirm the diagnosis of liver metastasis and provide information required to determine the most likely primary site.

## SURGICAL TREATMENT OF LIVER METASTASIS

*Is cancer curable after liver metastasis has developed?*

Some uncommon cancers that have spread to the liver, such as testicular cancer, are curable with chemotherapy. For the great majority of cancers, however, the only treatment available that can cure the cancer, is surgical removal ("surgical resection") of the areas of liver metastasis. The surgery to remove one or more areas of liver metastasis can be technically difficult, and requires the appropriate level of skill and experience from the physicians and other medical professionals who will provide care during and after the surgery.

## How do physicians evaluate the possibility that a person's cancer is curable by resection of all areas of liver metastasis?

Resection of liver metastasis can only cure a person's cancer if, after the surgery, all evident cancer has been eliminated from the body. For this reason, initial evaluation will focus on whether cancer has spread to areas of the body other than the liver, and whether this spread, as well as the liver metastasis, is curable with surgery. For example, if the MRI scan identifies both liver metastasis and lung metastasis, cure is still possible by surgically removing both the liver metastasis and lung metastasis. If, however, the cancer has spread beyond the liver in a way that is not curable by surgery, resection of the liver metastasis is unlikely to cure the cancer.

The liver has a remarkable ability to regenerate and repair itself after surgical removal of large portions of it. For this reason, extensive involvement of the liver may not prevent an attempt at potentially curative surgery. If the MRI scan, however, shows involvement of the major blood vessels feeding the liver or passing through the liver, surgical resection of liver metastasis may be difficult or impossible.

## Can chemotherapy reduce the size of the cancer, allowing a later attempt at surgical cure, when surgical resection appears to be difficult or impossible?

Chemotherapy, especially for liver metastasis from colon cancer, has the potential to reduce the size and extent of liver metastasis and "convert" liver metastasis from "unresectable" to "resectable" and curable with surgery.

### Do physicians recommend chemotherapy to prevent the return of cancer after the surgery?

Although the surgery may remove all evident cancer, microscopic areas of cancer may remain. For this reason, recurrence of the cancer after potentially curative surgeon commonly occurs.

In an attempt to prevent this recurrence, physicians commonly recommend that a person receive several months of chemotherapy after the surgery. The benefit of this chemotherapy and the optimum chemotherapy treatment for each form of cancer is still under evaluation.

## TREATMENT WHEN SURGICAL CURE IS NOT POSSIBLE

### What treatment is available if surgical resection is not an option?

If surgery is not an option, several available methods can treat a localized area of cancer in the liver. These methods involve destroying the cancer either with high heat or extreme cold, or with injection of various chemicals into the liver metastasis.

A relatively common method used at sophisticated medical centers is "radiofrequency ablation". This treatment involves inserting a probe into the liver metastasis that delivers a high frequency current. This current heats up and destroys the liver metastasis. Radiofrequency ablation is particularly useful if there are only a few areas of liver metastasis that are less than 1½ inches or so in diameter.

*What is the treatment of liver metastasis*
*when surgery, radiofrequency ablation or other*
*local treatments will not be appropriate or useful?*

When a person has liver metastasis that cannot be treated by local measures, or when liver metastasis are present along with metastasis elsewhere in the body, the treatment most likely to be useful will be chemotherapy or other forms of treatment, that can control cancer wherever it is in the body.

# LUNG METASTASIS

## DEFINITION

### What is lung metastasis?

Lung metastasis is the spread of a cancer that originated elsewhere in the body to one or both lungs.

## SYMPTOMS

### What are the symptoms of lung metastasis?

In its early stages, lung metastasis most often produces no symptoms. Symptoms, if present, might include cough, a vague pain in the chest, and some sense of shortness of breath.

## MAKING THE DIAGNOSIS

### What first raises the suspicion of lung metastasis?

When a person has had previous treatment for cancer, a chest x-ray, performed at regular intervals, remains one of the most simple and important tests that can identify evidence of cancer recurrence. If lung metastasis develops, it appears on the x-ray as discrete, somewhat round spots, referred to by physicians as "nodules". When only one such nodule is present, it is a "solitary pulmonary nodule".

A CT scan may provide additional vital information regarding the size, shape, location, and number of nodules in the lungs. The appearance of the nodules with the CT scan can confirm the likelihood that the nodules are lung metastasis, and assess whether surgery can remove all the nodules.

### Is a biopsy of the nodule necessary to confirm the diagnosis of lung metastasis?

Although a biopsy is the surest way to confirm a diagnosis of lung metastasis, there is risk, expense, and discomfort associated with the biopsy. A biopsy may not be necessary if the type of cancer for which a person has had previous treatment, its tendency to spread to the lung, and its response to previous treatment, makes the diagnosis of lung metastasis obvious.

An additional important consideration is whether the confirmation of lung metastasis will change a person's treatment. For example, if multiple lung nodules are present in a person already receiving chemotherapy for cancer elsewhere in the body, a biopsy to confirm lung metastasis is unlikely to change the treatment that is given.

### Is a biopsy necessary when a person with a previous history of cancer develops a "solitary pulmonary nodule"?

A solitary pulmonary nodule in a person with a previous history of cancer very commonly is a "primary lung cancer", that is, a new cancer that began in the lung. A solitary pulmonary nodule that is a primary lung cancer will require very different treatment than if that nodule is a lung metastasis. For this reason, the development of a solitary pulmonary nodule, in the absence of other evidence of spread of a person's previous cancer, requires appropriate evaluation, often including a biopsy of the nodule.

### How is the lung nodule biopsied?

The most common ways that the lung nodule is biopsied is either through "bronchoscopy", "CT directed needle biopsy", or though surgery. Discussion of "bronchoscopy" and "CT directed needle biopsy" as a method of making a lung cancer diagnosis is in the chapter of this book entitled "Lung Cancer".

## SURGICAL TREATMENT OF LUNG METASTASIS

### How is the decision regarding an attempt to cure a person's cancer by removing the lung metastasis made?

Removal of one or more areas of lung metastasis is a "metastasectomy". For this operation to be successful, the cancer from which the metastasis originated must be under control and must not have spread to other areas of the body. If, based upon the CT scan, the "thoracic surgeon" who would perform the operation believes that complete removal of the nodules can be accomplished, and that a person's underlying health is sufficient to withstand the surgery, consideration will be given to proceeding with the metastasectomy and attempting to cure the cancer.

## TREATMENT WHEN SURGICAL
## CURE IS NOT AN OPTION

*Besides surgery, what other treatments are available for lung metastasis?*

If a person has only a few areas of lung metastasis, a beam of radiation focused on the areas of lung metastasis can often shrink that local area of cancer and prevent its further growth. This focused radiation is "stereotactic body radiation therapy" and is administered in doses given over several days.

At some sophisticated medical centers, a treatment called "radiofrequency ablation" is available. This treatment involves inserting a probe delivering a high frequency current directly into the lung metastasis. This current heats up and destroys the lung metastasis. The FDA has issued a "Public Health Notification", indicating that radiofrequency ablation of lung tumors can cause death or serious injury and has not yet received specific FDA approval for the treatment of lung tumors. Despite this warning from the FDA, some physicians believe that radiofrequency ablation, if done correctly and by very experienced medical centers, can provide a great deal of benefit for some people with lung metastasis.

*What is the treatment of lung metastasis when surgery, radiation, or radiofrequency ablation will not be appropriate or useful?*

"Metastases" is the plural of "metastasis" and is the word used to describe more than one area of metastasis. When a person has many lung metastases involving one or both lungs, local measures such as surgery, radiation, or radiofrequency ablation are unlikely to be helpful. The treatment most likely to be useful will be chemotherapy or other forms of treatment that can control cancer wherever it is in the body.

# KIDNEY FAILURE AND MULTIPLE ORGAN FAILURE

# ACUTE KIDNEY INJURY

## DEFINITION

### *What role do the kidneys play in preserving health?*

The kidneys play a lead role in removing wastes and unnecessary fluid from the bloodstream and the body. The kidneys regulate the body's content of sodium, potassium and acid, and produce hormones that regulate blood pressure, stimulate the production of red blood cells, and help regulate the content of calcium in the bloodstream.

### *What is acute kidney injury?*

Acute kidney injury is a sudden and sustained failure of normal functioning of the kidneys. Acute kidney injury, which in the past, was more commonly and somewhat less accurately called "acute renal failure", is a common complication of many serious sudden illnesses, and is particularly common in critically ill people admitted to intensive care units.

### *How do the kidneys make urine?*

The heart pumps blood into the aorta, which, through its many arterial branches, supplies blood to all the organs of the body. The branches that supply the kidneys are the "renal arteries". Inside the kidney, the renal arteries break down into smaller and smaller branches until they become tiny blood vessels called a "glomerulus" (the plural of "glomerulus" is "glomeruli"). Blood enters the glomerulus where filtration of larger waste products occurs, and fluid that remains passes into a structure called the "renal tubule". In the renal tubule, depending on the body's needs, additional waste products, chemicals, or water are actively removed into the tubules or absorbed back into the body, The fluid that remains in the tubules is delivered into "collecting ducts" which empty into the center of the kidney in an area called the "renal pelvis". This fluid, which is now urine, moves to the ureters, which carry the urine downward to the bladder, then to the urethra, then out of the body.

## SYMPTOMS

### What are the symptoms of acute kidney injury?

The diagnosis of acute kidney failure can become apparent when a person with another serious illness has the typical abnormalities of acute kidney injury discovered through a routine blood test.

A person with acute kidney injury may notice a dramatic decrease in the volume of their urine. As acute kidney injury progresses, nausea, vomiting, shortness of breath, lethargy and confusion can develop.

## MAKING THE DIAGNOSIS

### How is the diagnosis of acute kidney injury made?

The diagnosis of acute kidney injury is generally made by a simple blood test which measures the level of "creatinine" in the bloodstream (called "serum creatinine") and by an assessment of the amount of urine a person is producing (the "urine output").

Assessment of the serum creatinine and the urine output allows physicians to make further important determinations with regard to the severity of the acute kidney injury. A common method by which hospital-based physicians judge the severity of acute kidney injury is the "RIFLE" criteria. "R" means that a person is at "Risk", because their creatinine is somewhat elevated and their urine output has dropped significantly for six hours or less. "I" means that "Injury" has occurred, that serum creatinine is even more elevated, and urine output has dropped for 12 hours. "F" means that the kidneys are failing, with yet higher levels of serum creatinine and an abnormally low urine output for over 24 hours, or no urine at all for 12 hours. The "L" and the "E" refer to long term outcome, with "L" meaning "Loss" of kidney function for over 4 weeks, and "E" meaning "End-stage kidney disease" with permanent loss of kidney function.

## THE CAUSES OF ACUTE KIDNEY INJURY

### What causes acute kidney injury?

To make urine three essential things must happen.

First, blood travels to the kidney where tiny capillaries called "glomeruli" filter waste products from the blood stream. Inadequate blood flow to the kidney causes "pre-renal acute kidney injury", also known as "pre-renal azotemia" ("azotemia" is the technical word for metabolic wastes in the bloodstream that collect because of kidney failure).

Second, the glomeruli and renal tubules described earlier in this chapter create the urine. Severe problems with production of urine within the kidney itself cause "intrinsic" or "intrarenal" acute kidney injury.

Third, urine must flow from the kidney to the ureters to the bladder to the urethra and then, to the outside world. Blockage of flow of urine from the kidney causes "post-renal acute kidney injury", also called "post-renal azotemia".

Because the treatment of each type of acute kidney injury is different, it is important to identify the cause of the acute kidney injury as quickly as possible. Prompt treatment of the specific cause of the acute kidney injury will give the best chance for recovery of kidney function.

## PRE-RENAL AZOTEMIA

### What causes pre-renal azotemia?

Pre-renal azotemia results from an inadequate flow of blood into the kidney. Sepsis and septic shock (see chapter entitled "Sepsis and Septic Shock") leading to pre-renal azotemia is the most common cause of acute kidney injury in people with cancer.

Three key factors can compromise blood flow to the kidneys and lead to pre-renal azotemia.

First, the heart must sustain proper blood flow to the kidneys. If the force with which the heart contracts is weakened by sepsis or septic shock or is weakened from other causes such as a heart attack, blood flow to the kidneys can be impaired and pre-renal azotemia can result.

Second, reduction of blood pressure or the volume of blood in the bloodstream can seriously compromise circulation of blood to the kidneys. Sepsis and septic shock can lower blood pressure, significantly impairing delivery of blood to the kidney. Massive internal bleeding, such as from upper GI bleeding (see chapter with that title) reduces blood volume. "Plasma", which is the liquid component of blood in which the blood cells are floating, constitutes about half of the volume of our blood and its loss, because of sepsis, vomiting, diarrhea, or diuretics, contracts the blood volume, reducing circulation to the kidneys.

Third, if the heart is pumping adequately, and the volume of blood is sufficient, an impediment to blood getting through the arteries feeding the kidneys can cause pre-renal azotemia. A number of medications can constrict the arteries feeding the kidneys and impair blood flow to them.

### How is the diagnosis of pre-renal azotemia made?

When acute kidney injury develops associated with a low blood pressure or major bleeding, the acute kidney injury is usually pre-renal azotemia.

Examination of the levels of electrolytes in the urine can help make the diagnosis of pre-renal azotemia. When blood pressure or blood volume is low, the body often compensates by actively absorbing sodium from the urine, which helps bring blood pressure back up. With some important exceptions, if the level of sodium in the urine decreases, it is suggestive of pre-renal azotemia. The test often performed to examine this is the "fractional excretion of sodium".

When there is doubt, a "fluid challenge", that is, extra fluid administered by vein, increases the production of urine (the "urine output") and points to a diagnosis of pre-renal azotemia.

### What is the treatment of pre-renal azotemia?

The treatment will depend on the cause and severity of the pre-renal azotemia.

If pre-renal azotemia is mild, and a consequence of loss of plasma as described above, fluid replacement with salt solutions such as "half-normal saline" or "normal saline" may be adequate to restore normal blood flow to the kidney and reverse the pre-renal azotemia. With changes in fluid administration, vigilance is required to assure that an inadvertent excess of fluid does not lead to blood volume overexpansion and heart failure or to dangerously high blood pressure.

Circulatory shock is a major reduction in blood pressure that diminishes the vital supply of blood to the kidney and other major body organs. If circulatory shock develops, intensive care is required.

### What treatment can restore kidney function if circulatory shock develops?

A first step often taken in the treatment of circulatory shock is to insert a catheter called a "Swan-Ganz catheter" through a vein in the arm, shoulder, or groin. From there, physicians advance the catheter through the circulatory system until it reaches the right side of the heart. The Swan-Ganz catheter can then transmit signals to a bedside computer and give precise measurements of pressures in various areas of the heart. These pressures provide the medical staff with information that guides treatment of circulatory shock.

Blood pressure monitoring with a catheter inserted in an artery (an "arterial line") also allows the medical staff to withdraw blood from the artery to see how well the lungs are providing oxygen to the bloodstream.

Determination of the extent to which the blood volume is diminished (a low blood volume is called "hypovolemia") is made by assessment of the blood pressure and by measurements of pressures of the blood inside the heart provided by the Swan-Ganz catheter. The treatment of hypovolemia is to give more fluid by vein and then closely monitor the effect of this administered fluid therapy on the blood pressure, the Swan-Ganz catheter measurements of pressures in the heart, and by measuring a person's production of urine (the "urine output").

If blood pressure is still very low after fluid treatment, several different intravenous medicines can bring the blood pressure up. Intravenous medicines that bring blood pressure up are "pressors". "Dopamine" and "dobutamine" and "norepinephrine" are the most common pressors which physicians prescribe when they attempt to raise the blood pressure of a person with circulatory shock.

# RENAL AZOTEMIA

## *What can cause renal azotemia?*

The principal kidney structures producing urine, described earlier in this chapter, are the "glomeruli" and "renal tubules". Glomeruli and tubules work together in a highly complex way to produce urine in adequate volume, and with an adequate composition to keep the body's fluid and electrolyte system in proper balance.

Prolonged lack of blood supply can cause severe damage to the kidney's microscopic tubules. This condition, called "acute tubular necrosis", can follow an episode of prolonged low blood pressure. Unusual reactions to medication can also damage these tubules. The radiologist's dye (called "contrast material") used to perform CT or MRI scans can damage the renal tubules and can rarely cause acute kidney injury. Antibiotics such as "gentamicin" or "amikacin" and "tobramycin" or chemotherapy with "cisplatin" may be essential and life saving, but also carry some risk of damaging these tubules and producing renal azotemia.

Contents of cancer cells, particularly the contents of lymphoma or leukemia cells, can be released into the bloodstream, after the destruction of these cells by chemotherapy. These contents can damage the kidney and cause renal azotemia.

## *What is the treatment of renal azotemia?*

Successful treatment of renal azotemia is largely dependent upon identifying and effectively treating or removing the precise factor or factors that caused the acute kidney injury, along with supportive measures used for any person with acute kidney injury (see below).

## POST-RENAL AZOTEMIA

### What causes post-renal azotemia?

The cause of post-renal azotemia is an obstruction of the flow of urine anywhere from the kidney downward to the ureter, bladder or urethra. Cancer, kidney stones, as well as blood clots can block the ureters from delivering urine from the kidney to the bladder.

### How is the cause of post-renal azotemia identified?

When there is an obstruction to the flow of urine at the level of the ureter or below, urine produced by the kidney backs up, and the ureter and the renal pelvis (see description earlier in this chapter) will enlarge. This enlargement of the renal pelvis is "hydronephrosis" and is visible with an ultrasound examination. To provide additional information about the exact cause of the post-renal azotemia, a physician may recommend that a person have a "retrograde pyelogram" in which a dye is put into the bladder and up into the ureters. This can give a clear image of any blockage that may be present in the ureters.

Before this initial testing, there may be a strong suspicion, based upon a person's symptoms and a rather sudden complete lack of urine output that an obstruction exists below the bladder. A catheter put up the urethra and into the bladder may get through this blockage, produce an enormous outflow of urine, and clear the obstruction.

## What is the treatment of post-renal azotemia?

If post-renal azotemia is caused by an obstruction between the urethra and the bladder, having a physician insert a catheter into the bladder relieves the obstruction and allows urine to drain.

If the obstruction is at the level of the "ureter", that is, the connection between the kidney and the bladder, a physician, using a scope that allows a clear view of the bladder and ureters, can insert a "stent", which is a tube, up into the ureter and across the obstruction. This props the obstructed area open, allowing urine to flow again down the ureter and into the bladder.

In very frail people with advanced cancer, or when there is severe compression of the ureters unlikely to be safely treated with a stent, a physician may recommend "percutaneous nephrostomy". Percutaneous nephrostomy means that, using ultrasound as a guide, a small plastic tube is put through the skin in the lower back into the kidney. This tube can then drain urine from the kidney into a drainage bag.

## TREATMENT OF PROBLEMS CAUSED BY ACUTE KIDNEY INJURY

### Besides identifying and treating the cause of the acute kidney injury, what treatment is helpful for a person with acute kidney injury?

One of the keys to successful treatment of acute kidney injury is close management of a person's fluid and electrolyte status. This involves closely monitoring the amount of fluid a person takes in by mouth and by vein, and monitoring the amount of fluid the person excretes in the urine and elsewhere (this is referred to as "input and output" or, by the abbreviation ("I and O"). A simple daily weight check can give some assessment of whether a person is retaining too much fluid. Blood tests will closely follow a person's blood levels of sodium, potassium, phosphate, bicarbonate, and calcium. Abnormalities of any of these electrolytes will be treated and corrected.

A special diet low in protein, high in carbohydrates and moderate in fats can help limit the body's accumulation of some waste products normally filtered by the kidneys.

### What happens if despite these measures, serious fluid and electrolyte problems persist and are difficult to control?

When fluid and electrolyte problems associated with acute kidney injury are uncontrolled by more conservative measures, dialysis may be necessary. Dialysis will remove abnormally high concentrations of potentially dangerous substances from the bloodstream. The hope will be that the kidney failure will clear and the need for dialysis will disappear.

### What other problems come up when treating people with acute kidney injury?

People with acute kidney injury have a weakened immune system and are susceptible to developing serious infections. Symptoms of sepsis (see chapter entitled "Sepsis and Septic Shock"), pneumonia (see chapter entitled "Hospital-Acquired Pneumonia"), or other infections require prompt evaluation and appropriate treatment.

Infection is a dangerous and occasionally fatal complication of acute kidney injury. Vigilance in identifying and treating infection is critical.

People with acute kidney injury can also develop gastrointestinal bleeding caused by bleeding ulcers in the stomach. These ulcers may slowly leak blood and gradually make the person anemic, or may bleed more rapidly and cause reddish or black stool, or vomiting of bright red blood. Blood tests can show rapidly worsening anemia and give the first indication of upper GI bleeding. (For more information, please see the chapter entitled "Upper GI Bleeding").

The kidneys produce a hormone called "erythropoietin" which is necessary for normal red blood cell production. With extensive kidney damage, the kidneys may not produce the adequate quantities of erythropoietin required to sustain the production of normal amounts red blood cells. This will lead to anemia. A synthetic form of erythropoietin is available but may not be very effective in reversing the anemia of acute kidney injury without a blood transfusion. Blood transfusion, at times, is necessary to treat the anemia when it is severe.

## *What is the outlook when a person develops acute kidney injury?*

People with cancer who develop acute kidney injury may have several life-threatening complications that are going on at the same time. Survival will depend upon the person's ability to recover from their other major complications, although the existence of acute kidney injury clearly puts life in further danger.

For people with "renal azotemia", the likelihood of recovery depends upon the prompt identification and successful removal of the cause of the intrinsic renal disease and the degree to which the kidney has already sustained damage.

People with post-renal azotemia that is promptly identified and treated generally recover their kidney function.

When kidney function does not recover, chronic dialysis may be considered, in the context of the outlook related to the extent of a person's cancer, its likely future response to treatment, and a person or family's desire for further aggressive treatment.

### *What is dialysis?*

Dialysis is an artificial way of removing wastes and excess fluid from the bloodstream and replacing some of the important functions of the kidney.

### *How does a person receive dialysis?*

Most of the time, dialysis takes the form of "hemodialysis". During hemodialysis, catheters and tubes divert the blood from the body into a machine containing membranes that can filter wastes and excess water out of the bloodstream. Once cleansed of these wastes, blood returns to the body. Dialysis centers repeat this treatment in approximately three-hour sessions three times weekly.

# MULTIPLE ORGAN DYSFUNCTION SYNDROME

## DEFINITION

### What is multiple organ dysfunction syndrome?

Multiple organ dysfunction syndrome is when two or more major organs have severely impaired function in a person who is critically ill. Organs involved can include the lungs, liver, kidneys, heart, brain and bone marrow. Multiple organ dysfunction syndrome is one of the major causes of death in an intensive care unit.

## THE CAUSES OF MULTIPLE ORGAN DYSFUNCTION SYNDROME

### Who develops multiple organ dysfunction syndrome?

Multiple organ dysfunction syndrome is most common after major trauma or after a major operation. Sepsis (see chapter entitled "Sepsis and Septic Shock"), acute pancreatitis (see chapter entitled "Acute Pancreatitis"), and many other acute, life-threatening illnesses or injuries can produce multiple organ dysfunction syndrome.

## What causes multiple organ dysfunction syndrome to develop?

When confronted by serious infection or other sudden serious illness, our body's natural defense will trigger an "inflammatory response" which seeks to counteract the internal injuries caused by the illness or, if there is infection, rid the body of the microscopic invader. This inflammatory response can, however, get out of control and trigger a "systemic inflammatory response syndrome" or "SIRS" in which inflammation involves the entire body. If complications of the underlying illness multiply, repeated insults to the body's defense system can trigger a highly overactive "inflammatory response" which results in a "severe SIRS". This severe inflammation can directly damage body organs, and produce "acute kidney injury", "adult respiratory distress syndrome", "coma", "heart failure" and "liver failure". These subjects are discussed in separate chapters with those titles, with the exception of liver failure that is discussed in the chapter entitled of "Hepatic Encephalopathy" and coma, discussed in the chapter entitled "Delirium, Stupor and Coma".

## TREATMENT

## What is the treatment of multiple organ dysfunction syndrome?

No specific treatment counteracts the systemic inflammatory response syndrome that is responsible for causing or perpetuating multiple organ dysfunction syndrome. When multiple organ dysfunction syndrome is triggered or worsened by low blood pressure, physicians will administer extra fluid along with medicines to keep blood pressure up in the normal range. Infections identified will be searched for and, if found, treated with antibiotics. Infection is common with multiple organ dysfunction syndrome and physicians may prescribe intravenous antibiotics even in the absence of clear evidence of an infection.

Continued delivery of nutrition can be helpful to the person with multiple organ dysfunction syndrome. Nutrition can be delivered intravenously or, when possible, by mouth or by a "NG" or "nasogastric" tube inserted via the nose into the stomach.

The organ failures are treated as they would be if the organs were failing individually. For information regarding specific treatments of organ failure, please see chapters entitled "Acute Kidney Injury", "Adult Respiratory Distress Syndrome", "Delirium, Stupor, and Coma", "Acute Pulmonary Edema" and "Hepatic Encephalopathy".

## **OUTLOOK**

*What is the outlook of multiple organ dysfunction syndrome?*

The outlook depends upon the survivability of the underlying disease that precipitated the multiple organ dysfunction syndrome, on the number of organs involved, and the length of time that has passed since organ failures began. Even with the best available treatment, multiple organ dysfunction syndrome is extremely dangerous and is a leading cause of death in the intensive care unit.

# METABOLIC
# COMPLICATIONS

# CANCER CACHEXIA

## DEFINITION

### What is cancer cachexia?

Cancer cachexia is a progressive involuntary loss of weight and muscle mass that is associated with advanced cancer. With cancer cachexia, the weight loss is associated with other symptoms, such as fatigue, nausea, early satiety, and loss of appetite. In contrast to starvation, the weight loss with cancer cachexia is most prominent from the muscles throughout the body.

## THE CAUSE OF CACHEXIA

### What is it about advanced cancer that can produce cancer cachexia?

Cancer cells release chemicals into the bloodstream that stimulate the body's metabolism to break down muscle cells, and, to a lesser extent, fat stores. The exact nature of these chemicals and methods of blocking them are still uncertain. The cancers most likely to produce cancer cachexia are cancers of the lung, pancreas, and stomach, although advanced cancer arising from any source commonly produces cancer cachexia.

*How do physicians and medical
professionals initially evaluate a person
with cancer cachexia?*

As an initial step, it will be important to determine whether the cancer cachexia is a direct consequence of the cancer, or whether other medical problems such as sores in the mouth, nausea and vomiting, or loss of taste for some forms of food or liquid are contributing to the weight loss. If such factors exist, initial treatment will attempt to correct this, and, by improving food intake, slow or stop the weight loss.

## **TREATMENT**

*What treatment is possible if there does not
appear to be a reversible cause of the cancer
cachexia, other than the cancer itself?*

There is no clear intervention, whether in the form of increased nutritional intake or medication, that has a significant effect in slowing the progressive weight loss and physical decline associated with cancer cachexia. Although it would seem logical to assume that increased intake of protein and other high quality nutrients would slow or stop muscle loss, muscle breakdown clearly proceeds despite nutritional intervention.

The only medications proven to have some effect on slowing weight loss with cancer cachexia are the medicine "Megace", and oral steroids such as "Decadron". Megace generally does not cause significant side effects, although its benefits, as related to muscle loss, are minor. Decadron, or other steroid medication, if taken for an extended period, has many unpleasant side effects that could outweigh whatever small benefit they may have in reducing weight loss in people with cancer cachexia.

# HEPATIC ENCEPHALOPATHY

## DEFINITION

### What is hepatic encephalopathy?

Hepatic encephalopathy is a serious disturbance of brain function caused by liver failure. One of the most important functions of the liver is to remove toxic substances from the bloodstream. When liver failure develops, these toxic substances accumulate in the blood and the brain, disrupting normal brain functioning and causing hepatic encephalopathy.

## SYMPTOMS

### What are the symptoms of hepatic encephalopathy?

The most prominent symptom of hepatic encephalopathy is a change in the person's personality or mental functioning. The nature of the change in personality can range from a confused, excited state, to a state of lethargy and coma. Drowsiness and a reversal of normal day-night sleeping patterns are other common early symptoms. There may be an inability to control normal body movements. As hepatic encephalopathy worsens, it can lead to complete disorientation, coma and death.

# CAUSE OF HEPATIC ENCEPHALOPATHY

*Why can a person with cancer*
*develop hepatic encephalopathy?*

Hepatic encephalopathy means that severe damage to the liver has occurred. When a person has cancer, this can mean that cancer itself has damaged the liver, that cancer treatments have damaged the liver, or that some other medical condition has developed that is damaging the liver and causing liver failure.

Extensive involvement of the liver by cancer can cause sufficient damage to the liver to produce liver failure. In addition, people with advanced cancer have a tendency to develop blood clots in dangerous places. One of these places is the vein called the "hepatic vein" that carries blood away from the liver and toward the heart. A clot in the hepatic vein causes the "Budd-Chiari syndrome", leading to life-threatening liver failure.

Chemotherapy and biological therapy medications, as well as radiation used to treat cancer, have the potential to cause serious toxicity to the liver.

People with cancer may have liver disease, either because of the cancer growing in the liver, or because of a previous illness such as hepatitis or cirrhosis. Medications such as sedatives or diuretics, as well as serious infections such as pneumonia or a urinary tract infection can worsen underlying liver disease and trigger an episode of hepatic encephalopathy.

*Does a personality change or a change in the level of consciousness in a person with cancer involving the liver or other underlying liver disease always indicate hepatic encephalopathy?*

People with cancer that involves the liver can develop personality changes because of several medical problems unrelated to hepatic encephalopathy. The liver normally metabolizes many tranquilizers and sedatives. When a person with liver disease uses tranquilizers or sedatives, even in very small doses, there may be accumulation of these drugs in the bloodstream and a profound change in the person's state of alertness.

People who are chronically ill may fall down, knock their heads, and get blood clots in or around the brain. Other diseases of the brain such as meningitis, brain metastasis, or stroke, certainly can develop in people with cancer who have liver disease.

New changes in personality in a person with cancer involving the liver or other underlying liver disease requires a thorough evaluation by the physician that may include a physical examination, blood tests, and, occasionally, a CT scan of the brain. With these tests, the diagnosis of hepatic encephalopathy (or of another medical problem) can be established or excluded.

## TREATMENT OF HEPATIC ENCEPHALOPATHY

*What is the treatment of hepatic encephalopathy?*

A first step in treating hepatic encephalopathy is to identify and begin treatment of any problem (such as infection or blood chemistry abnormality) which may have triggered the episode. If it appears that medications to treat cancer or other medications may be responsible, treatment with these medicines will discontinue.

Hepatic encephalopathy reflects the failing liver's inability to remove toxins from the bloodstream. Many of these toxins result from the interaction between the normal bacteria in the intestine and protein in the food. This interaction produces ammonia that accumulates in the bloodstream and is partially responsible for hepatic encephalopathy.

A medicine called "lactulose", taken by mouth or by enema, reduces the amount of ammonia in the bloodstream. A low protein diet and antibiotics such as "neomycin" and "metronidazole" may reduce protein in the intestine and reduce breakdown of protein into ammonia.

The antibiotic "rifaximin", (brand name is "Xifaxan", manufacturer's product website is www.xifaxan.com), is helpful in preventing recurrent episodes of hepatic encephalopathy and associated hospitalization. Xifaxan is an antibiotic taken by mouth that is barely absorbed into the bloodstream, but, instead, concentrates in the intestine. By doing so, it can kill a wide variety of bacteria that may produce toxins that stimulate hepatic encephalopathy.

# MALIGNANT HYPERCALCEMIA

## DEFINITION

### What is malignant hypercalcemia?

Hypercalcemia is an elevation in the level of calcium in the bloodstream. Malignant hypercalcemia refers to hypercalcemia caused by cancer.

## SYMPTOMS

### What are the symptoms of malignant hypercalcemia?

Most of the time, hypercalcemia is discovered with blood tests before it has produced symptoms. When symptoms develop, early symptoms of malignant hypercalcemia are fatigue, slight confusion, nausea, vomiting, an almost unquenchable thirst, and excessive urination. If not controlled, hypercalcemia can cause coma, as well as dangerous changes in the heartbeat, with the heart beating far too fast or far too slow.

Doctors in training remember the symptoms of hypercalcemia by the mnemonic "bones, stones, groans, and moans". "Bones" refers to pain in the bones, associated with bone metastasis that may be associated with hypercalcemia. "Stones" refers to kidney stones that may develop when blood calcium level is too high. "Groans" is for the groaning that goes along with pain in the abdomen, constipation, and nausea and vomiting. "Moans" relates to moaning associated with severe confusion.

## CANCERS THAT CAUSE HYPERCALCEMIA

### What cancers can cause hypercalcemia?

Most cancers can cause hypercalcemia. The cancers that most commonly cause hypercalcemia are breast cancer, lung cancer, and a cancer of the bone marrow called "multiple myeloma".

## THE REASON A PERSON WITH CANCER CAN DEVELOP MALIGNANT HYPERCALCEMIA

### How does the cancer produce malignant hypercalcemia?

Although cancer that has spread into bone can break down bone and liberate calcium into the bloodstream, the more important reason that cancers can cause malignant hypercalcemia is that cancer cells can manufacture a hormone that raises the blood calcium level.

### What is the hormone and why does it raise the blood calcium level?

The hormone, "parathyroid hormone-related peptide" raises the blood calcium level through two mechanisms. Parathyroid hormone-related peptide breaks down the bone, releasing calcium from the bone into the bloodstream, and, secondly, signals the kidney to retain too much calcium. These combined effects raise the blood level of calcium.

# TREATMENT

## *What is the treatment of malignant hypercalcemia?*

If the hypercalcemia just shows up as a number on a blood test without symptoms, physicians may do nothing other than urge a person to keep active, maintain a good intake of fluids, and be alert to symptoms of hypercalcemia, so that treatment can begin promptly if symptoms develop.

When treatment is required, the immediate goal of treatment will be to lower the blood level of calcium with fluid and medications. After the calcium is in the normal range, treatment will focus on preventing the hypercalcemia from recurring.

## *What type of fluid and medications can bring hypercalcemia down?*

People with malignant hypercalcemia who have symptoms are usually dehydrated. Intravenous infusion of large volumes of fluid can lower the concentration of calcium in the bloodstream and promote excretion of calcium in the urine.

The hormonal medicine "calcitonin" can inhibit the abnormal release of calcium from bone and increase the amount of calcium a person excretes into their urine. This will help clear the high levels of calcium from the bloodstream.

The family of medicines called "bisphosphonates" has emerged as the most effective medical treatment of hypercalcemia, although they take a few days to have an effect. The most commonly used bisphosphonates are "Zometa" (manufacturer's product website is www.zometa.com) and "pamidronate" (brand name is "Aredia").

The combined treatment of attention to proper hydration, calcitonin, and bisphosphonates is usually sufficient to keep the malignant hypercalcemia under control.

# CLINICAL TRIALS

## THE BIRTH OF A NEW DRUG

### *Where do new drugs come from?*

The development of the great majority of new drugs is a collaborative effort between pharmaceutical or biotechnology companies and academic medical centers. These drugs may be extracts of natural substances derived from plants or animals or may be synthetic substances made in laboratories.

### *What tests are required when researchers believe that they may have discovered a substance that has potential as a drug?*

First, extensive testing, conducted in the laboratory, both in non-animal models ("in vitro") and in animal models ("in vivo"), will seek evidence that the potential drug has the ability to work in the disease for which the drug is intended.

After tests are completed that indicate that the potential drug may be a treatment for a specific disease, toxicology testing will be done to determine the toxic effect of the drug in two or more species of animals. Usually, the United States Food and Drug Administration (the "FDA") and international regulatory authorities requires testing in mice or rats, and, depending on the nature of the drug, may require testing in animals other than mice or rats before the drug is tested in human beings. Drug companies or universities have no choice regarding animal testing prior to human clinical trials: the FDA and the rules of the "International Conference of Harmonization", by which almost every major country abides, require it.

## What happens after the drug has completed this laboratory testing?

When the company or academic center believes that there is sufficient data to justify clinical testing of the new drug, an "Investigational New Drug" application called an "IND" or its international equivalent is submitted to either the FDA or a foreign regulatory agency. This application contains comprehensive information about the chemical structure of the investigational medication, how it is manufactured, and the scientific rationale for its experimental use. Information submitted from animal studies will include safety data, as well as data regarding how the investigational medication is absorbed, distributed through the body, broken down ("metabolized") and excreted.

## PERMISSION TO TEST THE DRUG IN PEOPLE

## What does approval of an "IND" mean?

When the FDA approves an IND, it means that the company or medical center is permitted to test the safety and effectiveness of the experimental medication in people under the strict supervision of a protocol, local institutional committees, and reporting requirements to regulatory authorities.

# HOW CLINICAL TRIALS OF NEW MEDICINES ARE CONDUCTED

*What phases of testing must an experimental medicine go through before it is proven effective?*

There are three major phases of testing which drugs go through before they are available as marketed drugs.

The first phase, "Phase I" evaluates the safety of the drug at different doses. During phase I testing, tests called "pharmacokinetic" tests evaluate how long the drug stays in the bloodstream and how it is broken down ("metabolized") and excreted by the body. Even though the primary purpose of phase I testing is evaluation of safety, researchers will look for signs that the drug may have some effectiveness against the disease for which it is intended.

The second step, phase II, looks for evidence that the drug has effectiveness and will attempt to identify safe doses at which the drug has the highest degree of effectiveness.

In phase III, larger studies will attempt to establish definitive proof of the drug's effectiveness and will attempt to compare the effectiveness of the new drug with the effectiveness of other available medications, or, for untreatable diseases, will compare the effectiveness of the new drug with that of either no therapy or a placebo.

If large phase II or III trials clearly demonstrate a drug's effectiveness, an "NDA" or "New Drug Application" (for some types of drugs, this may be called a "BLA" or

"Biologics License Application") will be filed with the FDA. Upon approval of the NDA (or BLA), the drug will be made available throughout the country in hospitals, clinics, or in local pharmacies.

## FINDING A PROMISING CLINICAL TRIAL

*How does a person with a life-threatening disease identify promising clinical trials?*

Largely, this will depend on whether the disease is acutely life threatening, such as a brain hemorrhage or a myocardial infarction, or whether the disease is potentially life threatening, such as it is with cancer.

When the disease is acutely life threatening and the person is in the hospital, access to a clinical trial will depend upon whether the person is in a hospital where a clinical trial is already in place. If the person can survive transport to another hospital, and if there is no standard, effective therapy for the life-threatening illness, a physician may suggest transfer to a hospital that is evaluating an experimental treatment of the particular illness.

When a person has a disease that is not acutely life threatening, such as cancer, there is more time and freedom to make careful choices after a thorough exploration of options, usually with the help of the many resources available on the internet.

*Which website can help a person rapidly identify clinical trials that may be helpful?*

The National Institute of Health through the website www.clinicaltrials.gov maintains the most comprehensive registry of clinical trials. This website lists and provides information about every significant clinical trial in progress for life-threatening diseases. Each listing includes the name of the clinical trial, the purpose of the study, the criteria that make a person eligible to participate, the study locations, and information about how to contact the medical centers participating.

> **What first steps could a person with a life-threatening disease take when seeking a clinical trial?**

A first and important step may be to have a consultation with a physician in the home community and ask for information regarding clinical trials. Many communities, and especially communities within a 100-mile radius of a major medical center, have physicians with long-standing affiliations with the medical center. These physicians are often quite knowledgeable about the different experimental treatments available for people with diseases that fall within their area of expertise. On occasion, these physicians' offices may be "satellite sites" for a major clinical trial which is coordinated by a major medical center, but which permits people in distant communities to be enrolled in the trial and to be treated by their own physician. There may be no need to endure the inconvenience of a long trip to an academic center when the same experimental treatment is available close to home.

Some doctors are remarkably unhelpful in assisting a person who seeks experimental treatment programs outside of their community. In these circumstances, a person who wants to explore experimental treatment options will have to take the initiative and seek out the program with the assistance of family, friends and the internet.

## ENROLLING IN A CLINICAL TRIAL

### Can anyone with a disease enter a clinical trial?

As a first step, the person with a particular disease must find a medical center that is testing a particular drug. Only a few study centers participate in the clinical trials of most experimental medications.

Protocols set very strict "inclusion" and "exclusion" criteria that determine which people with a disease can or cannot enter a trial. People with very advanced disease, people who are bedridden, and people with cancer extensively treated with chemotherapy are excluded from many trials. The reason for this exclusion is the concern that such people are so weakened from a far-advanced disease that they are unlikely to respond to any therapy. This lack of response to treatment by people with far-advanced disease can falsely lead investigators to believe that the experimental medication is ineffective.

### How does a person enroll in an experimental program?

Once an experimental program of interest is identified, the goal will be to be evaluated by the medical center performing the innovative research as soon as possible.

An effective way to get the appointment for a prompt evaluation is by a physician referral. Major medical centers generally welcome self-referrals, although with a physician referral it may be more likely that a person will get a prompt appointment. Referral by the physician with current direct responsibility for providing medical care can also speed up the process by which medical information is shared between the two medical centers.

If necessary, self-referral can be accomplished by calling the medical center directly and making an appointment to see the physician running clinical trials. The name and contact information of the person coordinating the clinical trials of interest at a medical center can usually be found on the www.clinicaltrials.gov webpage.

## What preparations can be made prior to being seen at the medical center?

A complete package of information that gives a clear story of a person's medical illness can be very useful. Having this package of information completed and available can save a considerable amount of time in making an initial appointment at the specialized medical center. This complete package of information should be brought to the clinic at the time of the first appointment.

The center at which a person is evaluated for experimental treatment may give a person a checklist of what to bring to the appointment. This may include:

- A letter from the referring physician giving a detailed overview of the entire medical evaluation which has taken place and any treatments administered

- Radiologist's official reports of x-rays, CT scans, MRI scans, bone scans, and ultrasound examinations. If possible, it would be very useful to take a CD containing CT or MRI scans to the medical center at the time of the initial consultation

- The pathologist's report of all biopsies that established the diagnosis of the person's life-threatening disease. If possible, and if requested by the center to which a person is referred, the actual microscopic slides which established the diagnosis can be obtained and carried to the medical center at the time of the visit.

- Surgical reports of any operations which were performed to diagnose or treat the diseas

- Written reports of the findings of any endoscopy (such as gastroscopy, bronchoscopy, sigmoidoscopy, or colonoscopy) procedure performed to diagnose or treat the disease

- A list of all medications and doses of medications taken in the last six months

By having these documents, slides, and scans together at the time of the first visit, comprehensive evaluation can begin immediately, and decisions regarding the best treatment option can be made more quickly.

## How does a person make a decision about whether or not to enter a clinical trial?

This decision is made with a thorough understanding of standard treatments and experimental options.

When a disease such as cancer becomes far advanced, the chance of having a favorable response to experimental treatment becomes smaller. For people with these cancers, experimental treatment at a top medical center may be a critical and life-saving option.

## THE COST OF EXPERIMENTAL TREATMENT

### Who pays for the experimental treatment?

The experimental treatment itself should generally be free. Almost all true experimental treatment programs will pay for the experimental medication and for tests or procedures specifically used to determine whether the experimental treatment is working. Experimental trials do not usually pay for a person's overall medical care or for tests or procedures ordinarily done as part of the medical care of a person suffering from the same disease but not enrolled in the clinical trial.

When a clinic offers an "experimental treatment" for cash-only and for a very high price, a person should be very wary, since experimental treatment for a very high price is usually not associated with legitimate research.

## GIVING INFORMED CONSENT

### How is the experimental option explained?

The physician conducting the trial is responsible for giving a person full information about the precise nature of the experimental treatment to be given.

Before testing can begin, the person will have to sign a document called an "informed consent form". This document includes details regarding the nature of the treatment, the way it will be administered, the tests that will be conducted to determine the effects of the treatment, and potential side effects of the experimental treatment. The informed consent will also make it clear that the FDA and, often the biotechnology or pharmaceutical company which manufactures the experimental drug, will have a right to have access to the person's medical records so that the results of the testing can be clearly recorded and analyzed.

## OTHER BENEFITS OF ENROLLING IN A CLINICAL TRIAL

*Are there other benefits of enrolling in a clinical trial?*

Usually, the physicians running the trial are top quality physicians who have had extensive experience treating the disease for which the person is seeking experimental treatment.

# ABOUT THE AUTHOR

Stephen Garrett Marcus, M.D. is a physician who has focused his professional career on the development of new treatments for life-threatening and disabling diseases. Born and educated in New York City, Dr. Marcus received his medical degree from New York Medical College. After an internal medicine residency at Lenox Hill Hospital in New York, and oncology (cancer treatment) specialty training at the University of California in San Francisco, Dr. Marcus spent several years practicing emergency and critical care medicine and medical oncology.

In 1985, Dr. Marcus entered the biotechnology industry where he has been directly responsible or played a leadership role in the development of a number of important new medications. Dr. Marcus was the key figure in the development of beta interferon as the first effective treatment of multiple sclerosis and played a leadership role in the development of fludarabine for chronic lymphocytic leukemia. He has served as the leader of multinational teams of medical researchers developing new treatments of cancer, multiple sclerosis, as well as other life-threatening or disabling conditions.

At present, Dr. Marcus is the president and chief executive officer of a biotechnology company that is developing a new medication for the treatment of pancreatic cancer, cystic fibrosis, and other life-threatening diseases.

# INDEX

www.ingramcontent.com/pod-product-compliance
Lightning Source LLC
Chambersburg PA
CBHW071351170526
45165CB00001B/2